What To Eat When You're Expecting

❖ ❖ ❖

Arlene Eisenberg
Heidi E. Murkoff
Sandee E. Hathaway, R.N.

❖ ❖ ❖

Workman Publishing, New York

Library of Congress Cataloging-in-Publication Data
Eisenberg, Arlene.   What to eat when you're expecting.
Includes index.   1. Pregnancy—Nutritional aspects. 2. Mothers—Nutrition.
I. Murkoff, Heidi E. II. Hathaway, Sandee E. III. Title.
[DNLM: 1. Diet—in pregnancy—popular works.   WQ 150 E36w]
RG559.E43 1986   618.2'4   85-40903   ISBN 0-89480-015-9

Book Design: Susan Aronson Stirling
Cover Illustration: Judith Cheng

The following recipes originally appeared in *What to Expect When You're
Expecting* by Arlene Eisenberg, Heidi E. Murkoff, and Sandee
E. Hathaway: Whole-Wheat Buttermilk Pancakes, Bran Muffins, Cream
of Tomato Soup, Fig Bars, Fruity Oatmeal Cookies, Carob Brownies, Double-
the-Milk Shake, Innocent Sangria, and Mock Strawberry Daiquiri.

Workman books are available at special discounts when purchased in bulk for
premiums and sales promotions as well as for fund-raising or educational use.
Special editions or book excerpts can also be created to specification. For details,
contact the Special Sales Director at the address below.

Workman Publishing Company, Inc.,
708 Broadway
New York, NY 10003

Manufactured in the United States of America
First printing July 1986
20   19

DEDICATED TO:

Dr. Carl A. Zoll, who combined modern medicine with old-fashioned doctoring and whose lessons in nutrition more than 30 years ago laid the foundation for the Best-Odds Diet. We have him to thank, at least partially, for two generations of Best-Odds babies.

The newest crop of these babies—Emma, Rachel, and especially Wyatt, who was kind enough to stay put in his mother's womb until the last pages of this manuscript were delivered.

And all of the expectant parents who received What to Expect When You're Expecting *so enthusiastically and whose requests for more nutrition advice inspired this project.*

IN APPRECIATION

An author is lucky to have a good publishing team behind her once in a lifetime. We have already been so blessed twice. Among those we have to thank for their support, faith, and hard work are:

Our agents Elise and Arnold Goodman, whose confidence and encouragement continue to lead us to new and exciting projects.

Our editor, Suzanne Rafer, who lived through *What to Expect When You're Expecting* and was brave enough to come back for more with *What to Eat*, who ever keeps us on the straight and narrow, and who deserves our heartfelt thanks.

Our designer, Susan Aronson Stirling, whose good taste and sharp eye turned a mountain of unmanageable manuscript into a handsome book.

Our publisher, Peter Workman, and his entire staff, who have made working on any project with them more than pleasant.

Dr. Richard Aubry, one of those rare physicians who recognizes the value of good nutrition in pregnancy, who took time out of his busy schedule to read and comment on the manuscript and to write the foreword.

Our friends Chris Shayne and Ann Wimpfheimer, who waded through the manuscript and gave us their suggestions.

And especially our husbands. Behind every successful married author, there's an understanding spouse.

Erik, the model Best-Odds father, who made it (for the second time) almost effortless for Heidi to follow the Best-Odds Diet.

Tim, who this time gave up *both* his girls when work required Sandee to make the Boston–New York commute, and who has learned to love the Best-Odds changes in the family diet.

And Howard, the daddy and granddaddy of them all, who has been mentor as well as baby sitter and dish washer, and who was a willing taster during the years we were developing the Best-Odds Diet.

Contents

PART ONE

Making Healthy Babies

What Good   Nutrition Does • Why the Best-Odds Diet • What Controlled Weight Gain Does

Evaluating Your Eating Habits • The Best-Odds Quiz • Changing Your Eating Habits • *Forbidden Fruits/Less Than the Best* • The Best-Odds Nine Basic Principles • *Using a Best-Odds Menu Planner* • *Junk Food: What's in It for You and for Baby* • The Daily Dozen • Best-Odds Food Selection Groups • *Those Cruciferous Vegetables* • Shelf of Honor • *The Great Ice Cream War* • Best-Odds Approved Cheating • *Selections for Selective Cheating* • Monitoring Your Weight Gain • *Weight Gain and What It Is Made Up Of* • *Weight Gain: Low, Average, and High* • *Weighing In*

PART TWO

Getting Practical

What to Avoid When You're Expecting • *Kicking the Caffeine Habit* • What to Use with Care • *Know More About Food Safety* • What You Can Safely Eat • *Teratology Information Centers in the U.S.* • *Food Poisoning: The All-Natural Peril*

PART THREE
Best-Odds Recipes

A Best-Odds Cooking Primer • Cereals • Eggs and Pancakes • Breads and Muffins • Soups • Vegetarian Main Dishes • Main Courses • Vegetable Side Dishes • Salad Suggestions and Dressing Recipes • Puddings and Other Desserts • Pies • Cookies • Cakes • Frozen Desserts • Party Foods • Drinks • Quick Fixes

---

PART FOUR
Appendix

Putting It All Together • Junk Food: What's In it for You and Your Baby • Chemical Cuisine • Daily Mineral Needs for the Average Young Woman: Nonpregnant, Pregnant, and Lactating • Daily Nutrient Requirements for the Average Young Woman: Nonpregnant, Pregnant, and Lactating • Parlez-vous Best Odds? • Pregnancy Supplement Formula

A Word from the Doctor

BY GOLLY, THEY'VE DONE IT AGAIN! THE AUTHORS of *What to Expect When You're Expecting* have written another book that obstetricians can respect and expectant mothers can love.

We used to think of the fetus as a parasite contentedly draining what it needed from maternal nutritional stores. Now we know that during pregnancy the mother and baby share available nutrients, and that when there is an inadequate supply, both mother and baby suffer. Animal studies show that poorly nourished rats have litters of runts, and that with continued malnutrition the survival picture becomes bleaker for each generation. In human studies we've been able to show that improving the prenatal diet improves the pregnancy outcome for both mother and child. So, not surprisingly, most of us advise our patients: "Eat a healthful diet."

But just what does that mean to the pregnant woman? Often not much. She is bombarded at every turn with contradictory (and sometimes misleading) nutrition information—from family and friends, from books, magazines, and newspapers, and from the talk-show expert-of-the-week. Uncertain, confused, she needs a source she can trust. I believe *What to Eat When You're Expecting* is that source.

Not only is this book medically accurate, it's easy to follow and understand. The authors designed it to fit the lifestyle of the expectant mother—at home, at work, in a foreign country on holiday, on a vegetarian diet, or suffering from morning sickness. It doesn't just command, "Change your eating habits," it explains how to do it. The book provides nuts-and-bolts tips on shopping and cooking that I haven't seen anywhere else. It deals with drugs, alcohol, smoking, and chemical additives—the kinds of things that can sabotage even a good diet—in a constructive, sensible way. And, in its concern for what Dad and the kids eat as well, it doesn't forget that the expectant mother doesn't live in a vacuum; she usually lives in an expectant family.

In my opinion, the best birth-day gift a mother can give her baby is a good start in life. After years of working with expectant mothers and teaching medical students, ob/gyn residents, and practicing ob/gyn's, I'm convinced that good nutrition is vital in reaching that goal. And after reading *What to Eat When You're Expecting*, I'm convinced that this is the book that can best help you help your baby achieve it.

Richard Aubry, M.D.

Dr. Richard Aubry has been a member of the National Nutrition Committee of the American College of Obstetrics and Gynecology and has contributed to The International Journal on Nutrition. *He is professor of ob/gyn and director of obstetrics and maternal-fetal medicine at the Health Science Center of the State University of New York at Syracuse.*

How This Diet Was Born

THERE'S NEVER BEEN A BETTER—OR SAFER—TIME TO BE pregnant. That may be hard to believe. There is, after all, carbon monoxide in the air we breathe; toxic waste from neighborhood industrial sites contaminating our underground wells; radiation from microwave ovens leaking into our kitchens; poisonous fumes from the insecticides our communities use to kill gypsy moths polluting our yards.

And yet it's true. Even with so much in our environment out of our control, never before in the history of reproduction have babies had a better chance of being born alive and well. When the air was unpolluted and the wells were pure, when food was cooked over open fires, and insects lived in harmony with humans, survival for baby (and mother) was mostly a matter of chance, and the chances weren't encouraging. What was definitively known about making and delivering a healthy baby couldn't have filled one page of a modern obstetrical textbook.

Today, the environment may be against us, but its effect is overwhelmingly outweighed by the proliferation of knowledge on pregnancy and childbirth that now fills hundreds of textbooks and journals—and fills hospital nurseries with millions of healthy babies each year. Today, having a healthy baby is, most of the time, more up to us than up to chance. Though they capture much more of the media's—and thus the public's—attention, all of the negative environmental factors that are beyond our control have far less impact on the outcome of our pregnancies than the positive factors over which we have complete control.

In *What to Expect When You're Expecting*, we talked about increasing the odds of having a healthy baby by taking control of those factors we can influence and minimizing the risks (and worry) of those we can't. We explained the importance of improving fitness, getting optimum medical care, quitting smoking, drinking, and drug taking. We included a full chapter on eating, which, because we do it every day, at least three times a day, is an area in which there are enormous possibilities for control. This chapter introduced the Best-Odds Diet, one which is medically sound and, with some effort, can be any mother's first gift to her unborn child.

Although its name originated with its first publication, in *What to Expect When You're Expecting*, the Best-Odds Diet has, as a concept, existed for over 30 years in our family. When my mother, Arlene, was first pregnant, the rudiments were given to her by a family doctor who had cared for her from childhood. His advice was, at the time, revolutionary. Eat only whole grains, he ordered, plenty of protein and high-calcium foods; don't eat sugar. Like any mother-to-be eager to do the best for her baby-to-be, she obeyed.

The results were her payoff. Though during three pregnancies she gained as little as 13 pounds and never more than 17 herself (the medically accepted limit at the time), she produced three very healthy babies, weighing in at 6 pounds 5 ounces, 7 pounds 6 ounces, and 8 pounds. The babies were alert and developmentally advanced.

When I became pregnant, over a quarter of a century later, we discovered that scientific research had substantiated the doctor's advice on the value of a good diet during pregnancy. But we also discovered that according to today's standards my mother's weight gain had been inadequate. What struck us as significant was the fact that she was able to nourish her babies so well in the uterus on so few calories. Clearly the quality of the food she ate in pregnancy was at least as important as the quantity.

The Best-Odds Diet was refined in its second generation of use to include a more substantial weight gain (the generally recommended 20 to 30 pounds), but the idea of quality versus quantity in the selection of foods has remained paramount. I gained 20 pounds in each of my pregnancies eating only foods of the highest nutritional quality. My babies weighed in at 7 pounds 1 ounce and 7 pounds 8½ ounces respectively (and I weighed in at my prepregnancy weight within six weeks postpartum). My sister Sandee, too, followed the Best-Odds Diet and produced a 7 pound 7 ounce baby on a 24-pound weight gain. All three of the second-generation Best-Odds babies were exceptionally alert, strong, healthy, and quick in developing.

The pregnancies and deliveries were uncomplicated.

The chapter on the diet we presented in *What to Expect When You're Expecting* wasn't just based on family folklore—or on the family doctor's advice. It was based on the very latest in medical research on nutrition in pregnancy (of which there is too little) and on nutrition in general (of which there is more and more proving its importance). But though it provided a good outline for eating the best possible diet, the limitations of space prevented us from giving the kind of detail which can put a plan into action—and which many readers have since requested.

What to Eat When You're Expecting is devoted to such detail. And it is dedicated to the very important premise that diet has a statistically dramatic influence on the outcome of pregnancy. You probably know someone who junk-fooded her way through her pregnancy yet gave birth to a perfect baby, just as you probably know (or have heard of) someone who chain-smoked his way through an enviably healthy and hardy 90 years. Yet the chances of giving birth to a perfect baby are much greater for someone who's eaten well, as the chances of living to 90 are much greater for someone who doesn't smoke. Though eating the best possible diet doesn't unequivocally guarantee that a baby will be born in perfect health, and eating a poor diet doesn't absolutely condemn a baby to a lifetime of poor health, both increase the odds significantly.

Like *What to Expect When You're Expecting*, *What to Eat When You're Expecting* is a guide rather than a compendium of information— infinitely practical, unrelentingly realistic, easy to read, and easy to use. It is designed for today's pregnant women, taking into account that they don't live in a vacuum (or tied to a vacuum cleaner), that they often have families and careers, that they spend less time at home and more time traveling, and that they eat out almost as often as they eat in. It also gives full consideration to pregnant eaters with dietary eccentricities, those who have chosen to or, because of a medical condition, must eat differently than the rest.

As any one who has ever tried to make major alterations in her eating life-style knows, changing the way you eat is no small challenge. But when you're pregnant, planning to become pregnant, or nursing, the potential rewards of meeting that challenge—a healthier baby; a safer, more comfortable pregnancy and delivery; and a slimmer postpartum you—are great. And, we think you'll agree after you've read and eaten on, well worth your best efforts.

Heidi Eisenberg Murkoff

PART ONE

Making Healthy Babies

ONE

Turning Good Odds into Best Odds

Y OU HOPE YOUR BABY HAS DADDY'S BLUE EYES AND mommy's wavy dark hair; grandpa's sense of humor and grandma's beautiful singing voice. You may even have a secret (or not so secret) preference for a particular sex—a girl to dress in pinafores and Mary Janes, or a boy to go fishing with dad (mother-to-be daydreams are notoriously sexist). But you'd toss all these hopes out the delivery-room door in favor of your most fervent desire: a healthy baby.

What makes a healthy baby? In centuries past, "God's will" was thought the determining factor, though sometimes the superstitious believed even God's best intentions might be thwarted by the caprice of "evil spirits." In the early part of this century, scientists began to realize that there were genetic factors that helped to decide and, often, seal a baby's fate. In the middle of this century came the recognition that environmental factors—radiation from X-rays or other sources, infections, drugs, exposure to chemicals—also helped shape a baby's odds of being born alive and well.

Fortunately, God's will is benign and evil spirits are given credence by few today. Genetics usually does its work for good, and most of us escape serious exposure to environmental hazards.

Fortunately, too, we now know that there are other factors that go into making a healthy baby, factors that are neither so nebulous as God's will, nor as unpredictable as genetics or environmental exposure, factors very much under our control. One of the most significant is diet.[1] Not only are you what you eat, but your baby is, too.

---

1. The other major factor that affects your baby is also totally under the control of the informed expectant mother: getting good medical care early in the pregnancy.

WHAT GOOD NUTRITION DOES

Every day, scientific research is giving more support to the idea that what we put in our mouths matters. If we put in too much fat and cholesterol, we risk early demise from heart disease. If we put in too much fat and possibly animal protein, we risk certain types of cancer. If we put in lots of sugar, we can, among other things, expect our teeth to rot and our gums to recede. If we put in too much salt, we may find our blood pressure skyrocketing. If we put in too many calories, we face obesity with its attendant dangers.

What we don't put in is also significant. Too little calcium and our bones may grow old (and brittle) before their time. Too little roughage and we may develop not only constipation, hemorrhoids, and fissures, but intestinal cancer. Not enough vitamin C and our gums may bleed; none at all, and we may succumb to scurvy. A dearth of vitamin D when we are young, and rickets deforms our bones. Not enough chromium[2] and diabetes may develop.

---

2. Studies are presently under way to determine the connection of chromium deficiency to the development of gestational diabetes; studies have already shown that sugar depletes the body of this important trace metal.

The effects of nutrition on your body are endless and endlessly significant. But they are even more significant during pregnancy, when what you put in your mouth affects not only you, but your developing baby as well.

Your Baby Equals What You Eat

After your baby is born, the responsibility of feeding can be shared. Even if you elect to breastfeed, a sitter can see to the infant's nutritional needs with a supplementary bottle when you're out at a party. Or daddy can do it if you're down with the flu. During the nine months of gestation, however, you are your baby's only source of nourishment. You can't leave your uterus with a sitter while you're out on the town. Or have daddy pipe in nutrients when your appetite has flown with the flu. Every calorie, every gram of protein, every milligram of vitamin C, every trace of zinc and manganese your baby gets—or needs, and doesn't get—can only come from you. Not from stores in your body, for the most part, since few nutrients can be "saved up" for use by your baby, but from your diet.

In short, your fetus is what you eat—and what you don't eat. As you can probably guess, a baby made up of candy bars and colas is quite different from a baby made up of whole-grain breads and milk. A classic study done at Harvard many years ago and one done more recently in Montreal document this. In the Harvard study, women on poor diets had babies in poor health, women on average diets had babies in average health, and women on excellent diets had babies in excellent health. In Montreal, when nutritional education and supplementation (eggs, milk, oranges, and a vitamin/mineral supplement) were given to women who, because of poor diet and socioeconomic factors, were in a high-risk category, the rate of pregnancy complications, including stillbirths, perinatal mortality, and neonatal mortality dropped significantly—to a level lower than that in the rest of Canada.

Studies of women living under famine conditions point to a lower average birth weight for their babies and an increase in the incidence of miscarriages, stillbirths, neonatal deaths, and malformations. You aren't likely to be exposed to famine conditions, but nevertheless, what you eat or don't eat, will have tremendous impact on your baby:

Birth weight. Eating too little, or eating the wrong kinds of food, can keep your baby from growing; eating too much can make your baby grow too much. Two generations ago, to make delivery easier, doctors deemed it wise to limit the size of the baby by limiting caloric intake. We now know that babies who are small for the amount of time they've been in the uterus (small for gestational age) are far more subject to postnatal physiological problems than normal weight babies. But, very large babies *can* complicate delivery.

Ideally, your baby should weigh in somewhere between 6½ and 8½ pounds at birth.[3] You can't control your fetus' weight gain by putting him on the scale every morning, but *your* getting on the scale every morning can help (see page 76). So can monitoring your food intake for quality as well as quantity. Twenty pounds gained on the Best-Odds Diet can result in a bouncing 7-pound baby, while 50 gained on junk food can turn out a baby under five.

Miscarriage. In the first trimester, when cells begin differentiating into tiny organ systems, quality of food (nutrients) is more important than quantity (calories). Severe early deprivation of nutrients can result in fetal damage, and an impaired fetus is often spontaneously

---

3. Heredity is always a factor in fetal size. An Asian woman's 6-pounder can be as normal and healthy as a Nordic woman's 9-pounder.

aborted (miscarried) from the uterus. Fortunately, this kind of damage is rare on the typical American diet. Still, the earlier in pregnancy you start eating well, the better.

Organ development. During the early months of gestation, your baby's tiny heart, liver, lungs, kidneys, nervous system, and other organs are developing at a remarkable rate. The raw materials for this busy little organ factory are supplied by you through the rapidly growing placenta. Most of them come directly from what you eat.

Certain nutritional deficiencies are known, or believed, to cause specific malformations. A lack of vitamin D and calcium can interfere with bone and tooth formation. Lack of folic acid has been linked to spina bifida (a defect in the bony spine that leaves part of the spinal cord exposed and possibly damaged) and other defects in the formation of the neural tube, from which the brain and spinal cord develop. Too little zinc results in eye malformations in animals and may cause defects in humans. Lack of iodine can result in goiter, a defect of the endocrine system. A magnesium deficiency may be related to infant mortality and congenital malformations. The lack of a wide variety of nutrients, such as is common with gross malnutrition,

can result in retarded bone development and cardiovascular abnormalities.

As manager of the baby factory in your uterus, you are solely responsible for seeing that all vital raw materials are delivered to it daily.

Brain development. While the development of most organs is relatively complete midway through pregnancy, your baby's brain will have its greatest growth spurt during the last trimester. (The brain will continue to grow after birth, reaching its maximum number of cells sometime before baby's first birthday.) Protein and calories, which are particularly vital to brain development, need to be kept at optimum levels at this stage of pregnancy. Even if you begin to tire of eating for two, or if you find you've gained too much weight in your first six months, the last trimester will not be the time to cut back. And if you were less than faithful in meeting nutritional requirements in the early months (or prolonged morning sickness interfered with eating), the last trimester will be the time to start paying attention to the Daily Dozen.

You and Your Pregnancy Equal What You Eat

You hear so much about how important your diet is to your

baby during pregnancy that it's easy to forget the other person you're eating for: you. How you eat will have a profound effect on how you feel during your pregnancy, how well your body copes with and recovers from the stresses of both carrying a baby and delivering one, as well as on your general health now and in the future.

What you eat from the day the pregnancy test comes back positive (or even before) right on through delivery and breastfeeding will have a significant impact on many aspects of your life.

On your pregnancy. If you're well-nourished, you are much more likely to have an "easy pregnancy." Two of the most serious complications that can occur during these nine months, anemia[4] and preeclampsia/eclampsia[5] (also known as toxemia), are more common in the poorly nourished. Anemia can result from a deficiency of folic acid, but most often it is caused by too little iron in the diet. Though the mechanisms aren't clearly established, preeclampsia appears to develop in pregnant women whose diets are deficient in protein; vitamin and protein

therapy has been shown to reduce the incidence of this problem, which can rapidly progress to eclampsia, with its life-threatening convulsions, if not treated. It is suspected that a lack of the trace metal magnesium, which, as magnesium sulfate, is used in treating pre-eclampsia, may also contribute to the development of this pregnancy complication. Research has also suggested that another potentially serious pregnancy complication—gestational diabetes—is diet-related, possibly to a chromium deficiency common in Americans. Faithfully following the Daily Dozen daily will ensure that you have adequate intakes of all these important nutrients.

On your health and comfort. Fortunately, most of us don't experience the serious complications of pregnancy. However, it's the minor ones that often make our nine months miserable. Fatigue, morning sickness, constipation, varicose veins, tooth and gum problems, for example. Or nose bleeds, leg cramps, complexion problems, colds, flu, vaginitis, or other infections. And your susceptibility to all of these are affected to some extent by what you eat—or don't eat. A diet high in protein and complex carbohydrates can reduce fatigue and minimize morning sickness. One rich in fiber and fluids can

4. Anemia is characterized by a below-normal level of oxygen-carrying hemoglobin or red blood cells in the blood.

5. Preeclampsia is characterized by a rise in blood pressure accompanied by edema because of fluid retention and protein, or albumin, in the urine.

prevent or relieve constipation. Adequate intakes of foods rich in vitamin C can reduce the risk of varicose veins, bloody noses, and bleeding gums by keeping blood vessels healthy. Cutting down on sugar—or, better still, cutting it out entirely—can help protect teeth and gums from the ravages of bacteria that feast on the sweet and cause decay. The correct balance of phosphorus and calcium in your diet (see page 90) can lessen the chance that leg cramps will keep you awake nights. And infections of all sorts, as well as complexion insurrections, can often be kept at bay (or at least minimized) by overall good nutrition.

On labor and delivery. If eating (other than consommé, jello, and juice in the first phase, ice chips from then on) is taboo during labor and delivery, how can nutrition have an impact on childbirth? Because it isn't what you eat from when the first contraction strikes that counts, it's what you've eaten for the 40 or so weeks preceding it. First of all, a good pregnancy diet can prevent that lead-off labor pain from striking too early. Though all nutrients in a balanced diet are important in helping a woman carry to term, recent research has found zinc to be particularly significant, linking zinc deficiency directly to an increased risk of premature labor.

Second, childbirth requires a prodigious amount of energy. Though a well-nourished woman won't necessarily experience a shorter labor, she will cope more ably with her labor than the woman whose body lacks sufficient stores of energy and nutrients—in much the same way a well-nourished athlete will be able to perform better and endure longer than one who hasn't been eating properly.

On your emotional well-being. The normal hormonal changes of pregnancy can wreak havoc on your emotional state (and that of those around you), by turning premenstrual weepiness and mood swings from a three-day-a-month affair into a three- to nine-month ordeal. Though a good diet can't completely prevent prenatal emotional upheaval, it can help moderate it. Of particular influence on your emotional state are your intakes of caffeine (cut it out; see page 195), sugar (cut it down or out; see page 39), and the B vitamins (keep them adequate).

On your postpartum recovery. Whether you go through an enviably effortless three-hour labor and delivery or a pitiably trying 28-hour one, a planned cesarean or one that's an emergency, the stresses of childbirth will be enormous. After delivery, your body will need significant resources to recover from a variety of insults: stretching, pressing, and tearing; incisions and sutures; blood loss and sleep loss. The best way to speed healing and to bounce back as good as—or better than—new is to eat properly throughout pregnancy, and to do the same after you've delivered.

On your long-term health. Though a preoccupation with your diet during pregnancy is appropriate and desirable, good nutrition can have an impact on your life that goes far beyond the nine months of gestation. Its long-term effects, which will accumulate only if you continue to eat well after delivery (see page 17), are fast unfolding in scientific literature. By cutting back on all fats, particularly saturated fats and cholesterol, sugar, and salt, and increasing your intake of complex carbohydrates and high-fiber foods, you (and the other members of your family who share your good dietary habits) can reduce your risk of stroke, heart attack, some types of cancer, and, possibly, diabetes.[6] By continuing to consume calcium-rich foods after pregnancy, and by supplementing them, if necessary, with calcium tablets, you should be able to deter the postmenopausal scourge of osteoporosis, or brittle bones. (However, you should depend on low-fat sources of calcium—such as skim milk, low or nonfat yogurt, low-fat cottage cheese, ice milk, for example—rather than high-fat sources, which will court the previously mentioned ailments even as they fight osteoporosis.) By monitoring what you put in your mouth for the rest of your days, you can considerably extend their number, as well as their pleasure.

WHY THE BEST-ODDS DIET

The facts are in; the current clinical evidence has been placed before you. Now you know what good nutrition during pregnancy can do for you and your baby-to-be. What you don't know, and what you may be afraid to find out, is to what lengths you'll have to go in order to get that "good nutrition." Will you have to memorize charts of vitamins and minerals and their food sources? Carry a checklist of esoteric but essential nutrients to every meal?

No. Though you can, if you care to, memorize the nutrition charts in the appendix of this book and transcribe every gram and microgram of trace minerals into a daily diet diary, you needn't do either to ensure your

---

6. In addition to recent research indicating that sugar in the diet may lead to chromium deficiency which in turn can lead to diabetes, a diet high in fats and sugar and low in fiber is related to obesity which is also linked to diabetes.

body and your baby all they require. All you have to do is follow the Best-Odds Diet.

The Best-Odds Diet *is* good nutrition. It supplies you with the magnesium you need to help prevent preeclampsia, the extra protein you need to enhance your baby's brain development, the B vitamins you need to keep morning sickness and emotional instability in check, the zinc you need to ward off preterm labor, and every vitamin, mineral, and other nutrient you need to boost your odds of having an uncomplicated pregnancy, a safe delivery, and a healthy baby. It does it all in a scientifically sound but unscientifically presented manner that not only makes the diet easier to follow than most pregnancy diets, but easier to live with, too. And because enjoying your food is as important during pregnancy as at any other time, the Best-Odds Diet doesn't forget your taste buds while it's looking out for your—and your baby's—general well-being.

While it can't guarantee a perfect pregnancy, delivery, or baby, the Best-Odds Diet can give you the best possible odds for achieving them.

WHAT CONTROLLED WEIGHT GAIN DOES

Weight has long been a matter of fashion—though the proportions weren't always the same (witness the recently slimmed-down shape of the once full-figured White Rock girl). Today, as more and more studies begin to correlate a trim body with a longer and healthier life, weight has become a matter of fitness, too. But it's not enough, scientists are warning, to reach an ideal weight. In order to reap the long-term benefits of slimness, we must maintain our ideal weight—with as few dramatic ups and downs as possible— over a lifetime. What nutritionist Dr. Jean Mayer has dubbed the "rhythm-method of girth control"—loss, gain, loss, gain, ad infinitum—poses as much of a health threat as the obesity it struggles to conquer.

In pregnancy, weight is definitely not a matter of fashion. (How many bulging bellies adorn the pages of *Vogue*?) But, as researchers are documenting each day, it is definitely a matter of fitness—for both mother and fetus. Here, too, reaching an ideal weight (of 25 to 35 pounds above prepregnancy is not enough. To ensure optimum fetal growth and development, ward off pregnancy complications, and maintain maternal comfort, weight gain should be as steady as possible, with no precipitous drops or jumps (see page 70 for how to achieve such a weight gain).

The benefits—to both baby

and mother—of prudently monitoring weight gain are many.

A healthier baby. The recipe for a healthy baby includes not only good maternal nutrition, but adequate maternal weight gain as well. The size of your baby is related (though not precisely) to both of these factors,[7] and size is a significant determinant in newborn health. Undersize babies (whether premature or not) are more likely than normal-size babies to have health problems at birth and after. A woman who begins pregnancy close to her ideal weight and gains less than 25 pounds increases her risk of having a too-small baby, one suffering from intrauterine growth retardation (IUGR)—delayed growth and development in the uterus. In addition, if the mother's caloric intake is too low (a weight gain that is slow as compared to the norm on page 73 is the clue), her own body fat and muscle will be burned to fuel the baby's growth. The by-products of this metabolic process are chemical compounds called ketones. Excess quantities of these ketones transmitted via the placenta and released into the mother's blood can seriously hamper the development of the fetus. When calories from fats and carbohydrates

are deficient, protein in the diet will also be burned for fuel, which means it won't be available to the fetus for growth and brain development.

Baby is constantly growing during its nine-month stay in your uterus, and it therefore needs a regular supply of calories and nutrients. An uneven pattern of weight gain by the mother indicates an uneven supply to the fetus, which can put it at risk. For example, a woman who gains her 35-pound limit by the time she finishes her second trimester, and cuts back on calories so she won't gain too many in her third, is likely to have a too-small baby even though she's had an adequate total weight gain. Her inadequate calorie intake in the final months may also interfere with the baby's brain development. Reversing the imbalance—with a light gain in the second trimester and a heavy one to compensate in the third—isn't any better for baby. The woman who gains only 4 pounds in the second trimester is likely to increase the risk of delivering prematurely even if a 10-pound gain in the seventh month brings her to an adequate total weight gain.

A more comfortable pregnancy. There's some discomfort in every pregnancy, even if it's just from walking around with a watermelon for a belly. And an

---

7. Your baby's birth weight is also influenced by a variety of other factors, including heredity and your own birth weight.

overly large weight gain compounds almost every one of those discomforts. The extra pounds weigh heavy on your back, making backache more likely. They put pressure on the valves in your leg veins, increasing the risk of varicose veins, and on the stomach, aggravating heartburn. As anyone who has been overweight knows, when the numbers on the scale go up, energy levels go down; those who put on extra pounds now will find it more difficult not only to defeat the normal fatigue of pregnancy, but simply to get around.

A better-looking pregnancy and postpartum. Big may be beautiful during pregnancy, but it's more beautiful if it stays in the belly and breasts and doesn't stray much to arms, hips, and thighs. Not only will you feel better if your weight gain is well-controlled and evenly paced, but you will look better, too. And if your weight is gained on all the right foods, it's likely to end up in all the right places. A modest gain will also retreat faster after delivery, making for a better-looking postpartum period. (And since many women who put on excess pounds during pregnancy never manage to take them all off, a well-controlled weight gain can also make for a better-looking future.)

A too-much, too-fast weight gain can also exacerbate stretch marks (since skin stretches more gracefully if it's stretched gradually) and contribute to gestational doldrums (those who don't feel good about the way they look during pregnancy are apt to suffer from depression).

A less-complicated pregnancy and childbirth. Gaining too little or too much weight can seriously complicate the course of a pregnancy. When weight gain is low (which means you're not taking in enough calories), your baby factory must break down your own body fat and muscle to fuel production. And as pointed out, not only is that bad for you, it's dangerous for your baby. In addition, a low prenatal weight gain is associated with an increase in frequency of amniotic fluid infections, abruptio placenta (separation of the placenta from the uterus before delivery), premature rupture of fetal membranes, damage to the placenta, and placenta previa (abnormal location of the placenta)—all of which can lead to preterm labor and other complications. Though it isn't clear why there's a relationship between low weight gain and these serious conditions,[8] the fact that it does

8. One possible explanation for this relationship is that low weight gain may be related to inadequate maternal blood volume (the volume of your blood should increase about a liter during pregnancy), which in turn is responsible for retarded blood flow to the placenta.

exist is reason enough to increase your food intake when your weight gain curve falls below the normal range.

Excessive weight gain is not as potentially hazardous as too little, but it does present its share of pregnancy risks. It's associated with the development of pregnancy hypertension, usually of a nonthreatening type, and possibly with gestational diabetes. Layers of excess fat on the abdomen make assessing the baby's size and position—important if there is the possibility of a breech—more difficult. (If there is a breech, turning the baby by external manipulation may prove impossible because of the fat layers.) This excess abdominal fat can also interfere with surgery should a cesarean become necessary (it does in about 15 percent to 20 percent of deliveries); being overweight puts any surgical patient at additional risk.

TWO

What to Eat When You're Expecting

W E ARE ALL CREATURES OF HABIT. IT'S NOT THAT WE crave that bagel we smear with cream cheese every morning, or the pineapple Danish we munch at the coffee break, or the burger and Coke we down in a hurry so we can get some shopping done at lunchtime. We're just in the habit of eating them.

Habits, of course, aren't all bad. If you've made a habit of having a citrus fruit with your breakfast, that's good. If you're in the habit of having a salad every night with your dinner, that's good, too. To make the Best-Odds Diet work, you've got to examine the eating habits you've accumulated so far in your life, dispose of the bad ones, hold on to the good ones, and, unless your diet is already Best-Odds quality, add some new good ones. That's not to say that you'll have to kiss your bagels, Danish, and burgers goodbye forever, just that you'll have to begin eating them as part of a carefully conceived dietary plan.

One of the new good habits you'll have to cultivate—if you haven't already—is keeping a watchful eye on your weight. Your scale is a vital guide to what you should be eating when you're expecting.

EVALUATING YOUR EATING HABITS

Though few would claim theirs is a nutrition-textbook-perfect diet, and the occasional honest junk-food aficionado might even admit to total dietary folly, most of us think we eat pretty well. But while some of us do, many of us would be surprised to find out how far from the Recommended Dietary Allowance (RDA) tree our diets have fallen—even when we're being extra careful to feed our baby-to-be nutritiously.

Now, before embarking on the Best-Odds Diet, is a good time to test the accuracy of the notions you have about the way you eat by taking the Best-Odds Quiz.

THE BEST-ODDS QUIZ

On the pages that follow, note every bite of food, every drop of drink that goes into your mouth for the next three days. This may seem like a tiresome chore (particularly if you're as busy as most of us), but you will find it pays dividends. Not only will it help you discover how your dietary intake compares with the Best-Odds ideal, it will also force you to begin to actually notice what you eat every day, something few of us do. (You may be very surprised.) You start with one point for good luck; you may award or deduct partial credit for servings that are smaller than specified in the charts.

Protein

For each serving of *protein* food (page 53), give yourself one point; award half points for half servings. If you have four or five servings daily, add one additional point each day; if you have six or more, deduct one point daily (you are overdoing the protein). Fill in the number of servings for each day:

	Serving	+ or −	Total
Day 1			
Day 2			
Day 3			

Maximum possible protein score: 18
Your score: _____

Whole Grain or Complex Carbohydrate

For each *complex carbohydrate* food (page 59), give yourself one point; if you total four or five servings daily, add one point; award half points for half servings. If you have six or more servings in one day, deduct one point, unless you are very active, underweight, or a vegetarian. If you are sedentary or normal weight (or more), six carbohydrate servings may be providing too many calories and too much bulk (leaving no room for other foods).

	Serving	+ or −	Total
Day 1			
Day 2			
Day 3			

Maximum possible carbohydrate score: 18
Your score: _____

Calcium

For each *calcium* serving (page 56), give yourself one point; award half points for half servings. If you have four or five servings, add one point; if you have six or more servings, deduct one point unless you're a vegetarian. If you're a vegetarian don't count the same foods for protein and calcium allowances.

	Serving	+ or −	Total
Day 1			
Day 2			
Day 3			

Maximum possible calcium score: 18
Your score: _____

Vitamin C

Give yourself one point for each *vitamin C* food, up to two, daily. Additional vitamin C foods count as Other Vegetables or Fruits. (See page 55.)

	Serving	+ or −	Total
Day 1			
Day 2			
Day 3			

Maximum possible vitamin C score: 6
Your score: _____

Iron-Rich Food

Give yourself two points if you have at least one *iron-rich* food daily. (See page 60.)

	Serving	+ or −	Total
Day 1			
Day 2			
Day 3			

Maximum possible iron score: 6
Your score: _____

Fat

For each *fat* serving, up to two, give yourself one point; for every fat serving over two, deduct two points, unless you are underweight. (See page 61.)

	Serving	+ or −	Total
Day 1			
Day 2			
Day 3			

Maximum possible fat score: 6
Your score: _____

Green Leafy or Yellow Vegetables and Yellow Fruits

For each serving of *green leafy or yellow vegetable or fruit* up to three servings daily, give yourself one point. Ideally, you should have both green leafy *and* yellow daily. Additional green leafies or yellows, up to two, count as Other Vegetables or Fruits. (See page 57.)

	Serving	+ or −	Total
Day 1			
Day 2			
Day 3			

Maximum possible green leafy or yellow score: 9   Your score: _____

Other Vegetables or Fruits

For each serving of *other vegetables or fruits* (page 58) up to two, give yourself one point.

	Serving	+ or −	Total
Day 1			
Day 2			
Day 3			

Maximum possible other vegetables or fruits score: 6   **Your score:** _____

Fluid

For each eight ounces of *fluid* (not counting coffee, tea, other caffeinated beverages, or alcohol; see page 51), add half a point, up to 10 servings daily.

	Serving	+ or −	Total
Day 1			
Day 2	.		
Day 3			

Maximum possible fluid score: 15
Your score: _____

Less Than the Best

For each serving of *less than the best* foods (page 32) you've eaten, deduct one point. If you have eaten more than three in one day in this category, deduct one additional point for that day.

	Serving	Minus	Total
Day 1			
Day 2			
Day 3	.		

Your total less-than-best score: _____
Your score: _____

Forbidden Fruit

For each serving of *forbidden fruit* (page 32), deduct two points; if you have had more than two servings in this category on any one day, deduct three additional points for that day; if you had two or more on all three days, deduct a total of fifteen additional points.

	Serving	Minus	Total
Day 1			
Day 2			
Day 3			

Your score: _____
Your total three-day nutrition score (add together your positive and deduct your negative subtotals): _____

Evaluating Your Score

100 means you are doing everything right—at least for the three days in question. Congratulations and keep up the good work! You are getting your Daily Dozen (page 42) daily.

90 to 99 means you are well on your way to eating healthy. See in which areas your scores were below par and start compensating now.

80 to 89 means you don't have too far to go to start getting your dietary act together. Find the areas in which your scores were weak and start compensating now.

70 to 79 is just barely passing, nutritionally. You are probably deficient in several areas, all of which will need beefing up. Don't delay in turning your diet around.

Under 70 means you've let everything you've ever heard or read about nutrition pass you by. If you want a healthy baby and a comfortable and safe pregnancy, start taking the Daily Dozen as seriously as the Ten Commandments—*now.*

CHANGING YOUR EATING HABITS

It's one thing to acknowledge that there's room for improvement in your eating habits, but quite another to know how to go about filling that room. Fortunately, however, though habits that have been formed over a lifetime can't be changed without some effort, they *can* be changed—and changed for good. Using the same kind of behavior modification techniques used to alter any undesirable habit—smoking, for example—you can rid yourself of the worst in your diet while building up the best.

Don't put off till tomorrow what you can give up today. Quitting cold turkey is the only effective way to break a bad eating habit. For most sugar ad-

dicts, a little bit of sugar leads to a little bit more, and then, finally, a lot. Junk-food junkies who vow this bag of potato chips and can of cola will be their last, almost always have to eat—and drink—their words.

Think before you eat. Most dietary indiscretions aren't planned, they just happen. Would you pop a chocolate cream from your friend's coffee table into your mouth, guzzle a Coke on a hot afternoon, or order your tuna salad on white instead of whole wheat if you gave a moment's consideration to the consequences? Probably not.

So make the thought process preliminary to the eating process every time you are faced with food or drink. Does what you are about to consume offer your growing fetus something of important nutritional value, or does it take the place of something that would? If you answer "yes" to the latter, think again and make another choice. (If you're uncomfortable with on-the-spot decision making, plan your meals and snacks ahead of time.)

Think before you don't eat. If your major dietary problem is not what you eat, but what you don't eat (breakfast or lunch, for example), some changes are also warranted. (For an explanation of why skipping meals is un-

FORBIDDEN FRUIT

Sugar, corn syrup, honey
Commercial gelatin or pudding
Cake and cookie mixes
Icing and frosting mixes
Pancake syrups
Maple syrup
Chocolate syrups
Sundae toppings
Sweetened cocoa
Sweetened condensed milk
Sweetened fruit juices
Sugar or artificially sweetened
   soft drinks
Canned fruits in sugar syrup
Cookies or cakes baked with any
   type of sugar or honey
Pastries or pies baked with any
   type of sugar or honey

Commercial sweetened pie fillings
Doughnuts
Artificial whipped toppings
Commercial ice cream, ices,
   sherbets, frozen tofu desserts
Candy
Candied fruit
Maraschino cherries
Artificially-sweetened foods
Artifically or sugar sweetened
   cereals
Non-dairy creamers
Smoked fish or meats
Frankfurters, cold cuts
Commercial salad dressings (with
   sugar, chemicals, or artificial
   sweeteners)
Sweet relishes and pickles

LESS THAN THE BEST

Ice milk or frozen yogurt with
   sugar
Commercial flavored yogurts
Sour cream, sweet cream
Ketchup, barbecue sauce
Cornstarch or other starches
White bread, rolls, pitas, bagels,
   pancakes, biscuits

Instant dinners in a box
Canned soups or instant soup
   mixes (except "all natural"
   ones with no sugar and
   moderate salt content)
Commercial baked beans
White rice, white pastas

wise, see page 37.) The changes will depend on the reasons for meal skipping.

If lack of time is keeping you away from the breakfast table, try setting the alarm to go off earlier. Or, prepare breakfast the night before: a bowl of cold cereal and dry fruit ready to be covered with milk; a mound of cottage cheese to which canteloupe and a defrosted Bran Muffin can be added in the morning; or an egg-salad sandwich on whole wheat ready to down with a glass of milk. Try taking breakfast to work with you and eat it at your desk: a plastic container of cereal, raisins, and nonfat dry milk to which water—hot for oatmeal, cold for dry cereal—can be added; a container of plain yogurt with fresh or frozen unsweetened strawberries and wheat germ stirred in; sliced egg on whole-wheat bread, tomato on the side. If time constraints interfere with lunch, bring lunch to work, or, if you don't have time to fill a brown bag, make a habit of ordering in a sandwich a half hour before lunchtime (see page 117 for tips on healthy at-desk eating). Or, meet with business associates over lunch when possible (see page 108 for tips on healthy restaurant eating).

If you just don't like eating breakfast or lunch, make them more appealing. Ask your husband to eat a leisurely first meal of the day with you. Set the table attractively the night before, plan on serving something you love to eat, even if it's not traditional breakfast fare. (There's nothing wrong with a tuna sandwich first thing in the morning, or even a piece of cold chicken on brown rice.) Make lunch a pleasurable occasion by sharing it with a friend, your spouse, or a good book, or, in fine weather, eat al fresco in the backyard or park. If preparing lunch for one at home seems like a waste of energy, make a little extra at dinner and serve leftovers cold or reheated for lunch the next day. And don't forget: You're not really lunching for one, you're lunching for two!

If eating a big breakfast (or lunch or dinner) leaves you feeling uncomfortably full, don't skip the meal, split it. Have some yogurt or cottage cheese with fruit early on, then snack on a couple of Bran Muffins later. Or have half a bowl of cereal at 8:00, the other half at 9:00, a slice of whole-wheat toast at 10:30. You can easily apply the same split-meal principle to any meal that seems too filling.

Substitute like for like. Martyrs don't last long on special diets. So instead of giving up your midmorning jelly doughnuts and coffee for a slice of dry whole-wheat toast and a glass of skim milk, substitute naturally sweetened but sweet-tooth-satisfying Bran Muffins, slathered with fruit-only preserves or apple butter, and a cup of brewed decaffeinated coffee. Instead of trying to talk your sweet tooth into an apple for dessert when what it really would like to sink into is a nice thick slice of apple pie, help yourself to a nice thick (and guiltless) slice of Nature-Sweetened Apple Pie.

Avoid the scenes of your crimes. You're less likely to stray if you stay away from the places that have become associated with your bad food habits. If you can't resist the white and dark chocolate mousse at your favorite restaurant, resist the restaurant entirely during your pregnancy. If passing a pair of golden arches fills you with an irrepressible urge for a quarter-pounder and fries, take alternate routes during mealtimes. If late-night movies in the den have always been accompanied by late-night raids on the refrigerator, move the television into the bedroom.

Don't put your willpower to the test. At least in the early phases of breaking your bad habits, go out of your way to coddle your self-control. Don't thrust it into situations it might not be able to handle. Don't serve company sugar-filled bakery treats that might be left over to challenge your willpower to a duel the morning after. Your guests will appreciate your Best-Odds offerings just as much (maybe even more if they're watching their diets). When you're the guest at a party, don't even give the dessert table a glance. Ask your husband to fill a bowl with fresh fruit, if there is any, and keep thinking about the chewy Fudge Brownies or the slice of richly satisfying Angelic Devil's Food Cake that awaits you at home. In a restaurant, instead of letting the waiter reel off the list of 22 mouthwatering desserts he could bring you, or worse still, wheel the pastry cart over for your perusal, ask for the check and head home for your just—and justifiable—desserts.

Don't let short time or short money shortchange your diet. Two of the most commonly used alibis for sloppy eating habits—not enough time and not enough

money—are also two of the most invalid ones (see pages 92 and 94).

Don't let your emotions rule your appetite. If depression, anxiety, boredom, anger, or excitement lure you to the ice cream parlor or the candy store, find alternate ways to emotional satisfaction. Try relaxation techniques; exercise or dance classes; brisk strolls or bike rides; reading a good book; taking up a musical instrument, knitting, or a foreign language; baking nutritious Best-Odds treats (kneading bread is great for beating frustration); shopping for the baby. Instead of sending your husband out at night for a quart of mocha almond fudge, keep him home for a game of Monopoly, a soothing massage, a romantic bath (if you can still squeeze into the tub together), or a little lovemaking. If time is hanging heavy during your wait for the baby's arrival, take an adult education course, do volunteer work at a local hospital, learn CPR and baby safety techniques at the Red Cross.

Think positive. If you say at the outset "I'll never be able to stay on this diet for nine months," you probably won't. Walk into an Italian restaurant exclaiming "There's no way I'll be able to resist the fettuccine," and you'll undoubtedly order it. Insist that you can't make it through the morning without three cups of caffeinated coffee, and you'll talk yourself into a 10 o'clock sag the first day you try. Instead, boost your spirits and your willpower with a positive outlook. Walk into that Italian restaurant and tell yourself that not only will you resist that fettuccine (although you might take a bite from your dinner companion's dish), but you will really enjoy that Veal Piccata. Brew a pot of good-quality decaffeinated coffee in the morning, and linger over the fact that it's warm and satisfying instead of the fact that it's caffeine-free. Get your mind to work for you instead of against you. Tell yourself (and it's true!) that you *can* break your bad habits and take on better ones. You've never had a better reason.

Don't take two steps backward for every slip you make. Nobody's perfect, not even expectant mothers. If you occasionally slip up it doesn't mean you're a failure, just that you're human. Instead of railing against yourself, which will only push you further into the kind of mood that discourages control, or giving up entirely, learn from your mistake (next time you'll know better than to tell your husband it's okay to bring home a Boston cream pie "just this once") and get right back on the Best-Odds track.

THE BEST-ODDS NINE BASIC PRINCIPLES

These nine commandments for nine months of healthy eating don't have the lofty purpose or divine origin of the ten given at Mount Sinai. But following these guidelines religiously can give your baby the best odds for a healthy start in life—a pretty lofty objective in itself. Read them, study them, make them a way of pregnant life. If you don't have a pair of stone tablets handy, inscribe them on your refrigerator door. And don't forget to take them (but not the refrigerator door) along when you go to work, out to dinner, or on a trip.

Make every bite count. In the context of the several hundred bites taken every day, a single bite, that forkful of food which takes only seconds to go from plate to digestive tract, seems of little significance. Whereas you might think again about eating a whole slice of chocolate cake or an entire tray of lasagna, you probably wouldn't think twice about taking "just one bite" of either. Yet thinking about each and every bite of food is one of the most fundamental rules of Best-Odds eating. Because it ends up not just in your body, but in your baby's as well, the

USING A BEST-ODDS MENU PLANNER

If you find that gastronomic spontaneity—selecting the ingredients for your lunch after the first noon hunger pangs have struck, letting your culinary spirit move you through the supermarket aisles—is the recipe for dietary disaster, a little advance planning is in order. Using a pocket-size calendar or notebook, plot your Best-Odds menus— breakfast, lunch, dinner, and snacks, being careful to incorporate adequate doses of your Daily Dozen—a day, two days, or a week in advance. Draw up a shopping list from the menus, and stick to it when you're at the market.

Don't be fanatical about adhering to your menu planner. Pregnant women are notoriously prone to legitimate food moods—a sudden aversion to the planned fillet of sole or broccoli, a sudden craving for baked potatoes when rice has been scheduled. Follow these moods as long as they don't lead you down a pernicious path. And don't feel obligated to keep planning your meals in advance once eating and shopping healthily become habitual. (Believe it or not, they might.)

single bite *is* significant during pregnancy. It's an opportunity, repeated hundreds of times a day, to ship vital nutrients to your rapidly developing fetus.

You lose that opportunity when you reach for a white roll instead of a whole-grain one. Or when you order your potatoes fried (more fat, calories, and fewer vitamins) rather than baked in the skin. Or drink a ginger ale instead of a glass of fruit juice.

And because your stomach capacity will diminish as your growing uterus fills the abdominal cavity, leaving you feeling fuller on less food, lost opportunities to send nourishment to your fetus may not be recouped. You simply won't have room to supplement the unnutritious bites with more nutritious ones.

So before you bring a bite of food to your mouth, ask yourself: Is this the best bite I can give my baby? If it is, bite away. If it isn't, find a better one.

All calories are not created equal. In technical terms, a calorie is the amount of heat energy required to raise one kilogram of water one degree centigrade. So a calorie is a calorie; it'll raise that water temperature no matter what its source. But it makes a big difference—especially when you're pregnant—whether you get the calories to "heat" your body machinery from alcohol (which can be dangerous), from sugar (which is, at best, useless), or from a glass of milk (which is packed with protein, calcium, and other nutrients).

Your baby is less well-nourished when you eat a high-calorie diet in which the calories are furnished mostly by fat and sugar than when your caloric intake is just adequate but the calories are carefully selected to provide ample amounts of a variety of nutrients. So, select your calories for quality, not quantity. Don't consider your additional calorie allowance during pregnancy as a daily invitation to your favorite doughnut shop or hot dog stand. The 300 calories you invest in two nutritionally void crullers could buy your baby two Banana Muffins—providing one Whole-Grain and Other Fruit serving plus plenty of fiber. Likewise, the 300 calories you squander on a hot dog with ketchup on a bun (which gives your baby less than a third of a protein serving and only a few vitamins and minerals if the bun is enriched, not to mention a host of chemicals, sugars, and fats) could be far better spent on a chicken salad with tomato and lettuce on whole wheat (one full Protein serving, two Whole-Grain servings, a Vitamin C serving and some fiber).

Starve yourself, starve your baby. If you're an accomplished meal-skipper, accustomed to going 8 hours at a stretch (16 or more if you're skipping breakfast) with nary a nibble, not eating probably has little noticeable effect on you. Even if you don't skip meals on purpose, and miss one only because your alarm clock didn't go off or your appointment ran late, you're not likely to experience anything more debilitating than a headache and a few hunger pangs. Your fetus, however, can't weather missed meals as easily. He or she is growing all day, every day, and counts on a steady supply of building materials from you through the placenta. Skip or skimp on a meal, and he or she could run short of supplies at a critical moment. ("Combined" meals fall into this category, too. Brunch may be fashionable on Sundays, but fashion doesn't fill your stomach or your fetus' nutritional needs. Accept brunch invitations, but make sure you also eat a light, sustaining meal at your usual breakfast time.)

Intentionally fasting, for religious, philosophical, or other reasons, is also a pregnancy no-no. Fasting causes your body to release excess ketones into your blood, which, when they cross the placenta, can be harmful to your baby (see page 24).

It's true that the discomforts of pregnancy sometime interfere with your normal meal patterns: you're too queasy to eat; you have indigestion; your stomach capacity is reduced by pressure from the expanding uterus, making you feel uncomfortably full. These biologically motivated reasons for abstaining from meals may seem justifiable to you, but they aren't to your baby. He or she needs to eat whether you feel like it or not. Instead of succumbing to lack of appetite, look for ways to overcome it (see morning sickness, page 79; heartburn, page 85; and bloating and flatulence, page 84.

Become an efficiency expert. Squeezing the 28 servings of food and drink the Daily Dozen requires every day into three meals and a few snacks seems a task for Houdini. If the foods with which you fill your requirements are too dense with calories, you may get all your nutrients, but you'll also end up with too many pounds. Or, if the foods are too filling, you may not be able to fit all the servings in, and may find yourself short of requirements by day's end.

But you needn't become a magician to accomplish this 28-serving dietary feat, only an efficiency expert. Learn how to choose foods that will take you the farthest nutritionally for the fewest calories, and will take up the least amount of space in your increasingly crowded stomach. Get more than half a protein serving from a 90-calorie serving of low-fat cottage cheese, instead of a 120-calorie serving of high-fat cottage cheese; a full serving of protein from a 150-calorie grilled, skinless chicken breast, instead of a 350-calorie fried one. Don't regularly try to fill your protein requirements with high-calorie, more filling foods, such as baked beans (500 calories for 25 grams of protein) or peanut butter (500 calories for 23 grams). Instead, pick lower-calorie, more highly concentrated ones, such as water-packed tuna (150 calories for 24 grams). Don't choose ice cream (450 calories for each serving of calcium) or cream cheese (1,500 calories for each serving of calcium) as calcium sources; choose skim or low-fat milk (80 to 100 calories for each calcium serving) or low-fat yogurt (150 calories).

It's even more efficient, though not always possible, to fill two requirements for the caloric price of one. Use broccoli to fill your vitamin C, calcium, and green leafy requirements; at the same time you'll be getting a bonus of fiber. Yogurt (or milk or sardines) can be both a calcium and a protein food; wheat germ, a protein and a grain; orange, grapefruit, or tomato juice, a vitamin C food and a fluid; dried apricots, an iron source and a yellow fruit.

Carbohydrates are a complex issue. Once considered the nemesis of the waist watcher, carbohydrates are just now being cleared of the negative reputation they never really deserved. In fact, nutrition experts advise us that most of the calories in our diet should come from carbohydrates. Not just any carbohydrates, however, but complex carbohydrates like grains, potatoes, beans and peas, fruits, and vegetables. Complex carbohydrates are particularly useful for the person—pregnant or not—who finds she is hungry all the time. Because they provide a lot of bulk for the calories, they can keep a growling stomach satisfied more easily than can other types of food.

Unfortunately, though complex carbohydrates are all rich in nutrients when harvested, processing often depletes their benefits. Grains, usually subjected to refining, are the major losers in the processing game. Those folks who rely mainly on refined grains (in breads, pastas, cereals, and so on) are losers, too (see page 48). So are those who eat their potatoes in a processed flake, their vegetables from a can, and their fruits boiled in a sugary compote.

So, when you select your carbohydrates, pick the whole grains (whole wheat, whole rye, whole corn) over the refined ones (white flour, rye flour, degerminated cornmeal), the unprocessed (fresh potatoes or frozen fresh peas) over the processed (dehydrated instant potatoes or canned peas), and the complex (fruit and fruit juices) over the simple (sugar and honey).

Sweet nothings—nothing but trouble. Human beings had a sweet tooth long before sugar became available in five-pound bags. It was a gift from Mother Nature to ensure that we would search for sweet berries and tree fruits packed with vitamin C and valuable trace minerals—foods without which survival would have been impossible. It certainly was a wise gift, one that protected us from the scourge of scurvy. But then, along came a sweet without any vitamin C, without trace minerals, without anything, in fact, but calories: refined sugar. Our ancestors were fortunate that refined sugar didn't grow on trees. We are not so fortunate. Though it still doesn't grow on trees, it's more widely available in supermarkets than the fruits that do.

Nothing offers your baby less to grow on than sugar. Every calorie refined sugar supplies could better come from foods that yield a nutritional return, which is reason enough to offer it to your baby as rarely as possible. Add to this sugar's other proven and suspected drawbacks—it contributes to obesity, tooth decay, and gum disease (all of which are potential problems in pregnancy); it depletes the body of chromium and possibly other nutrients important in pregnancy; it is implicated in the development of diabetes (another possible, though usually temporary complication of pregnancy), heart disease, depression, and hyperactivity—and you'll have totalled the reasons why the Best-Odds Diet recommends avoiding sugar in all its forms during pregnancy. (To stay away from sugar, you need to know how to find it; see page 168.)

If you must, "cheat" on a "sugar food" once a week, but not more often (see page 68). And when you do, make it one that also contains ingredients of redeeming value—frozen yogurt instead of Italian ice, a slice of cheesecake rather than chocolate cake. (For some people, sugar, particularly when combined with chocolate, has an addictive effect, making once-a-week cheating impossible. If one sugar treat leads to another for you, you're probably well aware of it. And you'll probably find quitting sugar cold turkey—and satisfying your sweet tooth with a Best-Odds treat instead—a better solution.)

Eat foods that can remember where they came from. In the days when we went no farther than our own backyard (or the local farmer's fields) for our produce, fruits and vegetables (as-suming they weren't overcooked) generally appeared on our tables with most of their natural goodness intact. Today, when the harvests are taking place hundreds, even thousands of miles away, not just in other towns, but in other hemispheres, preserving the nutritional integrity of what appears on our tables is a challenge.

The best way to meet that challenge is to select foods that are as close to their natural form as possible, even when they aren't close to their native fields. Choose fresh fruits and vegetables over canned, bottled, or dehydrated, but don't assume that everything that appears in the "fresh produce" section of the market will supply those nutrients. Color, firmness, and overall condition are good clues to the freshness quotient. Broccoli that looks pale and tired from its journey across country (or was it that layover in the refrigerated warehouse?) isn't a good nutritional bet. Neither are carrots that have softened or split, asparagus that has gone to seed, or prematurely picked strawberries that weren't given the vine time they needed to develop a deep red blush. In cases like these, don't change your menu, just head to the frozen-food aisle. Today, since quick-freezing is done almost immediately after harvesting, when produce is at the height of its nutritive value, most frozen fruits and vegetables have as much or more to offer as their "fresh" counterparts. (Be careful, however, to pick frozens that are as close to their natural states as possible, with no added sauces, salts, butters, or chemicals; avoid packages that are covered with frost or otherwise look as though they have been refrozen.)

Carry this principle over to the other aisles of the market, too. Select fresh turkey over processed turkey breast, brown rice over refined white rice, rolled oats (that take five minutes to cook) over instant oatmeal, natural cheese over artificially-flavored cheese.

JUNK FOOD: WHAT'S IN IT FOR YOU AND FOR BABY

Picture a mother giving her baby a doughnut for breakfast, a hot dog and cola for lunch, and a fried-fish sandwich and fries for dinner. Not a pretty picture, but, sadly, a real one. Though no mother would feed her newborn a diet of junk food, many expectant mothers feed their unborn just that.

While you can eat what you choose to eat, a fetus has no choice. It eats what you've chosen, whether the selection serves its nutritional interests or not. It can't order in a bowl of shredded wheat to supplement your breakfast doughnut, or an extra serving of protein to augment that lunchtime hot dog. It can't leave the fries if it's surfeited with fat, or opt for a glass of milk instead of that cola when the craving is for calcium.

Eat junk food and fast food, and what are you giving your baby? In most cases, not very much to grow on. That doughnut, for example, has as many calories and scarcely a trace of the protein, vitamins, and minerals (particularly calcium) of a bowl of whole-grain cereal with skim milk and fruit. The hot dog on a refined bun has the same number of calories as a chicken salad sandwich on whole wheat but supplies less than half the protein and none of the trace minerals. The fast-food fried-fish sandwich, while containing anywhere from 2½ to 4 times the calories and 8 to 10 times the fat of a 4-ounce serving of broiled fish, contains less than half the protein.

Even when junk food and fast food do give your baby something to grow on (none will give your baby everything he or she needs), they usually provide you with so much unnecessary fat, calories, and sodium that you're also likely to grow—more than you'd like. See the chart on page 311 of the Appendix for a further breakdown of what junk foods do and don't contain.

Make good eating a family affair. While what your family eats during your pregnancy would seem less significant than what you eat, there are two good reasons to include them in your dietary retrenching. First, a Best-Odds family gives your diet the best odds for success. Making those you live with your allies, rather than the not-so-loyal opposition, will keep them from undermining your efforts, while supplying you with the encouragement and support everyone on a new eating regimen needs. Second, the Best-Odds Diet, when used as a foundation for permanent improvement in your family's nutritional life-style, gives all of them the best odds of longer, healthier, more productive lives (see page 183).

Don't sabotage your diet. Though it offers other positive side effects (keeping you from becoming obese, helping to reduce the discomforts of pregnancy), there's no doubt that your major motivation for following the Best-Odds Diet is to give your baby the best odds of being born healthy. The easiest way to thwart your efforts and reduce the odds of having a healthy baby is to smoke, drink, and/or abuse caffeine or other drugs during pregnancy.

THE DAILY DOZEN

Glancing over a chart of the vitamin and mineral requirements of a pregnant woman, you might begin to feel that you'll have to build a laboratory in your kitchen and never leave the house without a suitcase of Bunsen burners, vials, centrifuges, and slide rules. That you'll have to extract and measure the folic acid in your shredded wheat breakfast, analyze your Swiss cheese sandwich before deciding it's an acceptable lunch, and add up the traces of zinc in each meal on your pocket calculator to see if you've filled your daily quota.

But before you make the down payment on that laboratory (or, more likely, give up entirely on the possibility of feeding your fetus well), read on. The Best-Odds Diet has done the calculations for you, synthesizing what is known about maternal nutrition into a practical, portable, easy-to-follow, and difficult-to-fail daily program. It dispenses with micrograms and milligrams, relegating them to the appendix for the scientifically minded (and masochistic), and tells you only what you really need to know to feed your fetus well. (If, however, you find lists of vitamins and minerals, micrograms and milligrams, food sources and daily requirements fascinating, you're welcome to peruse the appendix.)

With the Best-Odds Daily Dozen, you don't need to know a micronutrient from a macronutrient, a vitamin from a mineral, a milligram from a microgram to fill every nutritional requirement of pregnancy to its fullest. All you need is to keep track of the following and whether you've eaten and drunk the prescribed number of portions from the Food Selection Groups (starting on page 53).

Calories

Eating for two doesn't mean taking the number of calories you need to live on and doubling it to accommodate the needs of your baby. Though he or she is working harder than you are, busily building bones, organs, and other tissues, your fetus, only a fraction of your weight, accomplishes it all on considerably less food energy—only about 300 calories a day. And for most pregnant women, those 300 calories are all that must be added to the number of calories required to maintain prepregnancy weight.[1] Some women, specifically those who begin pregnancy significantly underweight, who are carrying multiple fetuses, or

who are not gaining adequate weight, will need to add more calories (see page 72).

If a daily bonus of at least 300 calories seems like the opportunity of a food lover's lifetime, you're in for a letdown—unless you really love to drink milk. Remember, the calories are slotted for your baby's use in his or her marathon of growth, not for your personal pleasure. Add two extra cups of skim milk (or the equivalent) to your daily diet, and you've already consumed 180 of those 300 extra calories. Add the additional 50 grams or so of protein you need, and you've exceeded your allotted bonus. All of which means that instead of being able to add some fun frills to your diet during pregnancy, you'll probably have to trim most of them away.

Not getting enough calories in pregnancy has more serious consequences than getting too many. If you were snowed in at a ski lodge and ran out of wood for the fireplace, you would probably start burning everything in sight for fuel. Your body does much the same thing when it has insufficient fuel for baby making: It burns body fat and body protein. As a result, excess ketones are produced that can be hazardous not only to you, but to your baby. It will also burn the protein you eat, instead of allowing it to be used to build your baby's body. So, to protect your-

---

1. To determine how many calories you need to maintain your prepregnancy weight, multiply that weight by 12 if you're sedentary, 15 if you're moderately active, and up to 22 if you're extremely active.

self and your baby, be sure to get an adequate number of calories daily.

But now that you know how many calories you'll need every day for the rest of your pregnancy, forget it. Besides being a tedious chore, counting your calories is not an effective way of determining whether your baby is getting his or hers. So many factors go into whether a person loses or gains weight—for example, the level of activity and exercise, individual metabolism (which increases in pregnancy), the amount of fiber in the diet (fiber pushes some calories through the system before they can be burned for fuel)—that the extra 300 calories pregnant women need can only be used as a rough guide. Monitoring your weight gain, keeping it within the limits of the steady and moderate pattern described on page 70, is a much more effective way of keeping track of your baby's intake of calories. If you're not gaining weight quickly enough, then you're not getting your Daily Dozen of calories. If you're gaining too quickly, you're getting more than you need.

Protein—four servings daily

No one material is more essential to the building of a baby than protein's amino acids, the building blocks of human tissue. In fact, inadequate protein intake during pregnancy appears to be as closely connected to babies being born small as inadequate calorie intake.

Though a growing fetus doesn't require that you double your intake of calories, it does demand that you double your intake of protein. An average nonpregnant woman needs only 45 grams of protein a day, but an average pregnant woman should take in no fewer than 75 grams (three Best-Odds Protein Servings, page 53). The Best-Odds Diet recommends a full 100 grams (four Best-Odds Protein Servings), the amount usually prescribed in high-risk pregnancies. Not only may the extra protein serve to protect against some pregnancy complications, such as preeclampsia (page 20), but it will help to maximize fetal brain development, particularly in the last trimester.

A vegetarian who eats no animal proteins (not even eggs or milk), should have an extra protein serving—since vegetable protein is of a poorer quality than the animal variety.

To fill your protein requirement without overfilling your fat cells, try to choose high-efficiency protein sources—those with a high ratio of protein to fat or protein to carbohydrate. Select chicken, with skin removed, over fatty cuts of pork, lamb, and beef; broiled, baked, or poached fish over fried; low-fat cottage cheese over ricotta. Don't rely often on nuts (about 800 calories per protein serving), or exclusively on peas and beans (unless you're a strict vegetarian, since the 300 to 350 calories they offer per protein serving compares poorly to the roughly 125 calories in a protein serving of codfish).

Getting your four protein servings a day is a more easily attained goal than you'd think. Have just one serving at each meal (for example, a cheese omelet for breakfast, a large scoop of cottage cheese for lunch, and a chicken breast for dinner), plus three glasses of milk, and you're there. If you're having six meals a day, six half servings will substitute nicely. Or, if you prefer cereal (not a full protein portion) for breakfast, you can have a double portion of poultry or fish (just 6 or 7 ounces) for dinner to compensate. Remember, too, that you can get additional protein from whole-grain breads, wheat germ, pasta, and cereal. And that if on any day you should come in under four full protein servings, you can supplement with a couple of egg whites ("fried" in a nonstick pan coated with vegetable cooking spray and sprinkled with Parmesan cheese or hard boiled), which are pure protein (3 or 4 grams each) and very low in calories (15 to 20). A quarter cup of low-fat cottage cheese (7 grams of protein) for only 45 calories is another good protein filler.

Vitamin C Foods—two servings daily

This most widely known of vitamins has been proposed by some researchers as a cure for everything from the common cold to cancer. But these still-experimental uses for vitamin C are not as significant to you and your baby as its well-documented benefits. Adequate levels of vitamin C are necessary every day (the body doesn't store it) for growth, tissue repair, wound healing, bone and tooth development, and various metabolic processes, both fetal and maternal.

For a lot of people, the best thing about vitamin C is that it comes in foods that taste good and most Americans eat by choice: citrus fruits, tomatoes, strawberries, melons, peppers, potatoes (see page 55, for a complete list of vitamin C foods). And since you only need two vitamin C foods daily, chances are you won't have to make any alterations in your diet to ensure adequate intake.

As vitamins go, C is fairly fragile. Exposure to heat, light, and air destroys it over time. So it's best to get your vitamin C from foods that haven't been cooked, prepeeled, or precut. Section your grapefruit, squeeze your orange, slice your peppers, or blend your frozen juice just before serving whenever possible to preserve the maximum vitamin C. Potatoes retain the most C (and the most of everything else they contain) when cooked in their skins. All is not lost, however, if you can't always control the preparation of your C foods. First of all, some of the vitamin will surely survive no matter what kind of mistreatment the food receives. Second, you will get extra insurance from the small amounts of vitamin C in a wise variety of other fruits and vegetables and in your daily multivitamin supplement (see page 32).

Calcium Foods—four servings daily

When mother admonished us to drink our milk so we would get enough calcium for strong bones, she would have been wise to take her own advice. Scientists are now discovering that calcium is important not only for growing bones, but also for those that have already grown—particularly in women. It is also vital for heart, muscle, and nerve function, blood clotting, and enzyme activity. The four calcium servings an expectant mother needs every day are not just for the baby, they're for her own health as well. If she fails to meet this quota, both could be headed for trouble.

For some women, however, this requirement is easier said than drunk in the form of milk. Our mothers' threats, pleas, and cajoling when we were children left a sour taste for milk in some mouths. Fortunately, milk doesn't always have to be drunk, and when it is, it can be in delicious milk shakes, soups, even in decaffeinated coffee. It can also be eaten—in puddings, breads, cereals (hot and cold), meat and fish loaves, homemade frozen desserts, pancakes, casseroles, sauces, and more. (Look for Best-Odds recipes that are labeled Calcium Servings.)

Though milk is one of the most efficient mediums for meeting your calcium requirement, it's by no means the only one. You can get calcium from other dairy products, particularly yogurt and hard cheeses, or from such nondairy sources as canned fish with their bones and certain vegetables. (See the Food Selection Chart on page 56 for a complete listing of calcium foods, and if you can't tolerate milk or other dairy products at all, see tips for the milk intolerant on page 102.) Again, you will probably get a small insurance dose of calcium in your pregnancy vitamin supplement.

Protect your calcium intake

by avoiding or limiting those things that may interfere with absorption (most are not recommended in pregnancy anyway): alcohol, caffeine and its relatives in chocolate, laxatives, diuretic pills, excessive salt, and a high beef intake. And, since dietary fiber can rob your body of the calcium you eat before it has been absorbed, try not to take the bulk of your fiber along with the bulk of your calcium foods.

Green Leafy and Yellow Vegetables and Yellow Fruits—three servings daily

Peter Rabbit had the right idea when he made a bunny-line to the green and leafy section of Mr. MacGregor's garden. Green leafy vegetables and deep yellow ones, also bunny favorites, as well as deep yellow fruits, are rich sources of vitamin A, crucial for healthy cell growth (a fetus' cells are multiplying at an incredible rate), healthy skin, bones, and more. They are also excellent sources of vitamin E, riboflavin, folic acid, B_6, and numerous minerals. As an extra bonus for you, when eaten raw or cooked only lightly, greens and yellows (particularly the vegetables) supply plenty of constipation-countering fiber.

For those who don't share Peter's affection for green and yellow produce (particularly early in pregnancy, when aversions to certain vegetables are most common), a few palatable choices are likely to be found on the Green Leafy and Yellow Vegetables and Yellow Fruits Food Selection Chart (page 57). Some choices that aren't favored plain can be cleverly concealed under sauces (such as the high-calcium cheese sauce on page 261); added to soups (such as Broccoli-Cheese-Bread Soup); tossed into casseroles (such as Tuna Macaroni and Broccoli Casserole) and stuffings; and in fish, meat, and vegetable loaves (such as the Chickpea and Nut Loaf). Carrots, if sticks or steamed aren't appealing, can also be grated into fish, egg, and vegetable salads, and into a Carrot-Pineapple Cake that bears no taste resemblance to its vegetable namesake. Or try Pumpkin Pie or pumpkin-packed Harvest Pudding. If all greens and yellows offend your delicate early-pregnancy sensibilities, commercial or home-squeezed vegetable juices (not tomato, which is primarily a source of vitamin C) can stand in temporarily.

Use color as a guide to selecting your green and yellow vegetables: the deeper green or yellow, the higher the vitamin levels. Deep green romaine or chicory, for example, is a much better choice for your salad than barely green iceberg. Deep orange-yellow yams will provide more vitamin A than paler sweet potatoes, a sprightly hued carrot more than a faded one.

Try to have three servings (preferably one raw) from the Green Leafy and Yellow Vegetables and Yellow Fruits Food Selection Chart every day, ideally including one green and one yellow.

Other Vegetables and Fruits—one to two servings daily

Like Peter, who also indulged in radishes and green beans before beating a hasty retreat from Mr. MacGregor's fields, you should recognize the virtues of vegetables and fruits that aren't green leafy or yellow. Though they don't contain significant quantities of a single nutrient (vitamins A or C, for example), they do supply vital fiber, as well as healthy doses of other vitamins and minerals. And you needn't risk your cottontail to enjoy these benefits; just refer to the list of Other Vegetables and Fruits on page 58.

Whole Grains and Other Concentrated Complex Carbohydrates—six or more servings daily

Throughout most of the world, complex carbohydrates, in the form of breads—flat and raised, baked and fried—are considered the staff of life. They are also a mainstay of prenatal life. Grains (wheat, corn, rice, oats, rye, barley, millet, triticale) and the breads, cereals, pastas, and other dishes made from them, as well as legumes (dried beans and peas), contain a wealth of vitamins, particularly the B vitamins so essential for every part of your baby's developing body. They are rich in trace minerals, such as zinc, selenium, chromium, and magnesium, the importance of which, both pre- and postnatally, is only just being uncovered. And possibly most significant to some women in the early months of pregnancy, their starchiness can prove a comfort to queasy stomachs.

Though millions of people throughout the world are sustained primarily on whole grains, no one, including a laboratory rat, can live exclusively on refined grains: white rice, white wheat flour, degerminated cornmeal. Perhaps the best way to see why is to look at the label on a jar of wheat germ. A one-ounce quarter-cup serving of wheat germ contains 15 percent of the adult U.S. RDA for protein, vitamin E, and iron; 30 percent for thiamine; 10 percent for riboflavin and vitamin B_6; 20 percent for folic acid and magnesium; 35 percent for phosphorus; and 30 percent for zinc. Where did all this nutrition come from? It was taken out of all the refined breads, rolls, and cereals that most of America eats. And though many white bread manufacturers would have you believe that it's possible to duplicate nature's nutritional formula for whole grain and add it back to the refined products, it isn't. Enrichment tosses in a few of the vitamins and minerals found in the whole grain, but it leaves out many more—along with the naturally occurring fiber. And since a number of trace minerals were unknown when enrichment was first mandated, and others remain to be discovered, it's likely that laboratory re-creation of whole-grain nutrition in a loaf of white bread will remain an impossibility.

In our culture, we don't live by bread (or legumes) alone; complex carbohydrates are only one of the Daily Dozen. But because certain vitamins and minerals, as well as constipation-fighting fiber, are found in plentiful supply *only* in whole grains, it is crucial that each of your four or five daily servings be unrefined. (If you are on a special diet that prohibits whole grains, see page 105.)

Iron-Rich Foods—have some every day

Iron isn't important only when

your body is losing blood, as when you're menstruating, it's also important when you have to manufacture extra blood, as in pregnancy. In fact, your body's demand for iron will never be greater than it is now. To make sure the demand is met, and that an iron deficiency which could lead to anemia doesn't develop, adequate iron intake is essential. Since the iron requirement in pregnancy is so high, it's almost impossible to fill it through diet alone. So make sure your pregnancy supplement contains 30 to 60 milligrams of iron.[2] (Taking your supplement with orange or tomato juice will help your body utilize the iron, since the vitamin C enhances iron absorption.) Augment your supplement with those foods in which iron naturally occurs; consult the Iron-Rich Foods Selection Chart on page 60.

High-Fat Foods—two servings daily

Fat intake in pregnancy is a balancing act. You should stay within the recommended guidelines (no more than 30 percent of your calories from fat), but you shouldn't go much below it. That

2. Iron supplements can cause either diarrhea or constipation in some women. If yours seems to, talk to your practitioner. Switching formulas may help. Capsules that dissolve in the intestines instead of in the stomach may cause less distress, but they may also be less absorbable.

means if you weigh about 125 pounds and need about 2,100 calories, about 630 of them should come from fat. Since it takes 70 grams of fat (or as much fat as in a small burger, fries, and apple pie) to reach 630 calories, this requirement is not only easy to fill, it's easy to overfill. While you can safely add protein or complex carbohydrate servings (at 4 calories a gram) to your diet, excess fat (at 9 calories a gram) can defeat your efforts at weight control.

Keep track of your daily fat intake, being sure to count the butter you scramble your eggs in, the mayo in your tuna salad, the dressing on your salad, and the oil your chicken was browned in when you calculate your daily intake. If it seems you've exceeded the day's allowance already, you probably have. See Trimming the Fat, page 174, for tips on keeping added fat to a minimum. And remember that olive, canola, and polyunsaturated vegetable oils are better for the heart than fats from animal sources (such as butter, chicken fat, beef drippings, lard) or hardened, or hydrogenated, vegetable fats (see page 172).

If you are gaining weight too fast, you may have to cut back on your fat intake a little—by ½ serving to start with. If that doesn't work, cut down by 1 serving, but no more. Be sure there isn't a lot of hidden fat some-where in your daily meal plan. Don't cut your fat allowance out entirely, however, because your body and your baby need some fatty acids (that's why they're called "essential fatty acids") daily.

If you are gaining too slowly, you may be skimping on fat. Make certain you aren't. Try adding Whole-Grain and Other Complex Carbohydrate servings (up to a total of 11 a day) to increase weight gain. If you find the bulk excessive, or if you still don't gain rapidly enough, add an additional ½ to 1 fat serving to your daily quota.

Salty Foods—in moderation

Like weight gain, the issue of salt in pregnancy has made a full swing of the pendulum in the last 20 years. As with weight gain, most experts agree that the pendulum should be resting somewhere in the center instead of at either extreme. Your mother was probably advised to strictly limit her salt (like her weight gain) during pregnancy. If she developed edema (swelling) of ankles and feet, and sometimes of hands and face, in spite of dietary caution, she was given diuretics ("water pills") to flush out the extra fluid. Today, doctors recognize that mild swelling of the extremities is normal in pregnancy for many women (though many others don't notice such swelling) and that salt restriction and the use of diuretics can be hazardous. A few believe that excessive amounts of salt should be consumed by expectant mothers, and they encourage their patients to make a diet of such sodium-heavies as anchovies, herring, pickles, potato chips, and corned beef hash. Most, however, feel that too much salt is unhealthy for anyone, pregnant or not, and that it is closely linked to high blood pressure (though not apparently to preeclampsia), which can cause a variety of potentially dangerous complications in pregnancy, labor, and delivery.

The Best-Odds Diet, like the majority of practitioners and researchers, takes the middle point in the pendulum swing by recommending a moderate intake of salt during pregnancy. Avoid all high-sodium foods (they usually aren't the best sources of nutrients anyway and, since they're often processed, are likely to house a number of chemicals, too). Don't oversalt in the kitchen (this will help protect your husband and other family members from the perils of high blood pressure and heart disease). And salt only lightly at the table. Salting "to taste" is fine if you have a palate that hasn't been spoiled by years of fast-food and processed-food eating. A salt-spoiled palate, however, can't be trusted to tell you when you've oversalted.

To be sure of getting all the iodine you need, use only iodized salt at home.

Fluids—at least eight glasses a day

A person can live for days or even weeks without food, but only a few days without water. Water comprises one-half to three-fourths of the human body mass, is part of nearly all cells, and is necessary for almost every bodily function. During pregnancy, it is particularly vital. Between amniotic fluid, augmented maternal blood volume, and additional fluids in maternal tissue, 10 pounds of an average 30-pound pregnancy weight gain is comprised of liquids. It is needed for building the fetus' body cells, for the developing circulatory system, for the delivery of nutrients, and the excretion of wastes. Your body needs extra fluids during pregnancy, too, to help combat constipation, prevent dry skin, regulate body temperature, and to reduce the risk of urinary tract infection.

While the requirement for fluids doesn't change that much during pregnancy (everyone should drink six to eight glasses of liquids a day), the scrupulousness with which that requirement is met must. And if you're used to filling your tank with less-than-wholesome drinks, this should change, too. Switch from artificially and sugar-sweetened sodas, fruit drinks, and caffeinated coffees and teas to seltzer or club soda, fruit juices (and Best-Odds fruit sorbets; see page 289), vegetable juices, and naturally decaffeinated coffee. Don't forget to count milk (taken in liquid or frozen form, keeping in mind that milk is only two-thirds water), and soups and broths in your liquid tabulations. But *don't* count caffeinated or alcoholic beverages, which have a diuretic effect. (They're not recommended on the Best-Odds Diet.)

Particularly in early and late pregnancy, your frequent trips to the bathroom may tempt you into cutting back on fluids. Don't. The excreted urine is carrying out a vital task: removal of waste products from your system and your baby's.

Supplements—a pregnancy-formulated vitamin taken daily

Your intentions were good, but with your queasy stomach you just couldn't manage that portion of broccoli at dinner, leaving you short one green leafy for the day. Or you dined at your grandmother's, and the vegetables she served were so overcooked you knew barely a vitamin or mineral remained. Or you were held captive by the caterers at an all-day conference and couldn't track down a single whole grain or unsweetened citrus.

The point of taking vitamin supplements during pregnancy (or at any other time) isn't so you can let your diet slide, but to provide insurance in case it should slide inadvertently. It's also to keep you from being shortchanged should storage, cooking, or exposure to air rob foods of the vitamins and minerals you're counting on. In the case of nutrients that are difficult to obtain in adequate quantities from diet alone, such as iron (and, for strict vegetarians, calcium, vitamin D, B_{12}), a supplement makes the task easier. *But under no circumstance should a vitamin pill be used in place of a good diet.* Vitamins and minerals are best utilized by our bodies as they occur naturally in foods. Unprocessed foods also undoubtedly contain nutrients that haven't yet been discovered by scientists (many we recognize as important today were unknown 20 years ago) but are essential to human life.

The vitamin formula you take should be especially designed for pregnancy. Ask your practitioner to prescribe or suggest one, or select one yourself that contains the vitamins and minerals in approximately the same dosages as the formula on page 336. Do not take any other nutritional supplements without your doctor's approval. Some may be toxic in large doses. Taking megadoses of a single nutrient can also upset metabolism, increasing the need for other nutrients.

BEST-ODDS FOOD SELECTION GROUPS

Choose your Daily Dozen from these Food Selection Groups; they contain virtually every food worthy of inclusion. Absent, you will note, are sugar-sweetened sweets, refined breads and cereals, and soft drinks. Some foods appear on more than one list; these foods are rich in more than one type of nutrient. If you eat broccoli as a green leafy vegetable, it will also count as a vitamin C food. Similarly, cheese can provide both calcium and protein. Opt for double-duty foods often; they are nutritionally efficient.

Also nutritionally efficient are foods marked ↓. They contain a lot of nutrition for the calories, and are good choices if you are gaining weight too rapidly. (Slow gainers should include them, too; they're wholesome fare for everyone.) On the other hand, foods marked ↑ offer a lot of calories in small packages and are particularly good choices if you're gaining too slowly. Be wary of these if you're gaining weight too quickly.

You may want to measure portions at first, but once you get the feel for typical portion size, this should no longer be necessary. Portion precision is not required; educated estimates will work as well.

Protein Foods

Have four of the following protein servings a day, a combination of these foods equivalent to four servings, or have three servings from this list and one from the Vegetarian Protein Combinations on page 61. If you're a vegetarian, you may make more, or all, of your selections from the Vegetarian Protein Combinations. (If you eat only vegetable protein, you will need five protein servings daily.)

Each serving contains between 20 and 25 grams of protein; you need a minimum of 75 grams, preferably 100 grams, daily.

You will probably find that typical restaurant portions of meat and fish exceed a single Best-Odds serving, often equalling two, or even more, servings.

Dairy
2½ to 3 glasses (8 ounces each) skim or low-fat milk
2½ to 3 glasses (8 ounces each) low-fat buttermilk

2½ to 3 glasses (8 ounces each) whole milk (have rarely; see pages 38 and 207)

1¼ cups evaporated skim milk

1 cup nonfat dry milk

1¾ cups plain low-fat yogurt

¾ cup low-fat cottage cheese ↓

¾ cup full-fat (4 percent) cottage cheese (have rarely; see pages 38 and 207)

1¾ ounces (½ cup) grated Parmesan cheese

3 ounces part-skim milk mozzarella or other low-fat cheese

3 ounces Swiss cheese

3½ ounces Muenster cheese

3½ ounces low-cholesterol cheese

3½ ounces blue cheese or Roquefort

3 to 3½ ounces natural Cheddar

3 ounces any cheese with 7 or 8 grams of protein per ounce

3½ ounces any cheese with 6 grams of protein per ounce

Eggs
5 large egg whites ↓

2 large eggs plus 2 whites

Fish (cooked or canned weight; do not eat raw)

3 to 3½ ounces (drained) canned tuna, water packed ↓

3 to 3½ ounces (drained) canned tuna, oil packed

3½ ounces canned salmon or mackerel

3½ ounces (drained) canned Atlantic sardines

4½ ounces (drained) canned herring or Pacific sardines

3½ ounces fresh fish (bluefish, cod ↓, flounder ↓, haddock, halibut ↓, mackerel, salmon, shad, snapper ↓, sole ↓, swordfish or trout)

Seafood (cooked or canned weight unless otherwise specified; do not eat raw)

6 ounces clams, meat only ↓

5 ounces canned clams (drained) ↓

5 ounces (1 cup) canned crab meat ↓

5 ounces raw American eel ↑

4 to 4½ ounces lobster meat ↓

15 to 20 medium oysters

4 ounces scallops

3½ ounces shrimp ↓

Poultry (weights without bone; skin removed[3])

2½ ounces white meat chicken or turkey↓

3 ounces dark meat chicken or turkey

3½ to 4 ounces duck*

Meat (weights without bone)

3 ounces lean beef

3½ ounces beef, fatty cuts*

3 ounces lean lamb

3½ ounces lamb, fatty cuts*

4 ounces lamb chop, lean and fat*

3 ounces liver (see page 326)*

3 ounces lean pork

3½ ounces pork, lean and fat*

3 ounces veal

---

3. Chemical contaminants are stored in the fat and skin in poultry and the fat in meats, as well as in the liver and other organs; have the entries in these two sections that are marked with an asterisk rarely to avoid ingesting excessive amounts of such contaminants.

Miscellaneous

5 ounces frogs' legs

Vegetarian (nuts measured without shells)

⅔ cup miso (high in sodium)

5 to 6 ounces tofu (bean curd) ↓

1 serving texturized vegetable protein[4]

2½ ounces pine nuts (pignoli) ↑

3 ounces almonds or black walnuts ↑

3½ ounces sunflower seeds ↑

3⅓ ounces (⅝ cup) peanuts ↑

5 to 6 tablespoons peanut butter ↑

1 serving Complete Protein Combination (page 61) (Non-vegetarians should limit themselves to serving Dairy Protein Combination (page 62) CPC daily.)

Vitamin C Foods

Have two servings daily. Your body can't store this important vitamin, so be sure not to skip a day. Each serving listed contains approximately 40 to 50 milligrams of vitamin C. (Cooking will reduce the vitamin C content of these foods, so increase your portions accordingly.) You will also be getting smaller amounts of the vitamin in other fruits and vegetables.

4. Texturized vegetable protein is a meat analog (look-and-taste-alike) made from soybeans; the protein content varies, so check labels for brands that provide at least 20 grams of protein per serving.

Fruits

½ cup fresh strawberries or 3 ounces unsweetened frozen ↓

1⅓ cups blackberries, boysenberries, dewberries, loganberries, or red raspberries, fresh or unsweetened frozen

1½ cups blueberries

¼ cantaloupe ↓

⅛ small honeydew

1 cup raw red or white currants

½ medium grapefruit ↓

¾ cup fresh grapefruit sections ↓

½ cup grapefruit juice, fresh or frozen reconstituted, or ¾ cup canned ↓

1 large lemon ↓

½ cup fresh lemon juice, or ⅔ cup bottled ↓

2 large limes ↓

¾ cup fresh lime juice ↓

1 small orange ↓

½ cup orange juice, fresh or frozen reconstituted ↓

¾ cup canned orange juice

2 tablespoons undiluted frozen orange juice concentrate ↓

1 large tangerine

¾ cup fresh tangerine juice

½ large guava (amount of vitamin C varies)

⅔ medium kiwi fruit ↓

½ large mango

½ cup ½-inch cubes papaya

1 large plantain

Vegetables (raw, unless otherwise specified; cooked vegetables, which can be fresh or frozen, are measured after cooking)

1 cup or 10 spears cooked asparagus ↓

½ cup fresh broccoli, or ⅔ cup frozen, cooked ↓

½ cup fresh Brussels sprouts, or ⅔ cup frozen, cooked ↓

3¼- x 4½-inch wedge or 1½ cups shredded raw green cabbage, or 2 cups cooked ↓

1 cup cooked Chinese cabbage (bok choy) ↓

1 cup red cabbage ↓

⅔ cup fresh cauliflower florets, or ¾ cup frozen, cooked ↓

⅔ cup diced raw kohlrabi, or ¾ cup cooked ↓

1⅓ cups diced cooked rutabagas

1 cup cooked collard greens, ↓

2 cups cooked dandelion greens ↓

¾ cup fresh kale, or 1¼ cups frozen, cooked ↓

1¼ cups fresh mustard greens, or 1½ cups frozen, cooked ↓

1 cup fresh turnip greens, or 1¼ cups frozen, cooked ↓

3 cups raw spinach, or 2 cups cooked ↓

½ medium green bell pepper ↓

⅓ medium red bell pepper ↓

½ medium hot chile pepper ↓

1 large pimiento, canned ↓

2 small tomatoes ↓

½ cup cooked fresh or canned tomatoes, tomato paste or purée

1 cup tomato juice ↓

1¼ cups tomato sauce

¾ cup vegetable juice (vitamin C contents vary, check label) ↓

Calcium Foods

You need four servings a day during pregnancy, five during lactation. Each of the following contains one calcium serving, or about 300 milligrams of calcium. Many Best-Odds recipes also provide one or more calcium servings.

Dairy

¾ ounce (¼ cup) Parmesan cheese

1¼ ounces Swiss cheese

1⅓ ounces low-cholesterol cheese

1½ ounces Cheddar, provolone, or part-skim mozzarella

2 ounces blue cheese, camembert ↑, feta, whole milk mozzarella, Roquefort, processed American, or processed cheese spread (have processed cheeses rarely)

1¾ cups low-fat cottage cheese

1 cup skim ↓, nonfat ↓, or low-fat milk

1 cup low-fat buttermilk

1 cup low-fat or nonfat yogurt

⅔ cup calcium-added low-fat milk

½ cup evaporated skim milk ↓

⅓ cup nonfat dry milk ↓

Vegetarian (cooked vegetables are measured after cooking)

¾ cup almonds ↑

1¾ cups fresh broccoli florets ↓

1 cup cooked frozen chopped collard greens ↓

1½ cups cooked frozen chopped kale ↓

1½ cups fresh turnip greens, or 1¼ cups frozen, cooked ↓

3 tablespoons blackstrap molasses

THOSE CRUCIFEROUS VEGETABLES

Vegetables in the cabbage family (known officially as "cruciferous") may be instrumental in warding off cancer. So enjoy them several times a week. They include: broccoli, Brussels sprouts, cabbage, cauliflower, rutabagas, and turnips.

⅓ cup medium molasses
9 ounces tofu (bean curd), prepared with calcium
Soy milk and soy protein[5]

Seafood
4 ounces canned salmon or Pacific mackerel, with bones
3 ounces (drained) canned sardines, with bones
1⅓ cups or 18 to 25 oysters, meat only

Calcium Snacks

These snacks can all bring additional calcium to your daily diet.
Almonds ↑
Baked goods made with sesame seeds or soy flour
Best-Odds Ice Cream
Dried apricots and figs
Ripe olives

Green Leafy and Yellow Vegetables and Yellow Fruits

Have three of these daily, preferably at least one green and one yellow, and one should be raw.

---

5. The calcium content of these products vary. Read labels and use only those that provide between 270 and 300 milligrams of calcium for each 80 to 150 calories.

Generally, the deeper the color, the richer the nutrient content. Each of the following contains approximately 1,500 to 2,000 IU (International Units) of vitamin A; your requirement is about 5,000 IU daily during pregnancy and 6,000 when you're nursing. If you drink milk or eat cheese, you will get additional vitamin A from these sources, as well as from vegetables and fruits with smaller vitamin A contents.

Green leafy and yellow vegetables and yellow fruits also provide numerous other vitamins, minerals, trace metals, and fiber. Count the carrots in your soup, the broccoli dunked in a dip, the vegetable juice at a cocktail party, the tomato in your chicken sandwich, and the pumpkin in your Best-Odds Pumpkin Pie. Reaching your quota will be easy.

Fruits
2 medium raw apricots
½ cup juice-packed canned apricots
4 small halves dried apricots
⅛ 5-inch cantaloupe ↓
1 cup water-packed canned sour cherries

¼ large mango
2 medium nectarines
1 large yellow peach ↓
½ medium persimmon
1 medium plantain
1 cup juice-packed canned purple plums

Vegetables (raw, unless otherwise specified; cooked vegetables, which can be fresh or frozen, measured after cooking)
1 cup cooked asparagus or 12 spears ↓
½ cup bok choy ↓
¾ cup raw or cooked broccoli pieces ↓
1½ cups raw or cooked peas
⅓ cup cooked beet greens, kale, or Swiss chard ↓
¼ cup cooked dandelion leaves or turnip greens ↓
½ cup cooked mustard greens or collards ↓
1½ cups endive or escarole ↓
1½ cups or 10 large leaves green leafy lettuce (Boston, romaine, Bibb) ↓
⅓ cup packed chopped parsley ↓
½ cup raw spinach, or ¼ cup cooked ↓
½ small raw or cooked carrot ↓
1 tablespoon unsweetened canned pumpkin ↓
¼ cup boiled mashed winter squash, or 2 ounces baked
¼ small baked sweet potato or yam, or ⅛ cup unsweetened canned solid pack
1 large or 2 small tomatoes
¾ cup cooked or canned tomatoes or tomato purée

1½ cups tomato juice
6 ounces vegetable juice ↓
½ large red bell pepper or red chile pepper ↓

Other Fruits And Vegetables

Have one, or better still two, of the following daily. While they are not quite as rich in single nutrients as the green leafies and yellows, they nevertheless provide important vitamins, minerals, and fiber.

Fruits
1 medium apple
1 cup apple juice (less nutritious than orange juice)
¼ cup apple juice concentrate
½ cup unsweetened applesauce
1 small banana
⅔ cup sweet cherries, fresh or unsweetened frozen
1 cup cranberries (cook in fruit juice)
3 small fresh figs
⅔ cup grapes
1 medium white peach
1 medium pear
¾ cup diced pineapple or 1 medium slice, fresh or unsweetened canned
1 cup unsweetened pineapple juice
2 medium plums
⅔ cup black raspberries
¾ cup sliced rhubarb (cook in fruit juice)
2 cups (without rind) cubed watermelon

Dried fruits (unsweetened)
5 dates
3 figs
6 peach halves
2 pear halves
1 slice pineapple
5 large prunes
¾ cup prune juice
¼ cup apple rings
¼ cup raisins
¼ cup currants

Vegetables (can be eaten raw or cooked, unless otherwise specified; cooked vegetables, which can be fresh or frozen, measured after cooking)
5 or 6 asparagus spears, frozen or fresh ↓
½ medium avocado ↑
1 cup (drained) canned bamboo shoots ↓
¾ cup green or snap beans ↓
1 cup bean sprouts (alfalfa, mung, sesame, soybean) ↓
1 cup beets
1 cup shredded Savoy cabbage ↓
2 large ribs celery or 1 cup diced ↓
1 small ear cooked sweet corn (yellow preferred)
½ small cucumber (low in calories and nutrition) ↓
1 cup cooked eggplant ↓
1 cup sliced Jerusalem artichoke (sunchoke)
¼ head crisp lettuce (iceberg) ↓
½ cup sliced mushrooms
9 pods okra, cooked ↓
1 cup sliced onion, or 1 medium ↓
⅔ cup cooked parsnip
⅔ cup peas
⅔ cup snow peas
1 small potato, cooked
2 ounces seaweed or kelp, cooked ↓
½ cup summer squash (yellow or zucchini) ↓
4 to 6 radishes (low in calories and nutrition) ↓
1 cup diced turnip ↓
½ cup (drained) canned water chestnuts ↓

Whole Grains And Other Concentrated Complex Carbohydrates

Have four or five servings of the following daily. Do not count unenriched breads, cereals, or flours at all, and count enriched ones only rarely. Portions here are approximately equivalent, and if you have four or five, you will meet your needs.

Grains and flours (measured before cooking unless otherwise noted)
½ cup cooked brown rice
½ cup cooked wild rice
⅕ cup whole-wheat flour
⅕ cup soy flour
¼ cup whole rye flour
⅙ cup soy flour or grits
½ cup cooked millet, bulgur, or triticale
½ cup cooked kasha (buckwheat groats)
½ cup cooked unpearled barley

Cereals (measured before cooking unless otherwise noted)

¼ cup whole-grain (nondeger-minated) cornmeal

1 serving cooked whole-grain cereal (for example oatmeal, Wheatena, Ralston)

⅓ cup rolled oats, wheat flakes, or other flaked grains

1 ounce whole-grain, ready-to-eat cereal (Shredded Wheat, Nutrigrain, Grape Nuts, Cheerios, or any other with no more than 2 grams sugar per serving)

2 tablespoons wheat germ ↓

¼ cup unprocessed bran (this is probably too much roughage for most people)

Breads and other baked goods

1 serving Best-Odds home-baked bread

1 slice whole-wheat, whole rye, or other whole-grain or soy bread, preferably no sugar added

1 serving whole-grain corn bread

1 small (1 ounce) whole-wheat pita, or ½ large

½ whole-wheat bagel or English muffin

1 tortilla

1 serving Best-Odds baked goods (cake, cookies, or muffins)

2 to 6 whole-grain crackers (60 to 80 calories' worth)

2 brown rice cakes

6 to 8 small whole-wheat bread sticks

Legumes (cooked)

⅔ cup black-eyed peas or cow-peas, immature seeds

½ cup Great Northern, pea, pinto, or black beans

½ cup lentils or split peas

½ cup kidney beans or chick-peas (garbanzo beans)

⅔ cup lima beans

½ cup soybeans

Miscellaneous

1 ounce whole-wheat or high-protein pasta (Note: whole-wheat pasta has more fiber; high-protein pasta has more protein.)

2 cups air-popped popcorn, no butter ↓ (count no more than one popcorn serving a day as a whole-grain serving)

1 ounce pumpkin seeds

1 tablespoon brewer's yeast

Iron-Rich Foods

Small amounts of iron are found in most of the fruits, vegetables, grains, and meats you eat daily. Though you won't be able to get all the iron you need from your diet, the following foods will give you more iron than most.

Beef

Blackstrap molasses

Carob flour or powder; baked goods made with them

Chick-peas (garbanzos), split peas, and other dried beans and peas

Dried fruit (raisins, apricots, prunes, peaches, or currants)

Jerusalem artichokes

Liver and other organ meats (use infrequently because they

tend to be storage areas for chemicals)
Oysters (don't eat raw)
Pumpkin seeds
Sardines (drained, if canned)
Soy beans, soy products (tofu, miso); baked goods made with soy flour
Spinach
Spirulina (seaweed), dried

High-Fat Foods

There is some fat in most of the foods you eat. To be certain you are getting your essential fatty acids, in addition have two of the following daily; cut back to one if you're gaining weight too rapidly. Don't exceed this quota unless you are gaining too slowly.[6]

1 tablespoon polyunsaturated vegetable oil (for example, safflower or corn) †
1 tablespoon margarine high in polyunsaturates †*
1 tablespoon butter †*
1 tablespoon mayonnaise †*
½ small avocado †
3 tablespoons light cream †*
2 tablespoons heavy (whipping) cream †
2 tablespoons cream cheese †*
4 tablespoons sour cream or whipped cream †
3 tablespoons peanuts or pecan or walnut pieces †
2 tablespoons peanut butter †

6. The fats in the foods marked with an asterisk are saturated and/or high in cholesterol; they are not rich in essential fatty acids. Limit yourself to a total of 1 serving daily.

Complete Vegetable Protein Combinations for Vegetarians

When combined, the following legumes and grains are excellent choices for all pregnant women to eat. However, nonvegetarians should use only one combination a day as part of their protein allowance. Vegetarians should try to have five full combination servings daily (see page 44).

To make a complete protein serving, combine one portion, or combination of portions, from the Legumes column (10 to 13 grams protein) plus one portion, or combination of portions, from the Grains column (10 to 13 grams protein).

Legumes (measured cooked)
⅔ cup lentils or split peas
⅔ cup any pea or bean with 15 to 22 grams protein per cup
¾ cup soybeans
¾ cup mung, lima, or kidney beans
¾ cup chick-peas (garbanzos)
¾ cup any pea or bean with 13 to 18 grams protein per cup
1 cup small white, broad, or Great Northern beans
1 cup cowpeas or black-eyed peas
1 cup any pea or bean with 10 to 13 grams protein per cup
1⅓ cup green peas
½ cup miso
4 ounces tofu (bean curd)

Grains, Nuts, and Seeds (before cooking unless otherwise noted)[7]

2 ounces soy or high-protein pasta

2 to 4 ounces whole-wheat pasta (check nutrition label)

⅓ cup wheat germ

⅔ cup oats or whole-grain barley

1 cup wheat flakes

1 cup cooked wild rice

1½ cups cooked brown rice*

1½ cups cooked bulgur*, kasha (buckwheat groats)*, or millet*

4 slices whole-grain bread

2 whole-wheat pitas (6 inches each)

2 whole-wheat English muffins

½ cup soy flour

⅔ cup whole-wheat flour

¼ cup tahini (sesame-seed paste)

⅓ cup peanuts

2½ to 3 tablespoons peanut butter

⅓ cup black walnuts, or ⅔ cup English walnuts

½ cup almonds, Brazil nuts, or cashews

1½ ounces (⅓ cup) pine nuts (pignoli)

2 ounces sunflower seeds or pistachio nuts

¼ cup brewer's yeast

Complete Dairy Protein Combinations

Combine 1 portion, or combina-

7. The grains in this section that are marked with an asterisk are poor in protein; add 2 tablespoons wheat germ to each serving.

tion of portions (about 10 grams of protein), from the Legumes or Grains lists above with 1 portion, or combination of portions, from the Dairy foods below.

Dairy Foods

½ cup cottage cheese

1¼ cups skim milk

½ cup nonfat dry milk

1¼ cups low-fat buttermilk

⅔ cup evaporated skim milk

1¼ cups low-fat yogurt

2 whole eggs

1 egg plus one egg white

1½ ounces low-fat Cheddar or Swiss cheese

2 ounces blue cheese

¼ cup parmesan cheese

¼ recipe Best-Odds ice cream

1½ ounces any cheese with 7 grams protein per ounce

2 ounces any cheese with 5 grams protein per ounce

SHELF OF HONOR

Variety is not only the spice of gastronomic life, it is the key to a really well-balanced diet. As nutrient-crammed a vegetable as kale is, for example, you're better off alternating it with broccoli, romaine, and other green leafys than eating it every night. You're also playing it nutritionally safer if you vary your breakfast selection: oatmeal one day, shredded wheat the next, bulgur or corn cereal on the third.

But there are a few foods

that do stand daily repeating, that needn't be put aside every other day for variety's sake. Foods that are so superlative in their nutritive powers, and so· versatile in the ways they can be prepared and eaten, that they deserve at least a once-a-day slot in your menus. And though there are hundreds of wholesome, nourishing foods that merit a place in your Best-Odds kitchen, these five are on a shelf by themselves—the Shelf of Honor. Use them whenever and in whatever you can.

Wheat germ. In order to turn harvested wheat into white flour, refiners remove two parts of the grain: the bran (which contains the fiber) and the germ (the heart of the grain). Few of us (unless constipation is a chronic problem) regularly need the heavy-duty fiber power of the bran that's removed; a well-balanced diet that includes vegetables, fruits, and whole grains usually contains adequate roughage. But anyone—and, as usual, this goes double for pregnant women and their fetuses—can benefit from adding the concentrated nutrition of the germ of the wheat to even the best balanced diet.

No one food packs more of a vitamin, mineral, and protein punch into a single ounce. One-quarter cup (one ounce) of wheat germ supplies about 10 percent of an expectant mother's daily requirement of protein, plus an unparalleled host of essential nutrients, including many of the trace minerals that are scarce in most other foods. And unlike a prenatal supplement, which also contains a lot of vitamins and minerals (though no protein), wheat germ is not a bitter pill to swallow. It's a delicious food that, in a supporting role, imparts a nutty taste and crunchy texture to an almost endless variety of dishes, from morning pancakes and cereals to lunchtime yogurt and salad to dinner's breaded chicken and meat loaves. It enhances the flavor and boosts the nutritive value of just about anything you're baking, from muffins and breads to cakes and cookies (substitute ¼ cup of wheat germ for an equal quantity of flour in each cup). It restores most of the nutrients refined out of white breads, rolls, bagels, pizza crusts, and pastas when sprinkled generously over these foods before eating (carry some in a sandwich bag or a baby-food jar tucked into your pocketbook for emergency use when whole grains aren't readily available). And with just a splash of milk and a garnish of fruit, it makes a memorable starring appearance as a breakfast dish or snack.

Since wheat germ is a moderately perishable food, it should

be refrigerated after opening.[8] Carrying it in your handbag or travel tote without refrigeration is fine for a few days; if you won't have access to at least occasional refrigeration for longer than this (overnight, for instance), the wheat germ should be replaced every third day or so (more often in really hot weather) to prevent significant nutrient loss and spoilage.

Brewer's yeast rivals—often exceeds—wheat germ for protein and other nutrients. Unfortunately, few people find it palatable so it is not as widely used. If you find a variety that you can tolerate, by all means use it to supplement your diet.

Eggs. Just as the egg supplies nourishment for the developing chick, it can provide your growing fetus with outstanding nutrition (though unlike a chick, a human fetus needs more to live on). As far as protein quality is concerned, the egg comes first (yes, even before the chicken). The six grams of protein in the average large egg is of the highest quality, and coexists with substantial amounts of a number of other nutrients, including phosphorus, vitamin A, and many of the B vitamins.

For you, the egg offers other benefits. To most palates, one of them is taste. Whether they are scrambled, fried, poached, boiled, made into a frittata, omelette, or added to a salad, eggs can be as pleasing to the taste buds as they are useful to a fetus' developing body. But even those who don't like the taste of eggs straight won't mind them added to baked goods, pancakes, French toast, desserts, meat loaves, and soufflés.

Yes, eggs are a significant source of atherosclerosis-promoting cholesterol—more than 250 milligrams per egg, all in the yolk—but cholesterol is not a problem for healthy pregnant women. So unless your physician has discovered you have a cholesterol problem (which would probably be hereditary), feel free to have an egg or two daily. If you are put on a low-cholesterol diet, or when you are preparing meals for the family (all of whom can benefit from the reduction of cholesterol), using just the whites of the eggs will eliminate the cholesterol while retaining much of the protein and some of the vitamins. (Substituting 2 whites for 1 whole egg will not affect most recipes.) And since the whites have the additional advantage of providing good quality protein for very few calories, they can be used in quantities you wouldn't consider using for whole eggs. (See page 182 for tips on using egg whites.)

---

8. Wheat germ keeps at least six weeks in the refrigerator after opening, as long as six months in the freezer.

Milk. By putting their newborns to the breast, mothers all over the world show that they recognize the importance of milk for their babies after birth. But milk (or other foods equivalent in calcium) is just as important for babies before birth. It's a very rich source of calcium: Each 8-ounce glass provides a full 25 percent of a pregnant woman's daily calcium requirement. It is also naturally abundant in riboflavin and fortified with vitamins A and D. In addition, it is a fairly good protein source (three glasses or the equivalent in dry or evaporated milk can be counted as one protein serving).

Not every carton of milk belongs on the Best-Odds Shelf of Honor, however. Chocolate milk, of course, doesn't (not only does the large amount of added sugar in it tip the scales toward the nutritionally dishonorable, but the cocoa can interfere with your body's absorption of the milk's calcium). And whole milk, though it contains all of the desirable nutrients, also contains considerable amounts of undesirable fat, making it high in calories. Skim milk (80 to 100 calories per cup, to whole milk's 150) or 1 percent-fat milk (about 100 calories per cup) are far more efficient choices, as is low-fat buttermilk.

To some, a glass of cold milk with cookies (Best-Odds, naturally) or a warm cup at bedtime are the drinks of their dreams. To many others, milk from the carton is a nightmare for the palate.[9] For these milk-detesters, there are other options. Though mother heifer probably wouldn't recognize her product in these forms, powdered and evaporated milk are two of the best ways a human mother-to-be can supply her unborn baby with adequate calcium without ever drinking a glass of milk. Each third of a cup (or five tablespoons) of the dry variety (all the water has been removed) or half a cup of the evaporated (part of the water has been removed) is equivalent to an eight-ounce glass of full-fluid milk.

The concentrated character of these products makes it possible to pack milk's nutrition into sauces, soups, meat, fish, or vegetable loaves, baked goods, shakes, casseroles, cereals, beverages, pancakes, and desserts without offending the taste buds. (See page 178 for tips on using these Shelf-of-Honor items in your cooking. In the recipe section, look for recipes that indicate Calcium servings at the end.)

Low-fat cottage cheese. Anyone who's ever gone on a weight-reducing diet probably

9. For those for whom milk in any form is a digestive nightmare whether it's because of lactose intolerance or an allergy, there are nonmilk alternatives for obtaining milk's nutrients; see page 56.

THE GREAT ICE CREAM WAR

Makers of frozen desserts lure us from every angle: taste, richness, healthiness, and naturalness, but their lures are frequently baited with deception. What's touted as "good for you" isn't necessarily. Most of the carbohydrates in these foods are sugars, not the complex carbohydrates that you and your baby needs. And tofutti contains no calcium at all. The nutritional information below will help you get the most for your splurge when your chosen cheat is ice cream. (Percentages are of RDAs in pregnancy.)

	Calories	Protein/gm	Carbohydrates	Fat	Calcium
Approximate requirements	2,100	100 gm	282 gm	50 gm	1,200 mg
Haagen-Dazs Vanilla (4 oz)	267 (12%)	5 (5%)	24 (9%)	17 (34%)	152 (13%)
Tofu Glace Capuccino (4 oz)	210 (10%)	3.7 (3.7%)	21 (7%)	7 (14%)	24 (2%)
Light 'n Lively Triflavor (4 oz)	110 (5%)	3 (3%)	18 (6%)	3 (6%)	80 (7%)
Columbo Frozen Yogurt (soft; 5¼ oz)	130 (6%)	4 (4%)	23 (8%)	2.5 (5%)	134 (13%)
Sealtest Vanilla (4 oz)	140 (7%)	2 (2%)	16 (6%)	7 (14%)	80 (7%)
Breyers Vanilla (4 oz)	160 (8%)	3 (3%)	19 (7%)	8 (16%)	80 (7%)
Tuscan Frozen Yogurt (4 oz)	110 (5%)	4 (4%)	23 (8%)	1 (2%)	134 (13%)
Tofutti Wildberry (4 oz)	230 (11%)	3 (3%)	23 (8%)	14 (28%)	0 (0%)

has a less-than-flattering image of cottage cheese. And it's not surprising. Envision it as a dreary white mound on a faded green lettuce leaf, with no more to keep it company or pay it complement than dry melba toast and a glass of ice water, and you have painted a very unappetizing picture. But put your Scarsdales and Mayos in your past, and imagine cottage cheese melded with melted cheese and tomato sauce in lasagna, "creamed" in soups and hot cereal, blended with buttermilk and spices into tangy dips and salad dressings, folded into a richly nutritious cheesecake (see page 284), "sundaed" with fruit, nuts, and a dollop of all-fruit preserves—and the picture takes a change for the delicious.

A plus: cottage cheese is as

capable in the nutrition department as it is in the kitchen. Three-quarters of a cup of low-fat cottage cheese (and the emphasis is on "low-fat," since full-fat cottage cheese contains as many calories per half cup as some ice creams), while weighing in at a scant 135 calories, fills one full protein requirement and provides several of milk's nutrients. (Be aware, however, that cottage cheese does not contain milk's high level of calcium; three-quarters of a cup is only two-thirds of a calcium serving.)

Low-fat yogurt. Thought to be foreign, exotic, and esoteric by Americans 20 years ago, yogurt is today as American as apple pie. The problem is that in the form Americans often eat it—presweetened with preserves or frozen—yogurt can be almost as full of sugar as apple pie. Though it supplies many of the same nutrients as plain yogurt when fruited or flavored with vanilla or coffee (but less when frozen), its whopping sugar content makes this kind of yogurt a poor nutritional choice.

Plain low-fat yogurt is, however, a choice of great dietary distinction. High in protein (1½ cups equals 1 protein serving), low in calories, and, cup for cup, as rich in calcium (sometimes richer) and many other vitamins and minerals as milk, it should frequently find its way off your refrigerator shelf and into your meals. Like the other foods on the Shelf of Honor, plain yogurt is almost limitless in its talents, adding abundant nutrition and intriguing taste to breakfasts, lunches, dinners, and snacks. It combines with fruit (and, perhaps, a spoonful of fruit-only preserves) in a bowl to make a sugarless "sundae-style" treat, or in a blender to make a thick, satisfying shake or a delicious pancake topping. It stands in for mayonnaise and/or sour cream in dips and salad dressings or, mixed with chives, as a topping for potatoes, and stands out in a variety of desserts (including frozen desserts). Mixed with chopped raw vegetables (radishes, tomatoes, carrots, cucumber, scallions), it makes a cool summer lunch; blended with vegetables and stock it turns into a fine "creamed" soup; tossed with steamed new potatoes and chopped parsley or minced dill, it becomes an elegant accompaniment to many entrées.

BEST-ODDS APPROVED CHEATING

You're dedicated to giving your baby the best odds of being born healthy by eating the best possible diet while you're pregnant. You're resolved to make perma-

SELECTIONS FOR SELECTIVE CHEATING

Cheat no more than once a week with no more than one serving of one of the following:

❖ Roll, bagel, bread, English muffin made with refined flour (wheat, corn, rye, pumpernickel)—preferably enriched

❖ White pasta—preferably with a nourishing sauce, such as primavera or marinara

❖ White pancakes or waffles—preferably with fruit-only preserves rather than syrup

❖ Pizza—preferably with plenty of cheese plus peppers, mushrooms, or other vegetables

❖ Frozen yogurt—preferably not chocolate or coffee; preferably with toppings of nuts, raisins, wheat germ, or fresh fruit

❖ Bran or whole-grain (made with sugar or honey) muffin

❖ No-nitrate hot dog—preferably chicken or turkey, instead of beef or pork

❖ Pretzels or potato or corn chips—preferably all-natural, lightly salted or unsalted varieties (remember 10 chips are about 5 percent of your day's calorie allowance)

❖ French fries—preferably crispy, not greasy

❖ A fast-food burger on a bun (one chain offers a whole-grain bun, which may be appealing if you lose your taste for the refined)

nent changes for the better in the eating life-style of yourself and your family. You're determined to keep your weight gain moderate so your return to prepregnancy shape won't take as long as, or longer than, your pregnancy.

But, if you're like most expectant mothers, you're also only human. In spite of the best of intentions, you can't completely sublimate the occasional yearning for forbidden fruit (or,

more likely, fruit-flavored ice cream). And because the Best-Odds Diet is designed for human mothers-to-be, you don't have to. A guilt-free system for safe cheating, which allows you to satisfy your soul without sabotaging your body and your baby's, is built right into the Best-Odds Diet. Its guidelines are:

Don't feel obliged to cheat. Though cheating is permitted on the Best-Odds Diet, it's not man-

❖A fast-food chicken or fish sandwich (but remember, the calorie counts on these are way out of proportion to their food value)

Cheat no more than once a month with no more than one serving of one of the following:

❖Cake—preferably cheese, carrot, ice cream, banana, date-nut, or raisin-nut studded; preferably with whipped cream, cream cheese, or seafoam (egg whites) frosting instead of buttercream[10]

❖Pudding—preferably homemade rice, custard, or tapioca instead of commercial chocolate or butterscotch

❖Ice cream—preferably one made with a lot of milk instead of a lot of cream (see The Great Ice Cream War, page 66), preferably not chocolate or coffee, and preferably topped with wholesome items (see frozen yogurt, above) rather than sprinkles or sugary syrups

❖Pie—preferably homemade fruit, nut, or custard variety instead of cream

❖Cookies (two to three)—preferably homemade or noncommercial oatmeal, nut and raisin, date- or fig- (but not jelly-) filled

❖Candy bar—preferably one with nuts and raisins or granola, preferably milk chocolate instead of dark

❖Pastry—preferably a cheese, prune, or nut-and-raisin Danish instead of a doughnut

❖Refined muffin—preferably bran instead of blueberry

datory. If you're one of those who can fulfill all the fancies of her appetite on protein, whole grains, and fresh fruits and vegetables, don't feel duty-bound to ram an ice-cream cone down your throat every month or to force-feed yourself an onion bagel every Sunday morning. Just skip this page, and go back to your Daily Dozen. You can also skip this page if you're a Type-A dieter who'd rather resist than give in to temptation, or if you're the kind of junk-food addict who can't stop at "just one," making once-a-week and once-a-month cheating a mission impossible.

Treat without cheating when you can. Satisfy your treat-tooth cravings with Best-Odds variations most of the time. Best-

10. Bad news for those who love to wash their chocolate cake down with milk. Chocolate decreases the absorption of calcium by the body. If you cheat with chocolate, and must have that milk chaser, count only half the milk in your calcium allowance.

Odds bran muffins, cookies, cakes, pies, pastries, frozen desserts, puddings, and pancakes can be as tempting as anything you can cheat on, as can whole-grain pastas, bagels, and pizzas, when they're available. So save your cheats for when a Best-Odds option doesn't exist, such as in a restaurant or at a party.

Don't cheat your baby. A slice of cheesecake may have a smidgeon of calcium and a pinch of protein, but unless it's the Best-Odds Cheesecake you can't consider it a calcium or protein serving. A white dinner roll (which may or may not be enriched) lacks the fiber and trace minerals of a whole-grain one and shouldn't be applied toward your grain requirements. So when you're having your cake (or roll, or other cheating treat), make sure you're eating your Daily Dozen, too.

Be a discriminating cheater. All junk food is not created nutritionally equal. An oatmeal cookie, for example, while not worthy of regular appearances on your menu (unless it's a Chewy Raisin-Oatmeal Cookie), is not as worthless as a chocolate sandwich cookie. When you cheat, try to select the best of a bad lot, choosing items that have something to offer.

Keep your cheating in check. Be as disciplined about your

cheating as you should be about your diet. Stay within the guideline limits. If the system turns out to be unworkable for you—if one slice of pizza leads to two more, if a small fries leads you to crave a large, or if half a cup of ice cream leads to half a gallon—you are probably better off abandoning cheating entirely.

MONITORING YOUR WEIGHT GAIN

Weight gain. It's the most inevitable sign of pregnancy, and in our weight-obsessed society, often the most unsettling for an expectant mother. The body she's controlled (or, at least, tried to control) so carefully for so long suddenly seems to have taken over.

To an extent, the body knows what it's doing. Weight gain during pregnancy is not, as it may be at other times, a sign that something is wrong; it's telling you that some things are right: your baby is growing; a healthy support system of placenta, amniotic fluid, and enhanced blood supply is developing to nourish and protect him or her; and preparation is being made for lactation.

But though your body is operating in your baby's best interests, it can easily be led astray by an appetite fueled by emotional upset or weakened by morning sickness or indigestion, by psychically depressed willpower, by a misinterpreted craving or aversion. So while it isn't necessary, or wise, to completely wrest the control over your weight gain back from your body, it is important for you to share the responsibility of keeping your gain from missing the mark.

What is the mark? A generation ago, doctors strictly limited weight gain to between 15 and 18 pounds. But once the perils of insufficient weight gain (see page 23) were documented, the pendulum took a swing up the scale. For a few practitioners, who theorized that if more is good, a lot more is even better, it swung all the way up to 50 pounds. For most, however, who also recognized the potential problems attached to excessive weight gain, it settled sensibly in the middle.

The Best-Odds Diet recommends this sensible midpoint range—25 to 35 pounds—as a target gain for the average-weight woman during the average pregnancy.[11] This range allows for a 6- to 8-pound baby and for the necessary 14 to 24 pounds of baby-support system, including enough (but not more than enough) of the maternal fat stores needed for nursing. (The weight is distributed most effi-

ciently if it is gained on a diet of quality foods. When it is gained on a diet that is heavy on the junk food, the same amount of weight may be distributed in a way less beneficial to baby, with a higher proportion of maternal fat, a lower proportion of weight to the baby, and a weaker baby-support system.)

Not every pregnancy fits neatly into this "average" formula. The woman who is seriously underweight at the time of conception may be at a nutritional disadvantage before she starts. To avoid putting her baby at the same disadvantage, she should try to gain enough weight in the first trimester (before the baby's nutritional needs put a substantial drain on her reserves) to catch up to her "ideal" weight (see If You're Gaining Too Slowly, page 77). If she does catch up, she can continue to gain at an average rate (see page 74); if not, she will have to gain at a faster clip for the remainder of her pregnancy. In either case, a larger-than-average total weight gain, monitored carefully by her practitioner, is probably warranted.

The woman who is at least 10 percent to 20 percent over her "ideal" weight prepregnancy may also stray outside the average weight gain pattern; she can probably gain somewhat less weight safely. However, no matter how overweight she is, she

11. Women typically gain slightly more weight in first pregnancies than in subsequent ones.

WEIGHT GAIN AND WHAT IT IS MADE UP OF
(All weights are approximate)

Baby	7½ pounds
Placenta	1½ pounds
Amniotic fluid	2 pounds
Uterine enlargement	2 pounds
Maternal breast tissue	2 pounds
Maternal blood volume	4 pounds
Fluids in maternal tissue	4 pounds
Maternal fat stores	7 pounds
Total Average	30-pound overall weight gain

should *not* use pregnancy as a time for losing weight (if she waits until breastfeeding time, she will find weight easy to lose, particularly if she keeps up the good eating habits developed during her nine months on the Best-Odds Diet). Since the fetus can draw a small amount of energy from her excess fat stores, she will probably be able to cut back somewhat on calories (under the supervision of her practitioner), but not on anything else. The Daily Dozen are essential to her and her baby's nutritional well-being (but she can fill them most efficiently, by following the tips in If You're Gaining Too Fast). In most cases, however, her practitioner will want her to gain at least 20 pounds. Gaining too little, and relying on body fat to feed baby, can be extremely hazardous. When large amounts of fat are burned by the body, ketones accumulate (page 24),

presenting a risk to both mother and fetus.

The woman carrying multiple fetuses will gain more quickly than average right from the beginning. Not only will she have two (or more) babies growing apace, but she will usually (except when there is one large placenta for identical twins) have two placentas. She will also have additional blood and fluid supplies, a larger (and heavier) uterus, and more amniotic fluid. So though she needn't gain double the recommended weight for twins, triple for triplets, and so on, she does need to gain considerably more than the woman carrying just one baby. Physicians often recommend a gain of at least 50 percent more than for a single fetus, or roughly 37 to 55 pounds over the woman's ideal prepregnancy weight.

As important as gaining the right amount of weight is gain-

WEIGHT GAIN: LOW, AVERAGE, AND HIGH

(With room to plot your own)

Prepregnancy Weight_____

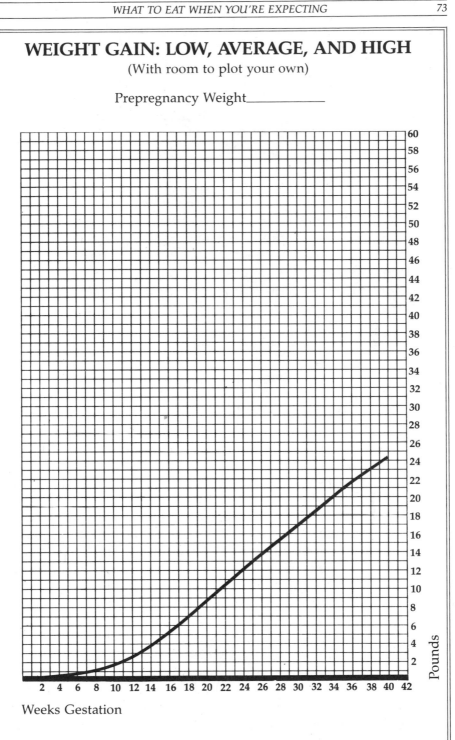

Weeks Gestation

Pounds

ing it at the right pace. The woman who plans to gain no more than 30 pounds and reaches that point at the end of six months shouldn't hold the line on added pounds for the next three, when fetal growth is at its maximum and nutritional needs are greatest, because she's already made her weight gain. Nor should the woman whose midtrimester gain falls victim to a summer-stifled appetite assume that she can make up those pounds in the final months of her pregnancy, when the weather has cooled.

Not only will your baby, who needs a continuous supply of nourishment, benefit from a well-paced weight gain, but you will, too. Your body will adjust more gracefully to the increased poundage, and the strains that come with it, if the weight is added gradually. There will be fewer stretch marks, less flab, and better distribution of the weight.

Steady doesn't mean spreading a 25-pound weight gain evenly over your 40 weeks of pregnancy. In the first trimester, most women need gain no more than two to four pounds (some, particularly those who are overweight, may not gain at all, while those who are underweight may gain considerably more). Weight gain should pick up to a rate of about one pound per week in months four

through eight, then drop off again in the ninth month to a pound or two, or even none at all (some women lose weight during the last two weeks). To be sure your weight gain stays within desirable limits, chart it weekly on page 73.

A steady weight gain doesn't mean a computer-precise rate that never strays from the recommended formula either. If in your fifth month you gain ¾ of a pound the first week, 1½ pounds the second, ½ a pound the third, and 1¼ pounds the last, you will average 1 pound a week without ever gaining exactly 1 pound in any week. And that's fine. You will also stay within the range of normal weight gain if you average slightly under or slightly over one pound a week. If you don't gain any weight at all for two weeks or more during the fourth to eighth month, however, or if you gain more than three pounds in any week in the second trimester or two pounds in any week in the third, check with your practitioner (also, read the information under If You're Gaining Too Fast, which follows).

On the Best-Odds Diet, watching your weight is as easy as watching your scale. It will tell you when you've eaten too much or too little, or when you're eating just about the right amounts.

If You're Gaining Too Fast

Check with your practitioner.
This is important if your weight
gain doesn't seem to be related
to overeating. In rare instances,
excessive weight gain may be the
result of undiagnosed multiple
fetuses. If you haven't already
had a sonogram (which can usually detect this possibility), your
practitioner may want to arrange
one, particularly if your uterus
appears large for your EDC (estimated date of confinement). It's
important to learn early on if you
are carrying more than one baby,
so that, among other things, you
can nourish them adequately. If
multiple fetuses are ruled out,
your practitioner may want to
assess your thyroid function to
determine if an imbalance in
your metabolism is at the root of
your weight-gain problem. Sudden rapid weight-gain (more
than three pounds in a week),
especially when accompanied by
swelling of hands and face,
headaches, and/or blurring of vi-
sion, should be reported to your
practitioner at once.

Cut back on fat. For those gaining too much weight, fat is the
first thing to trim. It's also the
only nutritional requirement
that can safely be reduced, from
two servings to one (do not eliminate this last serving; some
added fat in the diet is essential).
To fill, but not overfill, this requirement, be especially watchful of fat used in cooking. Once
you've used up that one tablespoon, there should be no oil in
your salad dressing; no oil, margarine, or butter in your eggs,
sauces, or sautéed dishes; and
none on your vegetables or potatoes. Fried foods, which often
take on more than one tablespoon of oil per serving, should
be avoided entirely. (See page
174 for tips on low-fat cooking.)

Be extra efficient. Choose
foods that yield the highest nutrition for the fewest calories.
Concentrate on the leanest
sources for your nutrients: fish,
poultry (with skin removed),
lean meats, low-fat cottage
cheese, and eggs instead of peanut butter, fatty meats, beans,
and peas for protein (unless
you're a strict vegetarian); skim
and low-fat milk products instead of full-fat for calcium; broccoli, kale, and carrots instead of
dried apricots, sweet potatoes,
and winter squash for your
green leafy and yellow vegetables. (Food selections and recipes which are not well-suited to
your caloric needs, and are best
avoided, are noted on the Food
Selection Tables with an †.)

Don't cheat. It's the frills that
fill you out in the wrong places—
while doing nothing good for
your baby. Drop even Best-Odds
cheating until your weight gain
stabilizes. Then try adding one

WEIGHING IN

Whether it's because of fear that they've gained too much weight, or anxiety that they haven't gained enough, the scale at the practitioner's office looms large and forbidding, and the approach of the monthly ritual of weighing in weighs heavy on the consciences of expectant mothers.

Surprisingly, the best way to fend off weighing-in phobia is not to make fewer appearances on the scale, but more frequent ones. Consult your scale daily. This way you'll be able to spot and correct an unwanted trend early, before it leads you too far off course.

To get the most out of a partnership with your scale, you have to understand the eccentricities of the weight gain it registers. Don't expect to gain one-seventh of a pound a day in order to gain one pound a week, or exactly one pound a week to gain four per month. Small fluctuations, or even larger, short-term fluctuations are a normal part of the weight-gain process of pregnancy. A salty meal, or one especially high in bulk and water, can move the scale up a shocking two pounds; a bout of loose bowel movements or an active day in the hot sun can make it slide back a pound or more.[12] Both reactions are temporary, and are likely to disappear in a day or two, once normal fluid balance returns. But remember, a certain amount of fluid retention—what you see as swelling of your ankles and feet, and sometimes of your hands—is perfectly normal.

When a large gain or loss stays with you for several days, it's probably not a fluke of fluctuation, but a sign that you may be eating too much or not eating enough. Consider it a call to action. A call to your doctor is wise, too.[13]

The Right Way to Weigh

❖Invest in a bathroom scale if you don't already have one. Most accurate are those that, like the doctor's scale, depend on weights, not springs. They're also the most expensive, and aren't necessary for monitoring pregnancy weight gain. A scale that is chronically "under" or "over," even by several pounds, may not give you an accurate weight, but it can still give you a day-to-day tally of losses and gains. Only a scale whose "zero balance" fluctuates unpredictably can't be used for reliable monitoring, and should be replaced.

❖Weigh yourself under the same conditions each day. Every morning before breakfast, for instance, naked, or with the same amount of clothing. It's also best to weigh yourself consistently before or after toileting.

permitted cheat a month. Then one every other week.

Turn on the burner. You may not be taking in too much fuel, you just may not be burning it fast enough. People with weight problems often don't eat more than thinner people, but they do sit more. With your practitioner's permission, and following his or her guidelines for safe exercise during pregnancy, get up and go—regularly. Ride a stationary bike. Take a brisk walk, an envigorating swim, or an exercise class especially designed for expectant mothers.

If You're Gaining Too Slowly

Check with your practitioner. This is important, especially if your slow weight gain doesn't seem related to undereating. A metabolic disorder or some other undiagnosed medical problem may be keeping you from achieving your weight-gain goals.

---

12. If your scale shows a sudden increase because of fluid retention, this is *not* a signal to cut out salt (though it's probably wise to avoid excessively salty foods) or cut down on fluids. If your weight drops suddenly because of dehydration, be sure to replace lost fluids quickly (see page 51).

13. A weight gain of more than three pounds per week in the second trimester or two in the third, especially when accompanied by edema (swelling) of hands and face, visual difficulties, and/or headache is a signal to call the practitioner immediately.

Do a diet audit. Are you actually getting your Daily Dozen every day? Or are you missing a serving here, two servings there, or, worse, entire requirements? Tally your totals and make a point of filling in all the blanks you've uncovered.

Fatten up your diet. Since pure fat is the most concentrated source of food energy, increasing your fat allowance to three or four servings a day will increase your calories without significantly decreasing your appetite. Don't multiply your fat intake further, however; because fat supplies little but calories, there are more nutritious ways to step up weight gain.

Don't be too efficient. Most pregnant women benefit from eating foods that supply them with the most nutrients for the fewest calories. If you're not gaining enough weight, such efficiency's likely to be counterproductive. To keep your scale on the upswing, favor foods with a more balanced ratio of nutrients to calories (examples of these foods are noted with an ↑ in the Food Selection Groups). If you're tangling with a sluggish appetite, take extra servings of wheat germ, one of the richest sources of appetite-stimulating B vitamins, and don't overdo on bulky, lower-calorie foods, such as green salads, which fill you up without filling you out. (But don't give them up altogether, particularly if constipation is a problem.) Focus instead on concentrated sources of calories and nutrients, such as avocados, nuts, hard cheeses, beans, and peas.

Launch a snack attack. Don't just sit there between meals—eat something. Build snack breaks (one midmorning, one midafternoon, and one before bedtime) into your schedule, and observe them faithfully. Make the snacks substantial in content, though not substantial enough in volume to sabotage your appetite for the next meal: a slice of whole-wheat bread or Best-Odds Zucchini Bread slathered generously with peanut butter and sliced banana; a handful of almonds and dates, washed down with a Double-the-Milk Shake; a chunk of cheese and some whole-grain crackers; a slice of whole-wheat pizza; Fig Bars or Chewy Oatmeal Cake and

milk—or any Best-Odds treat.

Don't jump in with junk food. Potato chips, ice cream, and chocolate cake may seem the obvious solution to slow weight gain. And, indeed, while you may gain plenty on a diet supplemented by junk food, your baby may come out a loser (see Junk Food: What's in It for You and Baby, page 41). Keep your junk food consumption within the limits allotted in Best-Odds Cheating (page 67).

Turn down the burner. If you're jogging or working out an hour a day, you may be burning up the calories you eat instead of using them to nourish your body and your baby. Try cutting back to no more than 15 minutes of strenuous exercise a day, as recommended by the American College of Obstetrics and Gynecology. And don't forget to compensate for the calories you do burn by heaping your plate extra high with healthy foods.

THREE

The Best Odds for a Comfortable Pregnancy

Even THE ORDINARILY EASY-TO-FEED CAN BECOME problem eaters during pregnancy. Nearly every pregnant woman experiences at least one of the common appetite-disrupting complaints of pregnancy: morning sickness, with its bouts of nausea and vomiting; indigestion and heartburn, promising discomfort after every meal; constipation, conferring perpetual "fullness"; cravings and aversions, confusing the appestat and confounding the body's natural gustatory instincts.

Not only can the Best-Odds Diet help the expectant mother eat well in spite of these maladies, but it also offers dietary strategies for minimizing the maladies so you can feed baby better and feel better yourself.

MORNING SICKNESS

Just when everyone tells her that she should be eating for two, the morning-sickness sufferer feels as though she can't even eat for one. If she's lucky, her morning sickness only keeps her away from the breakfast table; but if she's typical, her digestive sensitivity lasts through dinner. Her symptoms may be as mild as occasional queasiness, or as severe as frequent vomiting. They may disappear after the first trimester (they do in most cases), or persist into the third. Only in the rarest, most severe cases will they interfere with eating enough to seriously disrupt fetal nutrition.

In all cases, there are dietary measures that can reduce the severity of morning sickness (you may find some more effective than others) while minimizing its nutritional toll on the fetus.

Get the best odds with the Best-Odds Diet.

Because it's high in protein and complex carbohydrates, which tend to reduce nausea, the Best-Odds Diet gives you the best chance of fending off morning sickness. Being generally well nourished, which Best-Odds eating promotes, also helps to decrease symptoms.

Keep fluids flowing.

You'll need plenty of them, particularly if you're losing them through vomiting. They also make an effective short-term substitute for the nutrition in solids when you're having trouble keeping solids down. Opt for the fluids that least offend and are most likely to nourish: Double-the-Milk Shakes; fruit or vegetable juices; broths, either clear or puréed with vegetables, meat, or cottage cheese; or fruit soups made with juices instead of sugar syrup. Frozen fluids may work, too. And try Fruit Sorbets or Ice Cream.

If, on the other hand, you find solids easier to keep down than liquids, try to get your fluids in solid form, from foods that have high water contents, such as fruits and vegetables, particularly lettuce and other greens, melons, berries, and citrus.

Follow your stomach.

If your stomach cries out for sweets, and cries "foul!" at the sight or smell of anything remotely savory, take heed—but not by succumbing to the temptation of a couple of jelly doughnuts for breakfast, an ice cream for lunch, and chocolate cake and a milkshake for dinner. There's a better way to sweeten what you are eating.

Virtually any nutrient can come in a sweet package. Oatmeal blended with apple juice concentrate, cinnamon, and raisins or dates; cold cereal with fruit-only applesauce or preserves and/or fresh fruit; Bran Muffins; Whole-Wheat Buttermilk Pancakes with Fruited Yogurt; and a fruit-only jelly omelet can all sweeten your morning meal.

Fruit soups; fruit-and-nutted (include a yellow fruit, such as mango or melon) cottage cheese or yogurt sundaes served on a bed of green leafy lettuce; Sweet Cottage Cheese Pancakes; low-fat pot cheese mixed with cinnamon, chopped raisins, and a little apple juice concentrate on whole-wheat raisin bread; or carrot-raisin slaw or waldorf salad made with yogurt and apple juice concentrate—all can provide sweets for your noon meal.

Chicken or tuna salad with chunks of pineapple, red peppers, apple, raisins, and a dressing of pineapple and/or orange juice concentrate and yogurt; chicken breasts in a sweet and tangy lemon sauce or stuffed with apples and whole-wheat bread crumbs; turkey glazed with orange juice concentrate or fruit-only orange marmalade and served with a fruited brown rice stuffing; side dishes of orange or pineapple-sweetened carrots, baked sweet potatoes, or red-cabbage slaw can "sweet" you off your feet at dinner.

To some morning sickness sufferers, it's the sweet they can't eat. For them, it's easy to get the Daily Dozen in a savory setting. There is no nutrient— including vitamin C, which is plentiful in peppers, kale, broccoli, cauliflower, and tomatoes— that can't be had without a smidgeon of sweetness. Check the Food Selection Groups on pages 53 to 62.

If meat is a turnoff (it is for many women early in pregnancy), stick to fish and chicken. If even these are unpalatable, follow the tips for vegetarians on page 99 until you can again include flesh foods in your diet.

Most sensitive stomachs rebel against highly spiced, rich, or fatty foods. If yours is among them, side with your tummy, and drop these types of food from your diet.

See and smell no evil. Taste is not the only sense that can set a sensitive tummy into turmoil. In fact, those that precede it in the food preparation process, sight and smell, can be more offensive. If seeing a raw chicken breast or fish fillet sends shivers down your esophagus, have someone else see it into the broiling or baking pan. If the smell of frying onions or raw garlic repulses your innards, avoid using them in cooking (simply seasoned foods are more likely to sit well with a queasy stomach, anyway). Don't be a mother-to-be martyr, either, fixing favorite but odiously odorous favorites, like chicken livers or bacon for your family.

Beware the empty stomach. Believe it or not, one of the best measures for preventing and curing morning sickness is eating—often. An empty stomach produces acids that have nothing to dine on but stomach lining. One result: nausea. Long breaks between meals can also trigger a low blood sugar reaction, another accessory to morning sickness. Instead of three squares, try six mini meals (which are easier to digest, too) with snacks in between as needed. Best are complex carbohydrates (such as whole-wheat bread sticks or crackers, dried fruit, rice cakes) and/or high protein snacks (such as cheese or hard-boiled eggs).

Beat nausea to your stomach. Eat before queasiness strikes whenever possible, since that's when food will go down more easily and be more likely to stay down. Filling your stomach before an attack may also help to ward one off.

Open a bedside snack bar. Forget whatever your mother told you about eating in bed. It's one of the most effective approaches to dealing with morning sickness. Again, the idea is to keep the stomach happy by keeping it full, preventing irritating emptiness. When you retire, snuggle up with a good book (or a good mate) and a high protein/high carbohydrate snack (Fig Bars and milk or cheese and whole-wheat crackers, for example). Stock your snack bar with nonperishable carbohydrates (whole-grain bread sticks or crackers, dry cereal, raisins, dried apricots or figs) so you can reach for them if hunger hits in the middle of the night. Have them ready to reach out for, too, as soon as you open your eyes in the morning so you can line your stomach before you set a foot out of bed.

Don't eat for nothing. Making every bite count is particularly important for morning sickness sufferers, whose appetites for the Daily Dozen may be limited. Being efficient in your food selections—choosing foods that, bite for bite, provide the most concentrated nutrition—will help keep you from having to prolong your misery with extra bites, or worse, missing out on vital nutrition.

Secure your insurance. When you've got morning sickness, your prenatal vitamin supplement is insurance that you and your baby are getting your RDA of vitamins and minerals. Try to take yours when it's least likely to come back up. Your practitioner may recommend an additional ration of B_6 to calm your stomach, which seems to help some women. But do not take any medication or extra vitamins for nausea and vomiting unless prescribed by a physician who knows you are pregnant and has checked on the safety of the drug and the dose.

CONSTIPATION

Though the body, particularly the pregnant body, is a miraculous machine, it isn't a perfect one. Early in pregnancy it begins circulating hormones meant to relax the muscles that will be involved in childbirth, but which also incidentally relax the muscles of the digestive tract. There is a positive effect to this digestive relaxation: food stays in the intestines longer, allowing for absorption of nutrients. But there's also a negative effect: Feces that stay around too long may become hard, dry, and difficult to eliminate. In other words, constipation may occur.

Happily, you don't have to be a victim of your body's imperfections, or accept constipation as a normal and inevitable accompaniment of pregnancy. You can fight back, without resorting to laxatives or mineral oil[1] in these ways:

Rough up your diet. W.K. Kellogg, the founder of the cereal company, first suggested in the early part of this century that the bran or outer coating of the wheat grain could cure constipation. At the time, he was considered flakier than his cereals. Today, many millions of boxes of bran flakes later, his ideas are well-documented by scientific evidence. Bran and other forms of fiber (the material that surrounds and supports the cell walls of plants) move through the digestive tract essentially unchanged. But though the digestive system has little effect on fiber, fiber has a noticeable effect on the digestive tract. As it moves through the intestines, fiber absorbs water softening the stool and speeding its passage.

So take a tip from Kellogg (and from C.W. Post, another

early proponent of vegetarianism and high-fiber diets). When constipation makes you miserable, or preferably before it has a chance to develop, rough up your diet. The Best-Odds Diet is pretty rough to start with, but you can rough it up even more by concentrating on the highest fiber food choices. That means plenty of whole grains, fresh fruits and vegetables (some raw, some with skins left on, but well-scrubbed, when appropriate), dried legumes (beans and peas), nuts and seeds, but few highly processed foods. Prefer whole fruit over juices, crisp-cooked vegetables over mushy ones.

If you've been on the typical highly refined low-fiber American diet, don't go rough overnight. Instead, over a six-week period, gradually add foods with a higher fiber content to your diet. You may experience excessive flatulence (gassiness) at first, but this should disappear as your body adjusts to the new regimen.

Even if you're used to a high-fiber diet, don't overdo the fiber during pregnancy. (This is most likely to be a problem for vegetarians, who depend on legumes for their protein.) An excess of fiber can carry nutrients out of your system before they've had a chance to be absorbed for use by you and your baby. And because calcium is

---

1. Mineral oil should not be used at all during pregnancy (and only briefly under medical supervision at other times) because it interferes with the absorption of nutrients. Don't take laxatives, either, unless specifically prescribed for you during pregnancy by your practitioner.

particularly vulnerable to the effects of fiber, don't eat a lot of fiber at the same meal in which you're eating foods that are counting toward your calcium servings.

Wash it down. What makes fiber work is its attraction for water. By absorbing all available fluids, it keeps the stool soft and mobile. A lack of fluids could jam up the works. You should have at least your Daily Dozen quota of liquids (particularly water, and fruit and vegetable juices) every day, more if you add bran to your diet. A favorite health spa tonic, hot water with lemon juice (unsweetened), first thing in the morning often has an anticonstipation effect. Desperate cases may benefit from prune juice in small doses.

Give it time. Leave five minutes for your breakfast before you dash out of the house in the morning, and chances are you'll leave with your bathroom mission unaccomplished. Instead, rise earlier and try to breakfast at least half an hour before your departure. This will give your digestive tract the time it needs to move things along.

Give it a shake. Your digestive tract will move faster if you do. An inactive body encourages inactive bowels. So be sure to get some exercise daily, even if it's only a brisk 20-minute walk.

Give it bran, as a last resort. If after a few weeks on a high-fiber diet constipation still plagues you, try adding a daily heaping tablespoon of unprocessed bran to your diet. Don't add it to your cereal if you take your cereal with milk. Instead, have the bran as a snack, with unsweetened applesauce or cottage cheese (both of which bind the little flakes for easier swallowing), washed down with fluids, or in a glass of fruit juice.

If after a few days constipation is still a problem, add another tablespoon of bran. If that doesn't activate your GI tract, speak to your practitioner.

BLOATING AND FLATULENCE

For most pregnant women, the first time they can't button their skirts is less a sign that their fetus is outgrowing their waistlines than a sign that they're suffering from bloating caused by bowel distension. The bloating doesn't just necessitate an early switch to maternity clothes; it can be responsible for gassiness and discomfort that can last, in varying degrees, until delivery.

As distressing as they can prove for the expectant mother, bloating and flatulence are only threatening to the fetus if the constant feeling of fullness they impart keeps her from eating regularly. To make sure that it doesn't, beat the bloat with these tips:

Slow down. Eating on the run, gulping snacks, transacting stressful business over meals can all lead to air swallowing. The gulped air forms little pockets in the intestines that cause pressure and pain. So relax your pace. Make time for meals (see pages 37 and 94), take your snacks sitting down, don't mix business with lunch if it leaves you agitated.

Make your three squares into six. As with many of the dietarily connected complaints of pregnancy, large meals often compound bloating and flatulence. Eat a Thanksgiving-size feast, and you're bound to stagger away from the table feeling like a stuffed turkey—and to experience several hours of gastric rumblings uncomfortable enough to keep you from returning to the table for the next meal. (It may also interfere with your sleep, if you eat it at night.) Spread the nutritional content of those three large squares over six smaller meals, however, and your digestive tract won't be overloaded.

Don't ask for trouble. Eating foods to which you know your stomach reacts negatively is an invitation to bloating and flatulence. Don't extend the invita-

tion. Avoid anything that makes you gassy; potential culprits (they'll vary from stomach to stomach) include beans, onions, garlic, cabbage, Brussels sprouts, and fried and sugared foods (these aren't recommended for Best-Odds dieters, anyway). If a step-up of roughage in your diet seems to be causing or aggravating your stomach distress, don't yank yourself off the constipation-fighting regimen. Just increase fiber more slowly. After your body has adjusted to the increase in fiber (this will take a few weeks), bloating and flatulence should diminish dramatically.

Avoid constipation. Irregularity breeds contempt on the part of your stomach. The backup of uneliminated foods leads to bloating, gassiness, discomfort, and the feeling that there's no room for your next meal. See page 82 for tips on preventing and overcoming constipation.

HEARTBURN

Doctors term it "dyspepsia," television commercials dub it "sour stomach" and "gasid indigestion." Pregnant women who experience it, most commonly and painfully in the second and third trimesters, call it "miserable"—and sometimes they're not that polite.

The misery of heartburn (which seems to love company; at least 30 to 70 percent of all expectant mothers suffer from it) is misnamed. Though its major symptoms are a tightness and burning sensation midchest, it's the gastrointestinal system, and not the heart, that is implicated in this condition. The focus is the sphincter muscle that regulates the movement of food from esophagus to stomach. When the sphincter is weak (either naturally or because the hormones of pregnancy relax it as they do other muscle tissue), or when there is pressure on the stomach from below (as when one bends from the waist or when a burgeoning uterus presses upward), stomach acids may be pushed back up into the esophagus. These acids that "burn" the sensitive lining of the esophagus, causing the pain and discomfort of heartburn.

The best cure for heartburn is prevention. All of the following steps can help prevent or alleviate the condition.

Don't weigh yourself (and your stomach) down. The heavier you are, the more pressure you place on your esophageal sphincter. A moderate weight gain of 20 to 30 pounds is less likely to encourage heartburn than a gain of 40 to 50 pounds, so set your goals accordingly.

Favor your friends. A diet high in protein and low in fat is, according to many physicians, a heartburn-sufferer's best friend.

Avoid your foes. Identify and eliminate from your diet those foods that seem to lead to heartburn. The foods most likely to impair sphincter function are, with the exception of hot and highly seasoned foods, generally not recommended on the Best-Odds Diet: chocolate; coffee; processed meats (such as hot dogs, salami, bologna, and other luncheon meats, sausage, bacon); high-fat foods (either cooked with too much fat, such as fried foods, rich pastries and sauces, or naturally fatty, such as certain cuts of beef and pork, sweet and sour creams, butter and some cheeses); alcohol; and carbonated beverages (though Best-Odds does approve club soda and seltzers). Many people chew mint-flavored gum in order to reduce heartburn, but both peppermint and spearmint, like aspirin and tobacco, can affect sphincter function adversely by irritating the delicate esophageal lining. (Acetaminophen, such as Tylenol, will not contribute to indigestion, but, like aspirin, should not be taken without your physician's approval.)

Take it slow. Speed eating may save valuable time, but you're likely to pay the price in heartburn afterward. Gulping large mouthfuls of food without first chewing properly can contribute to discomfort (as well as interfere with optimum absorption of nutrients by the body). So take your time when you eat (allowing at least 20 minutes for a meal will also allow your appestat to signal when you are full), and a tip from etiquette experts: Cut your food into small bites and chew each thoroughly before taking another.

Take it easy. Like other digestive problems, heartburn is often directly related to emotional stress. That's why it's the weekday worker, not the weekend golfer, who's featured in those "gasid indigestion" commercials. Heartburn, which thrives in the nine-to-five world, often vanishes on vacation. (Of course, if your family is one of your jobs, the stress can be round the clock and round the calendar.) Though it may not be easy to achieve, relaxation should certainly be pursued, particularly while you're pregnant, and even more particularly during meals. Try a little yoga in the ladies room, the relaxation techniques you learned in childbirth class, or a leisurely walk after an especially trying meeting or a toddler's tantrum. Don't eat on the run or while on the phone with an irate customer; make meals a quiet time, if possible, a respite from the rest of your probably hectic life.

Keep your head up. Gravity helps your digestive tract keep food moving in the right direction. When you are flat on your back (not a good idea after the fourth month of pregnancy, anyway), indigestion is aggravated.

Go with the flowing. Constricting clothes around your middle can add to the pressure on your stomach. Be sure waistbands on skirts, slacks, and shorts have enough give as you grow (not all maternity clothes do). If they're leaving a ring around the belly, they're too tight.

FOOD CRAVINGS AND AVERSIONS

The pregnancy test hasn't even come back positive but your morning coffee suddenly tastes too bitter to swallow. You're trying to avoid refined sugar, but find yourself possessed nightly by a craving for fudge ripple ice cream (fortunately without pickles). Chicken has always been a mainstay of your diet; now you can't even look it in the breast.

Is your body trying to tell you something? Are food cravings and aversions accurate gauges of your nutritional needs? Sometimes. Many women, most often in first pregnancies and during the first trimester, develop aversions to things their bodies shouldn't have during pregnancy (such as coffee, alcohol, and cigarettes) and cravings for things their bodies need (cheese, grains, or fruit, for example). More often, however, the signals sent by the body get scrambled before they are interpreted by the brain, and the message we get is neither accurate nor worth heeding—as when it tries to entice us toward a bag of potato chips or away from anything green and leafy.

While you can't completely ignore food cravings and aversions, you needn't become a prisoner of them either. To keep them from compromising your nutritional position, you need to know when to humor them, and when to let them know who's boss.

Don't fight a healthy aversion. When your aversion is to something you're better off without, consider yourself lucky. It'll never be easier to give up coffee or alcohol than when they're distasteful.

Avert the harm of an unhealthy aversion. Even if your body says "no" to fish and chicken, you can still say "yes" to protein. Look for inoffensive protein equivalents on page 44. (Often, the aversion to flesh foods is less marked if the culprit isn't as easily recognizable; chicken off the bone and chunked in a casserole or stir-fried dish, fish flaked and tossed with pasta, may be less offensive than a chicken breast or a fish steak.) If it's green vegetables you're finding uninviting, opt for yellows until the greens are once again a welcome sight (fruits are fine substitutes, too) or drink vegetable juice.

Indulge your healthy cravings. Something you want badly isn't automatically unhealthy. Don't puritanically stifle a yearning for starchy carbohydrates, just direct it toward nutritious starches, such as whole-wheat bread, high-protein pasta, or baked potatoes. Even exceeding your four- to five-serving allotment for a few weeks won't disturb your dietary equilibrium, as long as you don't exceed it so far that you don't have room for the other 11 of the Daily Dozen or start gaining weight too rapidly. You can even satisfy a craving and some other nutritional requirements at the same time: getting your starch fix from peas and beans, which are a good protein combo, or having winter squash or yams, which make points with your requirement of yellows.

Substitute (or sublimate) and conquer unhealthy cravings. You'll feel better the morning after if you don't give in to cravings you know won't help, or may even hurt, your baby. But instead of attempting to quash them entirely, which probably won't work, try putting in a pinch-hitter. If chocolate is your heart's desire, bake a batch of Fudge Brownies, an Angelic Devil's Food Cake, or a Chocolate Pudding Cake. If potato chips strike your fancy, strike back with hollowed-out baked potato skins, sprinkled with Parmesan cheese and rebaked until crisp. If the object of your craving is a candy bar, pick up a no-sugar-or-honey-added carob bar (they come with toasted nuts, raisins, "crunch," and even minted) at your local health food store. If substitutions don't satisfy, try sublimation. Redirect your yen for unhealthy foods into healthy pursuits: exercise, dance, layette shopping, bootie knitting, sex. And, once in a while, give in to your cravings by using your cheating allowance (page 67); however, beware of cravings that aren't satisfied, but instead are stimulated, by giving in.

Don't confuse a craving for food with a craving for love. Sometimes food cravings are less a signal from the body than from the mind; you may be less starved for ice cream than for affection. Pregnant women, particularly in the first trimester, are extremely susceptible to the ebb and flow of their emotions. Often a request for a pizza at mid-night may really be a call for a little tender loving care. Talk this possibility over with your spouse; perhaps he can deliver a much-needed hug instead of that not-so-needed pie.

FATIGUE

Rare is the expectant mother who doesn't feel that her "get up and go" has gotten up and gone at least some time during her pregnancy. That's not surprising, considering the physical and emotional stresses on her body. In the early weeks, the placenta is developing, and this is a major manufacturing process (albeit one you can't see) that requires tremendous effort. Baby manufacturing is going on, too, and that continues for your entire gestation, making further demands on your energy levels. Later in pregnancy you begin toting a gradually increasing load of baby, amniotic fluid, and other pregnancy by-products, the equivalent of carrying a backpack on your stomach around the clock, day in and day out. As your belly burgeons, it can easily get between you and a good night's sleep.

Nothing can completely wipe out that wiped-out feeling. But the Best-Odds Diet (coupled with listening to your body when it tells you it needs some rest) can minimize it by providing the fuel you need to keep going. A well-nourished body—fed faithfully with the Daily Dozen—can cope with the stresses of pregnancy more effectively than an inadequately nourished one.

Candy bars, doughnuts, and Danish pastry won't do the job, despite advertising which promises an energy lift to get you through the morning (or afternoon). Any lift you get from sugar will be fleeting, and will be followed by a blood sugar crash that will leave you more exhausted than ever. Caffeine, too, provides only a temporary, chemically-induced lift; don't be tempted to enlist it in your fight against fatigue.

If your fatigue is severe, and is accompanied by fainting, pallor, breathlessness, and/or palpitations, anemia is a possible cause. Most often in pregnancy, anemia is caused by an iron deficiency—which can result even if you're eating iron-rich foods and taking a prenatal supplement which contains iron. Report severe fatigue to your practitioner and ask for a blood test to check for anemia.

LEG CRAMPS

Nothing can put a cramp in your sleeping style like leg cramps. Recent research has linked these painful spasms, that usually strike at night, to an excess of phosphorus in relation to calcium in the blood. Often, taking a calcium supplement (that doesn't contain phosphorus) can eliminate them entirely. If that doesn't work, your practitioner may recommend you cut back on high-phosphorus foods, such as meat and milk. See tips on meatless (page 101) and milkless diets (page 102) so you can be sure to get enough calcium and protein elsewhere. Persistent pain that doesn't respond to dietary change should be reported to your practitioner.

COMPLEXION COMPLICATIONS

While most of its major changes are taking place inside, pregnancy is skin deep, too. The hormonal alterations cause an increase in the secretion of skin oil. This is good for some women—usually those who start out with dry skin—whose complexions take on a radiant "glow" during pregnancy. For those who have oilier skin and/or who have a tendency to break out just before their menstrual periods, it isn't so good. Their skin takes on an "adolescent" look.

There's nothing you can do about the hormonal changes your body is experiencing (or that you would want to do; these changes are an essential part of baby making). But you can, as you can premenstrually, minimize the negative effects they have on your skin through diet. Healthier insides make for healthier outsides; the Daily Dozen (particularly pore-purifying fluids) can do at least as much for your complexion as a pharmacy full of expensive topical preparations. If your breakouts are disturbingly severe ask your practitioner about taking a 25 to 50 milligram supplement of vitamin B$_6$, which is sometimes very effective in the treatment of hormonally-triggered complexion problems.

Do not resort to vitamin A treatment, frequently used in severe acne, or to the use of drugs—either of which could be harmful.

If dry skin (particularly on your stretching abdomen) seems to be aggravated by pregnancy, moisturize outside with lotions and humidifiers (a pot of water left on a radiator, or simmering on the stove will do), and inside with plenty of fluids. Avoid overdoing the soap and hot water, and be sure that you're meeting your Daily Dozen requirements. If you haven't already, add wheat germ to your diet; it's rich in essential fatty acids, as well as in vitamin E and the B complex.

FOUR

The Best Odds for Everyone

YOU'D LIKE TO GIVE THE BEST-ODDS DIET YOUR BEST. But you're a vegetarian; how can you possibly get enough protein on a diet of plant foods? Or you have a lactose intolerance; how can you get enough calcium without consuming any milk or milk products? Or you have a gastrointestinal virus and you can't stomach any of the Daily Dozen. Or your job demands you eat most of your meals away from home. Or you're on a tight budget or a tight schedule and you can't figure out how the Best-Odds Diet can fit in. Or you're eating for three and you're wondering if the Daily Dozen should become the Daily Two Dozen—and if it should, how you'll be able to eat it all.

Fortunately, the Best-Odds Diet is designed not for the homogenized average, but for real pregnant women: pregnant women who get sick, pregnant women who are short on time or money, pregnant women who travel, pregnant women who've chosen different dietary paths or who have had different dietary paths paved for them by circumstance.

IN SPECIAL SITUATIONS

Toss your excuses out with the candy bars and the soda pop. Now is the time to change your eating ways—no matter what your special situation may be.

Best-Odds on a Budget

Watching your pennies shouldn't conflict with watching your diet. In fact, the two are surprisingly compatible. A few price comparisons will demonstrate how much cheaper it can be to eat well than to eat poorly. Convenience and fast foods are generally more expensive than those made at home (you're paying for advertising and packaging, not just food); soft drinks are more costly than juice or milk; a box of oatmeal, penny for penny, lasts a lot longer than a box of sugar-coated cereal; whole-wheat bread usually costs no more than white.

These basic principles can help keep costs down and nutrition up:

Be a no-frills shopper. Store brands and "no-frills" generic items may not be as pretty on the outside as more expensive name brands, but they are as nutritious on the inside. Often available are frozen vegetables, juices, unsweetened fruits, unsweetened applesauce, canned fruits packed in juice, cottage cheese and other dairy products, dry and evaporated skimmed milk, raisins and other dried fruits, nuts, and canned fish.

Choose frozen orange juice. It's less expensive and at least as nutritious as cartons of fresh or reconstituted juice.

Take your milk dry. Nonfat dry milk has all the calcium, protein, and essential vitamins of fresh milk; is more versatile; requires no refrigeration; and has a long shelf life. Purchased in the 20-quart size, store brand or no-frills, it costs less than half as

much as fresh milk quart for quart. A taste for reconstituted dry milk may need to be acquired if you're planning to drink it straight (it's not likely to bother you in shakes or cooking). To help acclimate your taste buds, mix the reconstituted with fresh milk, starting with one part each and gradually add more of the reconstituted as your palate becomes more accepting. Always use ice water for mixing, or chill the reconstituted mixture thoroughly before serving—either of which will improve the flavor.

Stay seasonal. Stick with what's seasonal in fruits and vegetables, and you'll be paying less while getting more nutrition. Grapefruits and oranges may be available year round, but they're freshest and cheapest in the winter months; green beans can be bought in December, but they'll have lost most of their nutrition as well as their attractively low summer price. When the season's over for a favorite fruit or vegetable, head for the frozen foods case, where the price and the nutrition are right. Again, skip over the nationally advertised brands and opt for the store or generic label.

Stock up and save. Fresh chicken, fish, and meat have no nutritional advantage over frozen. Buy large quantities of "specials," and freeze them in portion-size packages for easy thawing. But don't buy more than you can use within the safe storage period.

Keep it simple. Fancy cream and butter sauces add to the price and calorie count of a dish, not to its nutritional value (which is why they're not recommended on the Best-Odds Diet, anyway). Garnish inexpensively with chopped parsley and other greens, hard-boiled egg slices, carrot curls, radish or lemon roses, cherry tomatoes, and pepper rings in season.

When Time Is Tight

Between schedule demands on the job and at home, many expectant mothers feel as though they haven't the time for eating, much less eating right. Yet while careful eating does require more planning and dedication, it needn't require much more time. Once it becomes part of your routine, and with the help of the following tips, Best-Odds eating can become as convenient and speedy as fast-food restaurant-hopping.

Cook dinner for 10. Though it does take more time to cook from scratch Best-Odds style, your time can be well invested if you cook enough for two or more meals at once and tuck the extras, in meal-size portions, in the freezer for future use. (Plan cooking marathons for weekends when you have the time, and enlist your family's assistance.) Or roast a large turkey on Sunday, have warm turkey leftovers on Monday, turkey salad for lunch on Tuesday, turkey soup (with diced turkey) on Wednesday, and freeze turkey cacciatore for a week from Thursday. Make a double batch of broccoli, have it hot the first night, cold with a vinaigrette or warmed up in a pasta dish or casserole the second.

Bake for an army. Doubling and tripling recipes for muffins, cakes, and cookies takes little additional time, yet it yields enough baked goods to keep you and your family in sweets for weeks to come. Freeze them in air-tight bags and containers (cut cakes and breads to portion-size first).

Plan and shop ahead. Carry in your bag a pocket-size notebook for menu planning and shopping lists and jot down ideas whenever you have the time (on the bus, in the doctor's waiting room, while watching TV). It's more efficient to do a week's worth of staple shopping at once, supplemented by trips to the produce stand for fresh fruits and vegetables and to the fish market for fresh fillets.

Take shortcuts. Buy frozen vegetables instead of fresh; they're at least as nutritious and require no preparation for cooking. Buy ready-to-eat salad ingredients at your local salad bar (avoiding those that use sodium bisulfite to preserve freshness) instead of spending an hour washing and slicing. Use your microwave, if you have one, to quick-defrost frozen foods; quick-bake potatoes, yams, or squash (it's usually faster to steam other vegetables on the stove); and quick-cook main courses (poultry, particularly, will survive the rays best if not overcooked).

Ask for help. If you're not the only one doing the eating, you shouldn't be the only one doing the shopping, cooking, and cleaning up—especially now that you're also doing the baby carrying. Even if you married a man completely innocent in the ways of the supermarket and the kitchen, he doesn't have to remain that way. Train him and trust him with as many links on the food preparation chain as possible. Develop a system that works for you: you do the once-a-week marketing, he fills in the daily blanks on his way home from work; he washes the greens, you dry them; he peels the carrots, you julienne them; you put the fish in the broiler, he scrubs the pan afterward.

If you were lucky enough to marry a man who honed his skills in the kitchen before you ever met, take full advantage of his culinary talents. Let him do the cooking alternate nights, or more often if he wants to. But before you let him pick up a spatula or a skillet, make sure he's thoroughly versed in Best-Odds Cooking techniques. Have him read this entire book, or at least the section on Best-Odds Cooking (page 174). (Or, if you're putting him in charge of serious supermarketing, the section on Best-Odds Shopping, page 160.)

If Illness Strikes

Pregnancy is, in general, a time of radiant good health. But even the most glowing expectant mother is not immune to a circulating cold or flu virus, stomach-upsetting bacteria, a sore throat, or an aching tooth. (Though the Best-Odds Diet will help keep your resistance high and reduce the risk of illness.) If illness does strike, pregnancy is not the time to be your own doctor. Any illness, except for a mild cold, should be reported to your physician. Any tooth or gum problem should be reported to your dentist. A fever of over 102 degrees requires immediate treatment; ailments causing lower or no fever may require treatment if they persist. If your pregnancy is being handled by a midwife, call your family doctor or internist about your illness, but be sure to make it clear you are pregnant.

It's not just the glow that goes when illness strikes a pregnant woman—often it's the appetite and/or the ability to eat a regular diet, as well. Though a few days of toast and tea aren't usually of serious nutritional consequence when you're not pregnant, they can be when you are. Your stuffy nose and scratchy throat may be squelching your interest in food, but not your baby's. He or she needs the Daily Dozen on sick days as much as on well days. Fortunately, with some deft dietary alterations, it's possible to nurse your ailment and nourish your baby at the same time. (For extra insurance, be sure to take your pregnancy vitamin supplement faithfully.)

Colds and flu. Even when you're not pregnant, it isn't wise to starve a cold or a flu. Your body's recuperative powers are diminished when they're not fueled by food energy; if you have an elevated body temperature, you need additional food to compensate for the additional calories being burned. Still, when your nose is stuffy and your head achy, even your favorite foods taste like wood chips and usually tempting aromas might as well be kerosene fumes for all the appeal they hold.

Under these conditions, when you're obviously not living to eat, but eating to live (and to nourish your baby), the simplest and most compactly nutritious foods are usually the most palatable and practical. Think soothing, comforting, and warming—the dishes mother (or dad) used to make when you were sick, revised Best-Odds style: hot oatmeal or whole-grain cereal (fortified with wheat germ, powdered milk, cottage cheese, and/or grated cheese; see page 220); soft scrambled eggs (also calcium enriched with a sprinkling of cheese) with whole-wheat toast; chicken soup, made with plenty of carrots, celery, onion, parsnips, and parsley (puréed after cooking for an easy-to-swallow texture), and served with a full protein fix of diced chicken; Cream of Tomato Soup with cottage cheese and a whole-wheat English muffin; whole-wheat or high-protein noodles with a little butter and a lot of cottage cheese; a homey eggs florentine: creamed spinach and poached eggs served with mashed or baked potatoes; Cornmeal Mush; Brown Rice Pudding with unsweetened applesauce; Pure Fruit Gels.

At the height of congestion, milk may increase your mucus production. If it does, you can skip most, or even all, of your milk for a day or two. Take two 600-milligram calcium tablets daily instead and as many other high-calcium foods as you can tolerate (see page 56).

Liquids are not just important to fill your Daily Dozen now, but to replace fluids lost through a runny nose, sneezes, and fever, and promote a quicker recovery. They also keep your mucus secretions thin, which relieves congestion. Keep a thermos of hot grapefruit or orange-ade (½ cup unsweetened frozen juice concentrate to 1 quart of boiling water) next to your bed and drink at least a cupful every waking hour. Soups, juices (some say grape juice soothes a cough; grapefruit and orange juices provide valuable vitamin C), and water (but skip the ice, which can aggravate a cough) can also count toward this hourly quota. At least one study showed that the most effective liquid for colds and flu is chicken soup, with other hot beverages a close second, and cold beverages a somewhat more distant third.

Sore throat. Since swallowing is an essential part of eating, a sore throat that makes it painful to swallow can present a serious challenge to the expectant mother struggling to feed her fetus. Many of the cold-and-flu-coddling foods, specifically those that are soft enough to slide down the throat with a minimum of swallowing (puréed soups, thinned-out oatmeals and other whole-grain hot cereals (page 220), creamed spinach, Brown Rice Pudding, Apple-Banana Gel, for example) are also appropriate for the sore-throat sufferer. Stay away from throat-irritating acidic foods; drink orange and grapefruit juices well-diluted (see Colds and Flu, above), or switch to grape or apple juice. If this means you aren't getting your usual source of vitamin C, try another listed on page 45.

If you are running a fever, be sure to get plenty of fluids (at least 1 cup every waking hour; see above). Gargling with salt water may also reduce the soreness.

GI (gastrointestinal) distress. When the stomach bug hits, eating is not only unappealing, it is often impossible. If you do get something down, it often comes right up—or out. A "sick" stomach often needs nothing so much as a rest, and even in pregnancy, that may be the speediest route to recovery. Because rapid recovery is the goal (prolongation of diarrhea and/or vomiting could rob baby of vital nutrition), follow your physician's advice scrupulously. Most important to you and your baby in the short term (and most stomach viruses are blessedly brief) will be fluids. (Bedrest will help your body retain more of the fluids you take in.) Try to take a few sips of water, club soda or seltzer, or weak decaffeinated tea every 15 minutes if you are vomiting a lot. If even water won't stay down, suck on ice cubes. If diarrhea, not vomiting, is the problem, try drinking large glasses of fruit juice diluted with equal amounts of water as often as is comfortable. Don't eat anything for the first 12 hours unless you are very hungry. Then start adding undiluted fruit juices, clear broths or bouillon, thin cream of wheat or rice, and other soft bland foods. Avoid the remedies your mother probably recommended, such as ginger ale, colas, and commercial gelatin desserts, because sugar tends to prolong diarrhea.

As soon as you feel able, take in as many calories as you can in bland, inoffensive, fat-free foods, as prescribed by your doctor, such as white toast, boiled or steamed converted white rice, boiled or baked potatoes without the skin, cream of wheat or rice, bananas, applesauce, and gelatin desserts (page 268). Don't worry about the Daily Dozen during the worst days, just go back to them gradually once you're on the road to recovery—waiting until diarrhea has been in check for at least 48 hours, for instance, before starting up on significant roughage. If you're vomiting, take your vitamin supplement when it's least likely to come back up on you. And if your iron supple-ment seems to aggravate your stomach distress, skip it for a few days.

Dental problems. The chewing phase of the eating process is the one that may have to be eschewed if you've had dental work done, especially dental surgery. If you're put on a fluid-only diet for a day or two by your dentist, you can drink your Daily Dozen. Sip Double-the-Milk Shakes, juices (apple, grape, or prune if citrus or tomato burn), creamed soups (with chicken or cottage cheese and vegetables puréed in). When soft solids can be added, try the dishes recommended for sore throats, supplemented by cold softies such as small-curd cottage cheese mixed with mashed banana and applesauce, cold cereal that's been allowed to soak in milk until mushy, sorbet made with nonacidic fruits, and ice cream, unless affected teeth are sensitive to cold.

Chronic illness. Any woman with a chronic illness who is pregnant or who is planning to become pregnant should be under the care of an obstetrician who specializes in high-risk pregnancies, in coordination with her own internist, family doctor, or specialist. In virtually all chronic illnesses, good diet is an essential component of this care and treatment. This is particularly true of diabetes and high blood pressure, two of the more common conditions that must be monitored carefully during pregnancy. In diabetic women, strict dietary control can vastly improve pregnancy outcome; in women with high blood pressure it can prevent complications.

The Best-Odds Diet is naturally well-suited to these special regimens and, with some adjustments, can be adapted to either. If you are on a special diet, ask your practitioner about integrating it with the Best-Odds.

When You're Carrying Twins (or More)

The woman carrying twins, triplets, or more has at least twice as much to think about nutritionally as the woman carrying a single fetus. This doesn't mean she needs twice as many calories or that she needs twice as many nutrients. But, she does need more of some of the Daily Dozen, particularly calories, protein, calcium, and iron. For each additional baby she's carrying, a mother-to-be needs one additional protein serving (about 25 grams) and one additional calcium serving (about 300 milligrams). She should also have an additional whole-grain serving, which will provide needed calories as well as essential vitamins and trace minerals. Her daily nutritional supplement is of dou-bled importance, too; without it she may have difficulty meeting her RDA (particularly if she is suffering from morning sickness, which is more common and more commonly persistant among women carrying more than one fetus). The supplement should contain magnesium, since this trace mineral may help to prevent preeclampsia (also called toxemia), a complication more frequent among women with multiple gestations.

The Best-Odds Vegetarian

The meat-and-potato meal, once the mainstay of the American table, is rapidly becoming a dietary dinosaur. Today, 40 million Americans consider themselves semivegetarians (eat less meat than they used to), and 3.7 percent follow a fully vegetarian diet. Among these meat shunners there is a wide range of practice. There are those who eat no red meat but eat poultry and fish. Others who eat fish but no poultry. Ovo-lacto vegetarians eat eggs and dairy products (some eat only one or the other) but no flesh foods. Vegans, or strict vegetarians, limit themselves to plant foods. Those on the least rigid macrobiotic diet eat mostly whole grains (half their calories), supplemented by vegetables (a quarter), beans, sea vegetables, and broth (another quarter), and sometimes small amounts of fish. The most rigid, and most dangerous, macrobiotic diet consists almost entirely of brown rice.

Expectant mothers are no exception to the meat-minimizing trend. Fortunately, most of the dietary variations they're following present no problem at all for them or their babies. If you fall into one of the following groups, simply heed the related suggestions to be certain you and your baby fare well in the nine months to come.

Poultry and fish eaters. Since the Best-Odds Diet recommends the selection of poultry and fish over red meats as efficient protein foods (they have a higher proportion of protein to fat), the woman who eats poultry and fish, but no red meat, may have an easier time with Best-Odds eating than a meat-eating mom. There is nothing in the essential Daily Dozen that her special diet does not normally provide.

Fish-eating vegetarians. Pregnant women who avoid landlubbing animals in favor of fare from the sea are not strictly vegetarians, but often consider themselves to be. This growing group can feed their babies well since fish is the single most efficient source of protein, the nutrient so vital for fetal development, and offers the rest of the family (particularly father-to-be) protection against heart disease

in the form of atherosclerosis-combating fatty acids. A fish-eating vegetarian's diet also provides all the nutrients the fetus requires.

Ovo-lacto vegetarians. Expectant vegetarians who eat no flesh foods but plenty of eggs and dairy products can also give their babies all the nourishment they need, but they'll have to try harder. Though these women will have no difficulty with 11 of the Daily Dozen, the one remaining—protein—may present some challenge. Eggs and dairy products, while providing excellent protein, are not as efficient sources as fish and poultry. It takes only 3½ ounces of halibut to fill a protein serving requirement, but 3 glasses of milk, 4 medium eggs, 3 ounces of Swiss cheese, or 1¾ cups of yogurt to do the same. To get enough protein without taking in too many calories, an ovo-lacto vegetarian must be judicious in her selections. She should opt for low-fat dairy products whenever possible, since they often contain more protein and calcium than high-fat counterparts, as well as fewer calories. Low-fat cottage cheese, for example, which fills a full protein requirement with just one ¾-cup (135-calorie) serving, is at least as efficient a source of protein as fish. An expectant ovo-lacto vegetarian can also supplement her diet with strict vegetarian protein selections (see page 61).

Vegans or strict vegetarians. With current research recommending a de-emphasis on animal proteins and an emphasis on grains and vegetables in the diet, nonpregnant vegans have little to worry about nutritionally. Pregnant vegans, however, who require the same whopping amounts of protein as other pregnant women, do have cause for concern—and for very prudent diet planning. The list on page 61 suggests a variety of ways in which vegetable proteins can be combined to provide complete protein servings. Because vegetable protein is of a poorer quality than animal protein, vegans should have an extra protein serving daily. Soy products, such as tofu, make excellent protein choices for vegans, but beware those analogues (designed to look and taste like meat, fish, or chicken) that are low in protein and high in calories and sugar or other questionable additives. Check nutrition labels carefully. A serving should supply 20 to 25 grams of protein at under 350 calories. Soy flour or soy products can also be used to enrich baked goods and other dishes with protein.

Vegans will also have to make special efforts to fill their calcium, magnesium, vitamin B_{12}, and vitamin D requirements. The most important source of calcium in the American diet is dairy products, so vegans who abstain from them will have to choose alternates, such as dark green leafies, sesame seeds, and almonds. Soy products, including flour and baked goods, tofu coagulated with calcium (but not frozen tofu desserts, which contain little calcium or nutrition of any kind), tempeh (a fermented soy product), and some soy milks (but avoid those with added sugar or honey) are also fairly good sources of calcium. Check labels for calcium content (you need four 300- to-350-milligram servings daily), which varies from product to product. If you can't seem to make your 1,200 to 1,300 milligrams (or four Best-Odds servings) daily, ask your practitioner about taking a calcium supplement (see page 104) to fill the gap.

Strict vegetarians may also be deficient in magnesium because compounds in vegetable proteins can bind the mineral, thus making it useless. Since recent research shows that adequate intakes of magnesium (possibly above the present RDA) are essential in pregnancy, vegans should be sure their pregnancy supplement contains at least 100 milligrams. If yours is a high-risk pregnancy, your physician may want to check your blood magnesium levels.

Since vitamin B_{12} is found only in animal foods, all vegans, particularly those who are pregnant, should supplement their diets with this essential vitamin, as well as with folic acid and iron, which may also be in short supply in vegan diets. Check to be sure they're included in your prenatal pill.

The ultra-violet rays of the sun synthesize vitamin D from a form of cholesterol in skin oils, but unless we spend a lot of time outdoors in a climate that is sunny year round, sunshine is an unreliable way of getting this essential vitamin. That's why the federal government mandates that milk and many milk products be enriched with the vitamin. If you don't drink milk, you will have to get your D from your vitamin supplement. (Do not take any vitamin D beyond that prescribed by your practitioner; the vitamin can be toxic in even moderately large doses.)

Because many vegan sources of important nutrients, particularly those for protein, are bulkier and more filling than those that can be eaten by meat eaters, semivegetarians, and even ovo-lacto vegetarians, strict vegetarians will probably have to eat greater volumes of food in order to fill their Daily Dozen. But since vegetarian food is lower in fat than dairy and flesh foods, eating a lot of it shouldn't result in excessive weight gain.

(If the increased volume does prove overwhelming to the uterus-cramped digestive tract, see page 75.)

The macrobiotic dieter. The only way the true macrobiotic dieter can give her baby the best odds of being born healthy is to give up her diet from the time she discovers she is pregnant until she weans her baby. The macrobiotic regimen does not provide adequate quantities of protein and calcium, lacks the necessary nutrients found in fruit, and is fundamentally inappropriate for an expectant mother. That doesn't mean the pregnant macrobiotics follower has to abandon all her dietary principles and head for the nearest steak house. She can continue to eat plenty of whole grains and vegetables, but she must increase her intake of protein, calcium, and vitamin C. She can add fish, tofu, and fruit to her diet and take a calcium supplement; or, if that seems offensive, she can follow the recommendations for vegans.

Best-Odds for the Milk Intolerant

Cottage cheese, Swiss cheese, milk, yogurt, breakfast cereal—easily some of the best Best-Odds suppliers of calcium and protein. And easily capable of causing severe digestive distress in many people, including pregnant women. Lactose intolerance—the chronic, incurable disorder that makes digesting milk and milk products and foods containing them painfully difficult—is surprisingly common. Millions of adult Americans, especially those of Oriental, African, or Mediterranean descent, experience its symptoms: gas, bloating, indigestion, and cramping that can range from mild to severely uncomfortable.

Lactose intolerance may be diagnosed for the first time in some women during pregnancy when they suddenly begin drinking large quantities of milk daily (small amounts of milk and certain dairy products may not cause distress in some people),[1] though it may be difficult to distinguish from the normal gastrointestinal discomforts of pregnancy.

There's a simple test you can take to see if you are, indeed, lactose intolerant. When your stomach is empty (two to three hours after a meal or first thing in the morning), drink two to three glasses of skim milk. If you experience gas, bloating, indigestion, cramping, you may be lactose intolerant. You can get additional confirmation by abstaining from all dairy products

for two weeks. If all symptoms disappear, you have a pretty definite diagnosis. This kind of test is, of course, best done before conception, when pregnancy symptoms won't confuse the picture. If you try the second part of the test—abstinence from dairy products—during pregnancy, be sure to substitute adequate amounts of nondairy forms of calcium (see page 56) for the milk products you're cutting out. A calcium supplement will probably be necessary, too.

Even if you seem to have some degree of lactose intolerance, you may not have to give up all dairy products. Milk itself is usually the major culprit, and the closer a dairy product is to milk, the more likely it is to offend. Cream, ice cream or ice milk, cottage cheese, processed cheese foods, and foods containing these products or milk derivatives (such as whey, milk solids, or, especially, lactose) may have to be scratched off your eating list. But you may be able to handle aged cheeses (such as cheddar, Swiss, and Parmesan), fully cultured yogurt (not those to which fresh milk or milk solids have been added after processing), and butter. If you are only mildly intolerant, you may be able to take small quantities of milk. The best way to find out just how far your stomach will allow you to go is by putting it to the test. Try one

---

1. Since the ability to digest milk diminishes gradually after childhood, the problem may be more common in older mothers.

dairy product at a time, starting with the least likely to upset—aged cheese or yogurt, for example. If that passes through unprotested, try a small amount of cottage cheese or a quarter cup of milk. Continue adding in mini-increments until your stomach voices opposition. Then back down a few steps, and you should have found your tolerance level. In general, small quantities of the offending foods spread out during the day may cause less distress than one large dose; milk taken with food may also be more tolerable.

Because lactose intolerance is so prevalent, some dairy companies have begun producing lactose-reduced (70 percent of the lactose has been converted to a more digestible form) milks and cottage cheeses. If they are available in your area, test them out on your tummy. (Some now have added calcium, which means you can get your full calcium allowance with just 2½ glasses of low-fat milk.) If not, ask your pharmacist for a lactose-reducing formula, such as LactAid, which, when added to ordinary milk, can make the lactose easier to stomach.

If milk in any form, even lactose reduced, is intolerable, abandon the dairy case altogether. Screen for dairy products or derivatives in processed foods by reading labels carefully. The words *pareve* or *parve* indicates that a product contains no dairy at all; this can be particularly helpful in selecting margarines, many of which contain milk. Look elsewhere for the calcium and protein that dairy products would otherwise provide (see Calcium and Protein Food Selection Groups).

Since it's difficult to get adequate calcium without eating dairy products, ask your practitioner about prescribing a calcium supplement.[2] For best absorption of your calcium tablet, take it before going to bed. You should also be taking a prenatal supplement that contains vitamin D, since the prime source of this vitamin (other than sunshine) is fortified milk.

Best-Odds for the Allergic

What's a day without orange juice? If you're allergic to citrus fruits, a day without hives. A day without wheat, for those sensitive to the grain, may be a day without nasal congestion. And a day without eggs, for the

---

2. Calcium supplements vary. Calcium carbonate formulas are the most efficient; two tablets provide a full day's supply of calcium. They do, however, cause gassiness in some people. If you have discomfort after taking a calcium carbonate supplement, ask your doctor about prescribing one containing calcium phosphate, which appears to be less irritating. Dolomite tablets (containing calcium and magnesium) are not recommended because they often have been found to contain high levels of lead.

IF YOU CAN'T TAKE ROUGHAGE

Once almost all digestive disorders were treated with bland diets devoid of roughage. This is no longer true. Still there are a few people, even today, who must avoid dietary fiber for medical reasons. Although the Best-Odds Diet urges everyone who can to increase roughage and eat plenty of whole grains, it doesn't urge ignoring doctor's orders. If your physician has prescribed a bland diet, free of whole grains and raw fruits and vegetables, double-check to be sure it is necessary during pregnancy. If it is, you can still give your baby the best odds by following these guidelines:

❖Eat vegetables and fruits in larger quantities to compensate for nutrients lost to the long cooking your diet requires.

❖Be certain that all the breads and cereals you eat are enriched, since enrichment replaces some of the nutrients lost in refining.

❖Ask your physician if you can eat wheat germ, which is moderately high in dietary fiber, but less so than whole wheat with its bran content.

❖Supplement your grain intake with ¼ cup brewer's yeast daily, if you find it palatable. (It may be less objectionable baked into breads, meat loaves, or casseroles.) Brewer's yeast is very rich in many of the same nutrients found in whole grains.

❖Take a prescribed vitamin and mineral supplement (see formula, page 32).

❖For further information on your type of diet, contact the American Digestive Diseases Society, 7720 Wisconsin Avenue, Bethesda, MD 20814.

egg allergic, may be a day without breathing difficulties.

When you're pregnant, however, a day without orange juice, whole wheat, and eggs may also seem like a day without essential vitamin C, trace minerals, and protein. Happily, this needn't be the case. No food has a monopoly on a particular nutrient. From A to zinc, nature has wisely distributed each vital nutrient among dozens, even hundreds, of food sources. For the pregnant allergic, it's just a matter of finding suitable substitutes for the foods you're hypersensitive to.

Wheat. Ordering your chicken salad on whole wheat, pouring bite-size shredded wheat into your breakfast bowl, or sprinkling your yogurt with wheat germ may be some of the easiest ways of getting enough B vitamins and trace minerals while you're pregnant, but they aren't the only ways. Whole grains go by many names—corn (nondegerminated), rice (brown), rye (whole), bulgur, and oats, for example. And they can be supplemented by the other major sources of the nutrients found in whole wheat: dried legumes, including chick-peas, kidney beans, and lentils. (For a complete list of Whole Grains and Other Concentrated Complex Carbohydrates, many of which are wheat alternatives, see page 59. Note that triticale is not appropriate for the wheat sensitive because it is a wheat hybrid.)

As you probably know already, avoiding wheat requires scrupulous attention to the fine print on product labels and penetrating inquiries when ordering restaurant meals. Rye breads, oat cereals, meat loaves, and chicken breadings can all contain wheat, wheat starch, wheat germ, gluten, or bran. Finding breads, cereals, and other baked goods that are wheat-free is challenge enough; finding those that are both wheat-free and whole grain can be an ordeal. Your local health-food store is probably your most likely resource; to avoid long hours of label-reading, ask the manager to point you toward whole-grain, wheat-free products, including pastas made with Jerusalem artichoke, rice, or soy flour. If they're not already on the shelf, he or she may be willing to order some.

Of course, you can be surest of steering clear of wheat in your own baked goods. Substituting other whole-grain flours for whole wheat requires little effort (see box, opposite, for a list of substitutions) and can result in wholly delicious, as well as wholesome, breads, pancakes, cakes, and pastries.

Gluten. Even more limited than the wheat-allergic dieter is the gluten-allergic. Not only must she avoid everything the wheat-allergic dieter must avoid (except gluten-free wheat bread), but oats, barley, buckwheat, and rye, too, which makes most commercially prepared cereals off-limits. Whole-grain corn and rice cereals are acceptable substitutions; a hot "cornmeal mush," made from nondegerminated cornmeal, sweetened with raisins and cinnamon or made savory with salt, pepper, and cottage cheese and/or grated cheese, makes a satisfying and nutritious cold-weather breakfast. You may also be able to buy gluten-free wheat flour or bread. Like the wheat-allergic, the gluten-allergic expectant mom can fulfill her complex-carbohydrate quota with the addition of dried beans and peas.

FLOUR EQUIVALENTS

For each cup of white all-purpose flour substitute:

1 cup finely ground whole-wheat flour
1¼ cups rye flour
1 cup less 2 tablespoons rice flour
1 cup whole-grain cornmeal
13 tablespoons gluten flour
⅝ cup potato flour
½ cup barley flour
¼ cup buckwheat plus ¾ cup all-purpose flour
2 tablespoons soy flour plus ⅞ cup all-purpose flour
1 cup rolled oats
⅓ cup wheat germ plus ⅔ cup all-purpose flour
½ cup whole-wheat flour plus ¼ cup wheat germ (Best-Odds Mix for
    cakes and muffins)

Citrus. Though orange juice and grapefruit halves are America's most popular vitamin C sources, they're far from the only ones. A half of a medium red or green pepper, a quarter of a small canteloupe, or half a cup of cooked kale all provide as much or more vitamin C than either of these ubiquitous breakfast favorites. The citrus-allergic expectant mother has dozens of options when filling her vitamin C requirement (see page 55).

Milk. Unlike most milk-intolerants, the milk-allergic can suffer the consequences of even tiny traces of milk in her diet. But like the severely milk-intolerant, the milk-allergic can obtain her calcium and protein from other sources.

Oats. Since there's nothing that oats can do that another whole grain can't do as well, the pregnant oat-allergic suffers no dietary handicap. Commercial whole-wheat cereals, bulgur, raw wheat or barley flakes from the health-food store all make excellent hot breakfasts; the flakes substitute splendidly for oats in meat loaves, granolas, cookies, cakes, and breads (they add a somewhat crunchier texture to your baking).

Nuts. Nuts are a tasty and textureful addition to the Best-Odds Diet, but they are by no means a necessity. The "nutty" flavors of whole grains and wheat germ can simulate their taste, while cereals (such as Grape Nuts and crispy flakes) mimic their crunch. Wheat germ or finely ground whole-wheat matzoh or bread crumbs can replace ground nuts in baking, with more nutritious and less caloric results. Raisins can substitute for nuts in brownies and cookies; popcorn (particularly when flavored with curry, cheese, or chili) can stand in for them at parties.

Eggs. If you've been getting along without eggs until now, you can continue to get along without them on the Best-Odds Diet. Eggs are a very good source of protein, but not an indispensable one.

Fish. When all the fish in the sea are taboo, there are plenty of landlubbing protein foods to take their place.

EATING OUT AND ON THE GO

There was a time when pregnant women, like mother-to-be birds hatching their eggs, didn't stray far from their nests. That time, for most expectant humans, has long passed. Now that obstetrical science has officially shattered the eggshell-fragile image of pregnant women and their fetuses, expectant mothers are being seen far from the nest. At work, for instance—often up until delivery day. Or traveling, for business or pleasure, across the country or around the world. As a result,

they're also being seen less in their own kitchens and dining rooms, and more in restaurants, coffee shops, fast-food emporiums, and jet planes; at cocktail gatherings and dinner parties; and behind brown paper bags at their desks.

Can pregnant women eat on the go without sending their and their babies' nutritional interests out the window? Yes they can.

Eating Best-Odds in Restaurants

The average American family spends more than a third of its food dollars in restaurants. That's a lot of restaurant eating and, for expectant mothers, a lot of potential problems. Cook at home, and you're sure of what you're eating. Have someone else do the cooking for you, and you're going to be far less sure. Were those carrots steamed or boiled? Were those potatoes cooked in their skins before they were mashed? And how much butter were they mashed with? Does that cream of broccoli soup get its "cream" from calcium-rich milk or calcium-poor half-and-half? Is that buttermilk dressing really mostly mayonnaise? Will the chef's salad be piled high with nutrition-filled romaine and chicory, or nutritionless iceberg lettuce?

Fortunately, today's restaurateurs are rapidly becoming accustomed to such questions about their food preparation. Not just from expectant mothers concerned about feeding their babies well, but from men and women of all ages and conditions concerned with feeding themselves well—or too well. Waist watchers. The cholesterol-conscious. Diabetics and hypoglycemics. Vegetarians. Pritikin proselytes; the salt-restricted. With more diners on special diets than ever before, restaurants—from fast-food chains to four-star establishments—have no option but to be accommodating. Questions are answered and requests for special orders accepted by even the haughtiest *garçon* with a nonplussed nod instead of a disapproving scowl. From sole broiled dry (instead of sautéed with butter and blanketed with cream) to strawberries served plain (instead of suspended in zabaglione), "anything goes" is more likely to be the rule of the house than "no substitutions."

This relaxation of restaurant attitudes, which benefits every health-conscious diner, makes eating right when eating out during pregnancy almost easy. Depending on the type of restaurant you're dining in (see page 113 for tips on choosing a restaurant that will most likely be able to meet your dietary needs), it may be possible to have vegetables steamed instead of boiled or fried; to have salad dressings, gravies, and sauces served on the side (so you can control the amount you eat); to have fish and poultry broiled instead of pan-fried; to substitute broccoli for the french fries or a baked potato for the white rice your snapper provencale is usually served over.

To spend your share of restaurant dollars so that they most benefit you and your baby, follow these simple suggestions for Best-Odds dining out:

Start with the best restaurant. When possible, choose a restaurant that gives you and your baby the best odds of getting a meal that fits the nutritional bill.[3]

Don't turn down a drink. When the waiter asks whether you'd like something from the bar, don't refuse him. Instead, take the opportunity to start filling your fluid requirement with a glass of water, club soda, sparkling mineral water, tomato or vegetable juice, or fresh or frozen fruit juice. (Canned citrus juices are not ideal choices, since they've lost a lot of their vitamin C in processing.) If skim milk is not available, plan on filling your calcium requirement at

3. The American Heart Association chapter in some cities has prepared a list of restaurants at all price levels willing to accommodate patrons who want healthier food. Check with your local office to see if such a list is available in your area.

home or with other calcium foods, maybe with a fruit and cheese dessert.

Take a critical look at the bread basket. Before you plunge in and grab what's warmest and nearest, take a moment to inspect the contents. If you see white and only white, pass the basket—unless there's a favorite roll and your weekly cheat is still up for grabs. Ask the waiter if there are whole grain options available, perhaps whole-wheat sandwich bread; if not, plan on getting your grain servings at other meals or snacks. Be aware that all that is dark isn't whole grain; some of the darkest breads in the basket (pumpernickel, for instance) get their wholesome-looking hue from molasses or cocoa, not from whole-grain flours. These, and rye breads, corn breads that are made from degerminated cornmeal, and most muffins (which will also be highly sugared) are, in general, as nutritionally weak as white. To screen them out and differentiate them from whole-grain dark breads, ask your waiter to make inquiries in the kitchen. (He may not be able to obtain the answers; many restaurants order breads from bakeries and don't have access to their ingredient lists.)

There are, of course, exceptions to the better-unfed-than-white-bread rule that can be made when necessary. If you are unhealthily hungry, no whole-grain breads are available, and you haven't been able to round up an appetizer, take a piece of whatever is available. Try to make it the best of the bad choices—a roll that is sprinkled with nutritious sesame seeds, for instance.

Of course, even a basket filled with hearty whole grains isn't a license to overdo. Be careful to keep within your grain requirements. If you're having a sandwich, you may have to forgo the bread basket entirely. And remember to count not just the bread, but the spread; use butter or margarine sparingly.

Order a first course first thing. If you're hungry, don't wait while the rest of the party lingers over cocktails and a lengthy menu. It may be poor etiquette but good nutritional sense to ask for a first course immediately. (This is especially important if you haven't turned up anything worthwhile in the bread basket.) Salad (dark green leafy lettuces are best) or a vegetable in a vinaigrette are good ways to take the edge off the appetite while filling at least one vegetable requirement. A sliced mozzarella and tomato salad can meet both a calcium and a vitamin C requirement deliciously. Eggs à la Russe can provide a shot of protein (but don't down all the rich mayonnaise that covers them). Steamed, boiled, or poached (but not raw, smoked, fried, or pastry-covered) fish or seafood are also good starters that contribute protein; but you should limit cocktail sauces, which can contain a surprising amount of sugar, and butter and mayonnaise-based sauces, which can quickly push your fat intake over the edge.

Select soups carefully. Soups are not always what they seem. A milky-white chowder appearing to be a cache of calcium, may really be a cache of calories instead, having been made with cream instead of milk. A cold cucumber soup may have been thickened with low-fat, high-calcium yogurt, but might just as easily have obtained its body from high-fat, low-calcium sour cream. When a soup's ingredients are questionable, question your waiter for more details. In general, you'll be safe selecting plain broths, vegetable soups (though the vegetables are boiled, you'll be sipping the liquid in which their nutrients have been cooked), Manhattan-style chowders and other uncreamed fish soups, gazpacho, and cold vegetable soups made with a yogurt or milk base. Soups brimming with white rice, white noodles, or white bread or crouton toppings are better passed over. Pea, bean, or lentil soups,

though hearty in nutrition, are also hearty in calories, so take that into account when ordering the rest of the meal. A bonus from your bowl of soup: it provides approximately one fluid serving, more or less, depending on the ratio of liquids to solids.

Steer your main course in the right direction. Since most restaurant portions of fish, poultry, and lean meats[4] are large enough to provide 40 to 50 grams of protein, sometimes more, here's your chance to fill close to half your daily protein requirement at one sitting. However, if the protein comes breaded and fried or drowned in a rich sauce or gravy, it can also be your chance to overfill your fat allowance. To take the good without the bad, order your main course broiled, grilled, baked, or poached, and ask for sauces on the side. (To avoid the risk of toxoplasmosis and other parasitic diseases, do not order raw meat or fish. Meat should be cooked at least to "medium.") Avoid fish or poultry entrées that are served "stuffed," unless you've determined that the stuffing will be nutritious (wild rice, mushrooms, or spinach, for instance). Stuffings composed of white bread or cracker crumbs, white rice, or degerminated corn

4. Stick to lean meats; many restaurants serve well-marbled "prime" meats, which are prime sources of fat and thus lower in protein.

bread, and bound with much butter, margarine, or meat drippings, are best not ordered—unless you have the willpower to leave them over.

If your scale has been giving you a hard time, you can request your fish broiled dry, instead of in butter. Wine is an excellent substitute, since the alcohol evaporates but the flavor and moisture are retained. But tell the waiter that by "dry" you don't mean tasteless; you'd like the fish well-seasoned.

Get nutritional support on the side. Best supporting side-dish roles can be played by steamed, lightly sautéed, or stir-fried vegetables that appear in the Vegetable Food Selection Groups (page 57); by white or sweet potatoes baked, boiled, or steamed, and eaten in their skins (but not blanketed beneath fat allowance-exceeding amounts of butter or sour cream); or by brown or wild rice, bulgur or kasha, or whole-grain pasta. Should none of these nutritious bit players be available, glean what you can from boiled vegetables and potatoes, and small amounts of white rice (hopefully it will be converted rice, and thus more nutritious) or pasta. If all options are fried, and unless you are so underweight that the excess of fat won't present a problem, skip the side dishes altogether and ask if you can substitute a side salad or a dish of sliced tomatoes. Make up for the vegetables you've missed at your next meal.

Desert most desserts. Many restaurants are a desert when it comes to Best-Odds desserts. Cakes, pastries, and frozen confections are, with virtually no exception, made with sugar or honey and thus taboo (unless you're Best-Odds cheating; see page 67). But so are many fruit desserts, particularly compotes, cocktails, and marinated fruits (even if no sugar has been added, heavily sweetened liqueurs or wines often have been). Always ask if fresh, unsweetened fruit is available. Though sometimes not offered on the dessert cart, melon wedges and grapefruit halves slated as appetizers can stand in for a finishing course. Fruit and cheese platters are another option. If you'd like to indulge in a dollop of whipped cream on your fresh berries, feel free as long as you've made sure it's fresh and unsweetened, and as long as it's applied to your fat allowance.

Should no Best-Odds options exist, cleanse your palate with a club soda and lime or sip a cup of decaffeinated coffee, and wait until you get home for your sweet revenge—a slab of Best-Odds cake, some fresh fruit, or, better yet, both.

Best-Bets in Restaurants

It's not always possible to pick out your restaurant, particularly if you're not picking up the tab. But when you do have the choice, keep in mind that there are some cuisines which suit the Best-Odds diner better than others. Use the following as a general guide—the selection at your favorite restaurants may be very different.

Best. The best bets in Best-Odds dining are usually the places where culinary simplicity reigns, such as seafood, steak-house, American, and in many cases, continental restaurants. Particularly in the first three, broiled or grilled fresh seafood, poultry, and meats, all Best-Odds first choices, are the specialties of the house, and are often served with baked potatoes, fresh vegetables, and salads. (Though a shift toward the use of whole grains is slowly taking place in such establishments, most still provide only refined breads in their baskets, so be prepared to fill your grain requirements with whole-grain side dishes, if they're available, or at other meals.)

Indian cuisine, though far from simple, is a surprisingly good bet, too. Assuming the heavy use of spices doesn't offend your digestive tract, you can take advantage of many Indian specialties, including meats, fish, and poultry marinated (often in yogurt) and baked in Tandoori ovens; vegetable soups and salads made with yogurt; whole-grain roti, chapati, and paratha breads, sometimes stuffed with vegetables; and vegetable and vegetarian curries. (*Vegetarians note:* These dishes contain plenty of protein in the form of chickpeas and lentils.) Skip the fried dishes and white rice.

Next best. The second best bets are restaurants where you can get a Best-Odds meal if you select carefully, but where you can also be tempted into a less-than-best meal if you don't. Certain ethnic cuisines fit into this category, including:

Italian (particularly Northern Italian). Concentrate on fish, chicken, and veal dishes cooked in tomato sauces, lightly sautéed with lemon and butter, or grilled; vegetable side dishes (spinach, kale, arugula, and broccoli rabe—Italian favorites—are also among the most nutritious green leafies); and salads. Don't order your own pasta dish (a few nibbles from a neighbor's plate should satisfy). *Vegetarians note:* Lacto vegetarians can usually get adequate protein from the cheese in dishes such as eggplant Parmesan. A couple of spoonfuls of Parmesan cheese will add additional protein and calcium.

French. (particularly the nouvelle variety). Avoid rich sauces (ask for them on the side so you can "taste"), pastry shells ("en croute"), pâtés (they're held together with fat), and sausages (also prime sources of fat). Order a salad first course if vegetable portions are skimpy.

Jewish-style. Stay with the usually abundant poultry (especially roasted and boiled) and fish (but not gefilte fish, which may be made with questionably safe lake fish) main courses, clear consommes, vegetables (which may be overcooked but are better than nothing), and kasha, and away from the usually fatty meats, fried potato pancakes, noodle and potato puddings, highly sweetened carrot tzimmeses and blintzes, and stuffed derma (kishke).

Greek and Middle Eastern. Favor grilled and roasted fish, poultry, and lean meats (particularly shish kebob); stews that combine vegetables with fish or meat (moussaka, for instance); lentil and chick-pea dishes; yogurt-based soups; vegetable salads, and cooked whole grains such as bulgur. Avoid white rice and rice-stuffed dishes, fried and phyllo-wrapped specialties. *Vegetarians note:* the lentil, chickpea, yogurt, and bulgur dishes make this cuisine a good choice.

Cajun, or Louisiana-style cuisine. Eschew fatty pork chops and fried dishes for boiled, steamed, broiled, and "blackened" seafood and fish, and hearty seafood/poultry/vegetable stews such as jambalayas (go easy on the white rice) and gumbos.

Chinese. Once easily in the Least-Best class, today's Chinese restaurant food (at least in Szechuan and Hunan establishments) have jumped up to Next-Best. Though still high in sodium because of the liberal use of soy sauce, Chinese food features fish, meats, and vegetables that are quickly stir-fried and at the peak of nutrition. Many restaurants also offer no MSG either routinely or on request, will cook with little or no oil, and some even offer brown rice. Order dishes that have plenty of fish, poultry, meat, or bean curd (tofu) rather than those that are just garnished with protein foods; don't add soy sauce at the table; and avoid white rice, white noodles, and sweet-and-sour sauces. (It's worth asking whether the chef would be willing to reduce the soy sauce when he stir-fries your meal to order.) *Vegetarians note:* This type of restaurant is in the Best category for vegans since tofu is generally available and vegetables are plentiful.

Delis. Also next best, particularly at lunchtime. Hold the pickles and sauerkraut (too salty), the rye and pumpernickel breads, fatty and often nitrate-preserved fish, meats, and cold cuts (such as smoked salmon, white fish, pastrami, corned beef, frankfurters, salami, bologna, and tongue), and order sliced turkey or chicken (not turkey or chicken roll), or tuna, egg, or chicken salad on whole wheat, with side orders of cole slaw and sliced tomato.

Coffee shops are also good for lunch. You can usually get anything from broiled fish to poached eggs to fairly wholesome salads and sandwiches (on whole-wheat bread), although not often much in the way of fresh vegetables or fruits (they're frequently canned).

Fast-food restaurants are another next-best lunch choice. But only if they offer salad bars from which you can make a meal (an increasing number do) or a line of healthy menu selections, such as whole-grain buns.

Health food and vegetarian restaurants sound like they should be "best," and they are for vegetarians. But because animal protein may be scarce or nonexistent, they're less than perfect for most pregnant women. If the menu is meatless and fishless, order a dish prepared with plenty of protein-rich cheese or yogurt, or beans and brown rice. Enjoy the whole grains and the fresh vegetables. But be wary of desserts dubbed "sugarless" (they're probably made with sugar's health food alias, honey). *Vegetarians note:* This type of restaurant is in the Best category for nonflesh eaters.

Least Best. It's almost a sure bet you won't easily get a Best-Odds meal in the following types of restaurants, but when you haven't the choice, stay within these guidelines.

Japanese. In addition to high sodium in the form of soy sauce and miso in some dishes, most Japanese restaurants today specialize in sushi (raw fish), which is taboo for expectant mothers, and tempura (deep-fried) dishes, which should be taboo for everybody most of the time. Stick to teriyaki or grilled poultry, fish, or meat, and limit yourself to just a couple of pieces of tempura. *Vegetarians note:* Unless the restaurant has at least one tofu dish, there may be nothing nutritious for nonmeat eaters.

German, Russian, and Middle European. These cooking styles are traditionally heavy on breadings, dumplings, noodles, and high-nitrate, high-fat sausages and wursts, and light on nutritiously cooked vegetables and broiled fish and meats. Some more contemporary eateries will offer lightly broiled fish and poultry for the health conscious. When they don't, scan the menu for anything broiled (chops, chicken, steak) or for a meat-

and-vegetable stew like goulash or paprikash. Kasha or potatoes make good side dishes.

Mexican and Tex-Mex. Most menus are composed primarily of taco- and enchilada-style dishes, which offer little protein and plenty of fat. In some restaurants you'll be able to order a chicken dish that isn't fried (chicken mole in a Mexican establishment, for instance, or barbecued chicken in a Tex-Mex). A few may even offer grilled fish or chicken. You're not likely to find much in the way of fresh vegetables (often fried in Tex-Mex) or salads, but you may be able to drink your salad in the form of gazpacho. Stay away from the white rice, taco chips, and refried beans (the latter are laced heavily with lard), and order plain red beans, if available, for a starch.

Southern. Old South cooks like to fry most things, and tend to put bacon and fatback in everything else. Most starches— biscuits, corn bread (unless it's made with nondegerminated cornmeal), dumplings, and stuffings—are nutritionally superfluous. If you're lucky, you'll be able to find a cook who'll broil your fish (make sure it's not a suspect lake or river fish), or a menu that includes barbecued chicken. Side dishes are tricky (hush puppies are fried, as are many vegetables; potatoes are frequently mashed with plenty

of butter), but cole slaw is often available. When steamed or stir-fried, Southern vegetable specialties such as turnip or collard greens are bountiful in nutrients; unfortunately, they appear too often in Southern restaurants boiled or simmered with fatback—which may be better than nothing (if you count the fat in your fat allowance).

Spanish. This fare includes many stews, such as paella, which feature chicken and seafood, though little else of nutritive value (white rice, bits of onion and tomato), and some fairly simply prepared seafood and fish dishes. Again, select beans over rice as a starch, and fill your grain and vegetable requirements at another meal.

Fast-food restaurants that don't have salad bars or special "healthy" menus. These should be frequented as infrequently as possible. When you must fast-food it, try to bring along a whole-grain bun for your burger (at least one major chain— Wendy's—already offers them), order cole slaw and sliced tomatoes if they're available. Sample a few fries from a friendly companion's bag, but don't order your own (if baked potatoes are featured, take advantage, particularly if they are topped with vegetables and cheese), and drink unsweetened juice (not juice "drinks," sodas, or shakes), milk, water, or a Best-

Odds beverage brought from home. Fried fish and chicken should be ordered rarely since their astronomic fat and calorie content far outweigh the protein they supply. Two slices of whole-wheat crusted pizza, on the other hand, can be ordered more often. They generally provide a full protein serving, two complex carbohydrate servings, and a vitamin C food for a not unreasonable 400 calories (more or less). Unfortunately, whole-wheat pizza is hard to find; when it's not available, two slices of ordinary pizza with peppers and mushrooms (avoid pepperoni and other sausage toppings) isn't a bad nutritional buy and is better still (and even tastier) sprinkled with wheat germ carried from home. *Vegetarians note:* Pizza is an excellent fast-food choice for those who eat milk products.

On the Job

Working nine to five can take a toll on an expectant mother's nutritional status, particularly when "nine to five" turns into a quarter to eight until seven-thirty. In the frenzy of a workday it's easy to devote all of your concentration to your job, leaving none for your diet. Without thinking, it's easy to forget to eat (has lunchtime slipped by again?), to eat what's available rather than what's appropriate (a

drumstick from the bucket of fried chicken the office manager brought in, instead of the tuna on whole wheat you'd have to send out for), or to succumb, halfway through a long afternoon, to temptation (the Danish from the box on your neighbor's desk, the marble cake on the coffee wagon).

Unless you're a food critic for the local paper, you can't make a full-time occupation out of eating, spending your working hours thinking about and planning for your next meal or snack. But with just a little extra organization, preparation, and forethought, you can take Best-Odds care of your baby's nutritional needs without neglecting the needs of your job.

Stock up on office supplies. An expectant working mother needs more on-the-job supplies than staplers, note pads, pencils, and paper clips. She needs ready access to nutritious snacks and beverages to round out her Daily Dozen and ward off between-meal hunger pangs and coffee-wagon temptation. If there's a refrigerator in your workplace, keep it stocked, space permitting, with one or more of the following: skim milk, unsweetened fruit juice, seltzer, fresh fruit, a jar of wheat germ (for sprinkling on yogurt or cottage cheese and for enriching the pizza you didn't resist or the bagel you're stuck with at a morning meeting), a container of plain yogurt, a chunk of cheese, even some fruit-only preserves or peanut butter (for spreading on Best-Odds Bran Muffins or whole-wheat bread). Your desk drawer or locker can hold such unperishable supplies as: whole-grain crackers, bread sticks, or matzoh, a ready-to-munch whole-grain cereal (such as bite-size shredded wheat), some dried fruit, a jar of naturally decaffeinated instant coffee or a box of decaffeinated tea bags, and a container of nonfat dry milk for enriching coffee, tea, and cereals. To facilitate your desktop eating and snacking, also stash plastic cutlery; paper napkins, plates, and cups; and individual-serving peppers and salts pocketed from fast-food restaurants and cafeterias.

Bring care packages from home. You can't bring a kitchen's worth with you each day, but you can pack your brown bag with enough food to ensure adequate breakfasts, lunches, and snacks while you're at work.

If you don't have time for breakfast at home or in a coffee shop, and don't care to order in (see Research Your Local Resources, below, if you do), bring any of the following (or anything else nutritious that appeals to you) for your first meal of the day: a container filled with yogurt and/or cottage cheese, and either a mélange of fresh seasonal fruits, unsweetened applesauce, raisins, cinnamon, and nuts (sprinkle wheat germ from your pocketbook stash just before eating); or a variety of cut raw vegetables, such as tomatoes, radishes, scallions, and cucumbers; a container of unsweetened plain instant oatmeal or dry cereal mixed with nonfat dry milk and your favorite toppings, ready to add hot or cold water to; a sandwich (see lunch suggestions); Best-Odds muffins, already spread with peanut butter and/or fruit-only preserves; whole-grain breads, bagels, or rolls with cheese and fruit; hard-boiled eggs.

Brown-bag lunchers can prepare sandwiches on whole-grain bread, rolls, or pita, with such fillings as tuna, salmon, seafood, chicken, turkey, or egg salad; sliced leftover turkey or chicken, sliced roast beef, veal, and lamb (have these less often than poultry); cheese, sliced hard-boiled eggs (don't forget a few extra whites), and cold meat loaf. Filling flavors can be enhanced by mustard, a yogurt dressing, sliced or chopped tomato and/or cucumber, dark green leafy lettuce, alfalfa or bean sprouts (these are particularly convenient for sandwich-making, since they don't need to be washed), and avocado. An-

HANDBAGGING IT

Expectant mothers don't just get hungry in the kitchen, at their desks, or in restaurants. They get hungry on subways, in department stores, at playgrounds, and lots of other places where food isn't available. Which is why a roomy, well-stocked handbag is a pregnant woman's most important accessory. Fill yours with any of the following—in tightly covered containers or zip-locked or well-tied plastic bags—and don't leave home without it:

❖ Whole-grain crackers, bread sticks, or bread ❖ Best-Odds muffins or cookies ❖ dried fruit (with nuts, if you're not gaining weight quickly enough) ❖ fresh fruit ❖ small cubes of hard cheese (avoid the processed varieties) ❖ hard-boiled eggs (they will hold several hours without refrigeration) ❖ a thermos of juice or milk ❖ a mini-jar or plastic sandwich bag of wheat germ (this should be refrigerated when not being carried in your handbag)

other good brown-bag choice: leftovers from dinner that are good cold (to guarantee you'll have leftovers, make a point of cooking extra), such as poultry and fish (bring along a container of Buttermilk-Dill Dressing), Tuna-Pasta Primavera, and side dishes of marinated vegetables. Also good brought from home: a large container filled with Pregnant Chef's Salad or a Salad Niçoise, with the salad dressing of your choice (page 264) carried separately so the salad won't wilt before lunch; or any of the breakfast selections, such as yogurt and cottage cheese combos, which appeal to you at lunch. Good accompaniments include crudités, fresh fruit, a thermos of a hot or cold beverage or soup.

Even if brown bags aren't your style, and you prefer to take your breakfast at home and your lunch from the local sandwich takeout, you'll still need to keep a supply of snacks in your handbag ready for between-meal fortification (see Handbagging It, above).

Research your local resources. Does the little deli down the street carry half-pint containers of skim milk and containers of plain yogurt? Does the take-out shop you order from make sandwiches on whole-wheat bread? Does the little greengrocer on your way to work sport an extensive salad bar that doesn't use chemical preservatives? Are the restaurants you generally take clients to or meet friends at on the Best, Next Best, or Least Best list? Is there a produce stand nearby where you can pick up a piece of fresh fruit on your way back to the office?

Now that you're an expectant working woman, you'll need to make it your business to find out everything you can about the nutritional resources near your job. Getting the information may take a little fancy footwork and a few phone calls, but it will make feeding yourself and your baby during the rest of your working months a lot easier.

On the Social Circuit

Being unable to stay up past 10:00 P.M. and unable to fit into any of your favorite party frocks can cut into your social life somewhat. But following the Best-Odds Diet shouldn't.

Cocktail parties, formal dinners, brunches, barbecues—you can't just kick up your heels (or, more sensibly, your flats) and go. But with a little planning, you *can* enjoy the pregnant high life without lowering your dietary standards. Here's how:

Don't go hungry. Unless you are absolutely certain that there's a complete Best-Odds buffet waiting for you at your hosts' home, protect your nutritional interests by making a deposit before you go. Eat just enough to take the edge off your appetite without ruining it entirely. Good preparty snacks include: hard-boiled eggs, a slice of whole-wheat bread with peanut butter or an ounce of cheese, half a cup of cottage cheese, a Best-Odds muffin, or a Double-the-Milk Shake.

Bring emergency rations. It's rare that you'll find yourself at a party where there's nary a baby-benefiting bite. But for the occasional exception, or when food isn't served right away or isn't served at all (such as when "cocktails" means cocktails, and nothing else), be prepared with your trusty handbag snack bar. See page 119 for tips, but avoid bringing foods that might overpower your perfume, such as hard-boiled eggs or strong-smelling cheeses.

Peruse, pick, and choose. There's almost always something you can eat. All you have to do is locate it among the array of comestibles. At cocktails, for example, while you're cruising with your club soda-and-twist or Virgin Mary, be on the lookout for raw vegetables, cheeses, chicken wings, or meatballs. If there are no whole grains, have your cheese or other spreads on available vegetables or on the best of the batch of crackers. Depending on your weight situation (you know it best), take small to moderate portions of such delicacies as chicken or vegetable crepes, quiche, or deep-fried vegetables. Avoid smoked fish and cold cuts as well as greasy hors d'oeuvres, especially the nitrated pigs-in-blankets and fatty ribs. Allow exceptions only for occasional bites of the most tempting morsels making the rounds (fold uneaten portions discreetly in your napkin, or share them with a companion). If you're unable to find more satisfactory sustenance, nibble from a bowl of nuts (keep these to a minimum if you're gaining weight too quickly) and raisins.

At buffets, do a careful start-to-finish survey of the options before you begin filling your plate (there may be a chafing dish of chicken breasts down the way from that fettuccine Alfredo, steamed asparagus opposite the fried zucchini, or a bowl of fresh fruit salad sitting modestly alongside a glaring assortment of pastries). Take heaping portions of foods your baby would appreciate most (proteins, salads, simply prepared vegetables, unsweetened fruits, and any whole grains), and just taste-size servings of less wholesome items you can't resist.

At sit-down affairs, you can't peruse until the food is upon you and your picking power is minimal, but you still have some control over what you end up eating. If the opportunity arises, ask for smaller servings, or none at all, of foods that are nutritionally questionable. If your plate is set before you already filled, simply take a nibble or two of the perilous portions and concentrate on what's good for baby. If it is clear that your hostess will be offended if you turn down her chocolate mousse, explain you can only take a taste because of your pregnancy diet. Proclaim it wonderful after one bite ("I wish I could eat more!"), and you will satisfy her needs without compromising yours.

Take inventory when the party's over. Once you've kicked off your shoes and put up your feet, figure how far your partying has left you from fulfilling your daily dozen. Then try to make up the difference before you retire (see Quick Fixes, page 302).

Reciprocate in Best-Odds style. Serve unto others what you would have them serve unto you. Your guests don't have to be pregnant to enjoy nutritious dining—they don't even have to be the wiser. Chances are they won't notice anything "different" about what they're eating (no need to tell them), except that it's especially delicious).

On the Road

You see her everywhere. In airline terminals, on trains, in cars crammed with camping gear. En route to a convention in Las Vegas, a sales meeting in New

KEEPING THE HOLIDAY SPIRIT

Stick to the Best-Odds Diet on the holidays? Bah humbug, you might scoff. Scrooge had a better chance of enjoying himself at a holiday celebration than a pregnant woman who has to watch what she eats.

Not so. Unlike Scrooge, Best-Odds dieters needn't rely on cold gruel to kindle their holiday spirits. The Thanksgiving turkey, the Easter lamb, the Fourth of July burgers, the Rosh Hashanah roast all have a place at the Best-Odds holiday table, as do many other festive favorites. And with a few adept alterations in their recipes, most holiday trimmings—from stuffing and gravy to sweet potatoes and cranberry molds to Fruitcake and Hot Cross Buns—can make the transition from taboo to table, too.

There are, of course, some traditions that may have to be broken, or at least bent, this year. But though a certain amount of sacrifice will be necessary to ensure that your baby benefits from holiday eating at least as much as you enjoy it, you can stay on the Best-Odds Diet without dampening your holiday spirit. Here's how:

Don't take a holiday from regular meals. If you traditionally skip breakfast on Thanksgiving so you can stuff yourself with turkey-and-trimmings later, take a break from tradition this year. Eat a breakfast that is lighter in calories (you'll likely be overloading on these at dinner) but doesn't shortchange baby of his morning supply of the Daily Dozen. Cereal and fruit or eggs and whole-wheat toast should do the trick.

Don't be the guest of Christmases past. Before you go over the river and through the woods to grandmother's house (or anyone else's who's hosting a holiday feast), prepare yourself by reading On the Social Circuit (page 120). An ideal holiday gift for the hostess who has everything (except, possibly, something you can eat for dessert) is a Best-Odds sweet you've made yourself: a Fruitcake, a batch of Fudge Brownies, or Cranberry Crunch Bars, a basket of Hot Cross Buns. Everyone is likely to enjoy every serving of your gift—and no one needs to know how *self*-serving it really is.

York, a merger in Houston, a visit to grandma in Tampa, a vacation almost any place in the world. The expectant mother of today is nobody's homebody.

But the pregnant peripatetic life presents a predicament: how to keep the diet from wandering when you are. How to get meals regularly when your schedule's so irregular. How to handle hunger that strikes in midair, halfway between train stations, or 100 miles from the nearest high-

Be the hostess with the bestest. Again, serving the best nutritional interests of yourself and your baby shouldn't interfere with serving the best-tasting meals to your guests at holiday time. Few holiday favorites don't translate into Best-Odds fare, and most translate so well and so easily that little of the traditional taste will be lost in the translation. Your great-aunt's stuffing will be, perhaps, even greater made with whole-wheat bread (or nondegerminated corn bread or brown or wild rice) or whole-wheat matzah crumbs. Guests will relish your cranberry relish every bit as much when it is sweetened with concentrated apple and orange juices instead of sugar, and your mushroom gravy when you've skimmed the fat off the drippings. And both the creamed oyster bisque and the creamed onions will taste just as creamy when prepared with evaporated skimmed milk instead of heavy cream. (For details on Best-Odds cooking substitutions, see page 174.)

Treat yourself without mistreating your baby. There's no better time to cheat than holiday time. And as long as you remain faithful to your Daily Dozen, your baby won't suffer from a few bites of yule log, a couple of spoonfuls of sweet potato pie (though if made Best-Odds style with juice concentrates, fresh yams, and a whole-wheat crust you can help yourself to a whole slice), or a sliver of honey cake. So indulge in moderation. Limit your cheating to foods that, while they might not do baby any good, aren't likely to do any harm, either. Alcohol does not fit in this category. A few sips of champagne or spiked punch are as far as you should permit yourself to stray. Do your serious toasting with Innocent Sangria, Sparkling Punch, Mock Daiquiris, nonalcoholic Holiday Wassail Bowl, Eggnog, or any other unspirited (and unsugared) holiday beverage.

Remember there's always next year. The holidays will come again—when you're not pregnant. In fact, unless you're planning to claim the most-babies-born-to-one-mother slot in the *Guinness Book of World Records,* more unpregnant holidays lie ahead for you than pregnant ones. Be satisfied with those little tastes of holiday cheer, and know that you'll be able to take bigger bites next year.

way exit. How to fill your Daily Dozen when you can't drink the water, eat the salads, or track down as much as a crumb of whole-grain bread?

You needn't cancel your travel plans to avoid canceling your participation in the Best-Odds Diet. But you do need to include your dietary considerations in your plans, and a few essential extra items in your suitcase. Before you go, it's a good idea to attend to the following:

Check ahead. What kinds of meals and snacks will be offered on the plane? Can you special order? (On most airlines, you can ask for a broiled fish or poultry entrée for dinner or a cheese omelet, cottage cheese and fruit platter, or other ovo-lacto vegetarian meal for lunch; many will also provide whole-grain bread and fresh fruit for dessert if requested.) Does the train you are taking have a dining car (which will usually serve simple, but complete meals) or just a snack bar—or no food facilities at all? Are there frequent rest stops on the interstate you are planning to drive? Do they offer full restaurant meals or just snacks and fast foods? (Travel guides, road atlases, automobile associations, and state tourist boards can provide you with such information.)

If you are traveling out of the U.S. you will also want to check ahead about the safety of water, raw vegetables and fruits, seafood, or other food contamination in the areas you're planning to visit. The American College of Obstetrics and Gynecology, One East Wacker Drive, Chicago, IL 60601, can provide such information, as well as important data on immunization for pregnant women. Specify "travel information" on the envelope.

Pack a Best-Odds survival kit. Once you leave familiar surroundings (even if you're venturing just 200 miles from home for a sales conference), you can't be sure of finding the foods that are the foundation of your Best-Odds Diet. So pack a Best-Odds bag for insurance. What you put in this nutrition survival pack will depend on where you're headed and for how long. All kits should include instant nonfat dry milk in packets (unless you can't tolerate milk, in which case take a calcium supplement along), a small jar of wheat germ (since wheat germ is moderately perishable, it's best to replenish your supply at least once a week, unless you can keep it on ice or refrigerate it periodically), small packs of raisins, and whole-grain crackers. If you are going to be away for more than a day, pack enough of your prenatal supplements to last the trip; if you are going abroad, ask your practitioner to prescribe or recommend a pregnancy-safe medication to treat traveler's stomach. If constipation is a problem, pack a plastic bagful of unprocessed bran or dried prunes, whichever you find more effective in overcoming irregularity. Also handy are a combination bottle/can opener and small knife and spoon. (A camping utensil may provide all these in one easy-to-carry item.)

Fix an en-route snack pack. When hunger hits en route to your destination, you can't always yell, "Stop the car (or plane or train), I want to get off and get something to eat." But you can pull out the en-route snack pack you cleverly prepared in advance and stave off starvation until you reach the next rest stop, until the flight attendant finishes serving cocktails and starts serving lunch, or until the dining car opens.

Snack packs can include more substantial fare (sandwiches, yogurt, cottage cheese, even cold chicken and small containers of salads or crudités) if the road you're taking will be restaurant-free for many miles or if there's no dining car on the train (snack cars usually don't offer much more than hot dogs, hamburgers, skimpy pizzas, sandwiches on refined bread, sweetened yogurts, potato chips, sodas, and other less nourishing fare, though you may be able to get a chicken salad on whole-wheat bread). If the food you bring is perishable and you won't be eating it for more than four hours, store it in a mini-cooler or an insulated bag packed with a tightly closed plastic bag of ice or a prefrozen cold pack.

If you know you'll be stopping for meals, or will be offered a full meal on the train or plane, a good handbag selection of snacks will probably satisfy your stomach in between meals (see page 119). Include something whole grain, and possibly some cut-up raw vegetables, since road stops, train dining cars, and airline menus rarely offer these items. And since drinking is as important as eating, particularly in hot weather, be sure to bring some liquid refreshment along if you're traveling by car. Club soda and some canned juices are usually available in train snack cars and on airplane beverage carts; skim milk usually isn't. (The dehydrating effect of flying should be compensated for with extra fluid intake, so ask your flight attendant to make your club soda or juice "a double.")

Here's how you can keep your baby well fed at your destination:

Stay on schedule. As important as being in Belgium on Tuesday, Holland on Wednesday, and Luxembourg on Thursday, is eating breakfast in the morning, lunch at midday, and dinner in the evening—regularly, every day. Don't let the irregularity of touring or meeting schedules, or the eccentricities of foreign gastronomic habits upset the rhythm of your eating routine. As tempted as you might be to skip breakfast or lunch so you can "save up" for a more lavish supper, resist. Your fetus won't be impressed by a four-star, five-course dinner at Maxim's, but certainly will be distressed by missing a meal. When in Rome (or anywhere else where continental breakfasts are the vogue) don't do what the Romans do. Supplement your roll (lightly buttered, and sprinkled lavishly with wheat germ if it's white) or croissant and juice with an order of "American" eggs or cereal, if available. (If eggs aren't regularly available, you may be able to persuade the chef to hard boil some for you.) In Spain and other countries where the dining hour is fashionably—and for pregnant women unhealthily—late, make a point of having a substantial snack (which includes some protein) around your usual mealtime to hold you and your fetus, and then eat less heavily at dinner (heavy meals at any time, but particularly before bed, can overload the digestive tract, causing indigestion). And whenever you know you're going to be at the mercy of a tour guide (or a business associate or convention program) who's not likely to pay heed to your grumbling stomach, make your first stop of the day a local market and purchase a sustaining supply of Best-Odds snacks for your handbag or tote.

Don't go dry when you can't drink the water. Your body and your baby need fluids even when the water is undrinkable for tourists. So when you are warned "Don't drink the water" (see Check Ahead, page 124), find something else to drink: bottled water, canned or bottled fruit juices, club soda or sparkling mineral water, hot soups (or soups that were boiled before chilling). Use bottled water, if necessary, for brushing your teeth and rinsing your mouth.

Stay on Montezuma's good side. The symptoms of "Montezuma's revenge" (highlighted by diarrhea and stomach cramps) don't only show up in travelers visiting his home turf. Drinking impure water, eating exotic or spicy foods your innards are unaccustomed to, or foods that are prepared under unsanitary conditions or stored without proper refrigeration can result in traveler's tummy anywhere in the world. Since this malady can not only spoil your trip, but rob your baby of vital nutrition, taking steps to avoid it should be part of your travel regimen. These tips should help:

❖ Don't drink the water (or brush your teeth with it) or eat raw vegetables or fruits—if they haven't gotten a clean bill of health. When in doubt, peel fruits and vegetables, skip raw salads, avoid ice cubes and reconstituted juices or milks unless made with bottled, boiled, or sterilized water.

❖ Forgo the unfamiliar. The digestive tract of a Spanish mother-to-be will probably have no trouble with the spicy cuisine in Madrid; yours, on the other hand, may explode with discomfort. Save such gastronomic experimentation for a future trip, when you won't be sharing meals with the fussy fellow traveler in your belly. Whenever possible, opt for the simplest and most familiar dishes on a menu. If you're not competent enough in the local language to translate a menu, try eating in restaurants where English is spoken so that you'll be able to find out what you'll be eating before it's too late. The sauce-on-the-side approach (see "Parlez-Vous Best Odds?") may give your taste buds the opportunity to enjoy an exotic flavor without punishing your stomach.

❖ Stay on the beaten restaurant path. Little out-of-the-way native restaurants touted by the cognoscenti of local cuisine may offer authentic food, but they may also serve up an unhealthy dose of stomach-distressing germs. When there are signs that little attention is paid to sanitation head for the nearest Howard Johnson's (or reasonable regional fascimile). Also to be on the safe side, forgo food sold by street vendors.

❖ Don't let spoiled food spoil your trip. If roasted ducks are piled in a clearly unrefrigerated storefront window or cream pies and sandwiches are arrayed on a countertop, it's a sure bet that food handling in the restaurant is careless. Unrefrigerated foods can build up hazardous bacteria counts. Try to avoid such blatant violators of basic food storage principals, but be alert for tainted food everywhere you eat (an unrefrigerated cart of whipped cream mousses in a ritzy hotel restaurant may be just as risky). Though spoiled food does not always have an unpleasant smell or off taste (particularly if it's spicy or covered with sauce), food that doesn't smell or taste right is probably spoiled. Play it safe to avoid being sorry; if a food is questionable, send it back or leave it over.

❖ When in doubt, don't eat out—that is, not in restaurants. If the local eating establishments all show a disregard for common cleanliness, disregard them. Instead, dine on bread and cheese, yogurt or cottage cheese, or tins of salmon, tuna, sardines, or herrings from a food market. (Again, don't buy perishable foods, such as meats and salads, that are not refrigerated.) Be sure all dairy products you consume, in restaurants or out, are pasteurized.

Be a regular traveler. You don't have to be expecting to have problems with constipation on the road. Erratic schedules, un-familiar, communal, and some-times unavailable or nonexistent bathrooms, and alterations in eating agendas can contribute to traveler's irregularity in anyone. Add the pregnant body's natural susceptibility to constipation and you have a potentially trip-ruining problem. To fend it off, make certain to get plenty of the three major constipation comba-ters: fiber (especially raw fruits and vegetables, and whole grains; if the first two are taboo in the country you're visiting, concentrate on the last), fluids (when you can't drink the water, see page 126), and exercise (walking is perfect; plan to do at least some of your sightseeing by foot, take a 15-minute stroll when the meeting is breaking for coffee, walk all walkable dis-tances to restaurants, hotels, and stores instead of taking taxis). Also try to keep to as reg-ular a schedule as possible; try not to leave your hotel room in the morning until after you've been able to use the toilet (eat breakfast a half hour earlier if need be). A small can of spray or liquid disinfectant for cleaning shared bathrooms is a wise addi-tion to your travel tote, one that may relieve some of the psycho-logically triggered barriers your bowels may encounter.

Learn the language of healthy eating. If you're traveling within the U.S. you certainly won't have trouble asking for or identifying your nutritional standbys in the native tongue. And except in perhaps the small-est of towns, you probably won't even have trouble finding them. Such Best-Odds basics as whole grains, wheat germ, and skim or lowfat milk products are becom-ing increasingly available out-side the U.S., too, but unless you're fluent in the language, tracking them down may prove impossible. Call the country's national tourist board before you leave home and ask them for the translations you'll need. Or see Parlez Vous Best Odds, page 334.

FIVE

What to Eat When You're Nursing

Y OU POP THE CORK ON A BOTTLE OF CHAMPAGNE, dig, with guiltless abandon, into a celebratory ice-cream cake, and, contemplating your still sizable belly, begin planning how to return to your old sylphlike self in a hurry. The cord cut, the placenta delivered, your baby's nutritional dependency on you has ended.

Or has it? For a growing number of women, those who choose to breastfeed, the answer is "no." For them, baby's nutritional dependency will continue through weaning.

Does that mean the cork goes back in the bottle, the ice-cream cake to the freezer, and the weight-loss campaign to the back burner for the duration? Fortunately, the answer again is "no." The nutritional responsibilities of breastfeeding, though significant, are not as restrictive or demanding as the nutritional responsibilities of pregnancy. They allow (though in moderation) for the champagne, the ice-cream cake, the after-cake cup of coffee or diet soda, and other dietary indulgences you've missed during pregnancy. And they permit you to lose weight—at a satisfyingly steady pace.

Anyone who's ever seen a photo of a sunken-eyed famine victim breastfeeding an infant might assume that a mother's ability to nurse her baby has little to do with whether or not she herself is adequately nourished. But such pictures don't tell the whole story. Although a starving woman may continue to produce milk, it is usually inadequate both in quantity and quality. Eventually, unless she begins to eat, her milk dries up.

In the U.S., famine is not a major concern for the typical middle-class woman who wants to breastfeed her baby. But self-inflicted starvation (in the form of overzealous dieting) or self-inflicted mal-nourishment (in the form of a junk-food-centered eating life-style) are and frequently reduce a woman's ability to produce milk in sufficient quality and quantity.

The Best-Odds Breastfeeding Diet, while allowing more dietary latitude than the pregnancy diet, assures an adequate intake of calories, nutrients, and fluids, all of which are essential in the production of an ample supply of perfectly formulated breast milk.

NINE BASIC DIET PRINCIPLES FOR THE BREASTFEEDING MOTHER

If you've lived by the Nine Basic Principles of the Best-Odds Pregnancy Diet for nine months, they've probably become second nature to you by now. Though eating right might have been an effort in the early weeks, chances are by the time you were ready to deliver you were doing it without thinking.

Now is not the time to abandon these hard-won habits. Instead, with the following modifications, continue to live by them while you're nursing. (You can, in fact, benefit by continuing to live by them for the rest of your life.)

Make most bites count. You're no longer sharing every bite with your baby. But, in order to produce an adequate supply of grade-A milk, speed your recovery from the trauma of child-birth, maintain the levels of energy needed to meet the demands of new motherhood, and lose the excess poundage of pregnancy at a respectable rate, you'll still have to make the most of every bite you take. Occasional bites (or even full servings) of foods that count for little but calories (chocolate cake, white bread, candy bars, Danish pastries, and so on) won't jeopardize your milk, your recovery, your energy levels, or even your chances of getting back into shape—as long as the rest of your bites count toward good nutrition. But if the worthless bites begin to replace the necessary ones or, worse still, start to outnumber them, you and your baby are headed for trouble.

All calories are not created equal. This dietary credo is always true, and always worth remembering. Whether you're pregnant, nursing, or just trying to eat well, the 1,490 calories of *one* typical fast-food meal (a Big Mac, fries, chocolate shake, and apple pie), besides being loaded with saturated fats, excessive salt and sugar, and chemicals, are not nutritionally equal to the 1,490 calories in *two* well-balanced meals (tuna salad sandwich on whole wheat with lettuce and tomato, side of cole slaw, glass of skim milk, and half a cantaloupe; veal chop, large baked potato with sour cream, steamed broccoli, and slice of Nature-Sweetened Apple Pie). The first meal provides very few of the Daily Dozen (except calories, fat, and protein); the second two provide nearly all.

Starve yourself, starve your baby. Fasting, semifasting, even missing a meal can, to varying extents, reduce your milk supply. But unless you're living under famine conditions or on a crash diet, your baby's not likely to starve with you. In occasional meal-skipping or meal-skimping, you're the one who's more likely to suffer. Producing milk, in and of itself, is a draining physiological experience. Add the strain of caring for a newborn—particularly without much sleep—and the experience can be debilitating if you don't keep enough food fuel on the fire. Extensive dieting, in which large quantities of your body fat are burned for fuel or for milk, can cause the concentration of ketones in your milk, which can be hazardous to your baby. For the sake of yourself and your family, don't fast or skip meals while you're nursing. (Except for religious reasons or under medical supervision, fasting is never advisable—even if you're neither pregnant nor nursing. Nor is consistent meal skipping, which has been linked indirectly to a shortened life span.)

Stay an efficiency expert. Efficient food selection is the key to gaining, losing, or maintaining weight while assuring adequate nutrition during pregnancy, lactation, or any time in your life. When you want to gain weight, getting the most calories and nutrients for the least bulk is the most efficient eating strategy: For example, a bowl of a nutrient-and-calorie-dense, highly concentrated cereal, such as Grape Nuts (220 calories in half a cup), is a better choice than a lighter, airy cereal, such as Cheerios (110 calories in a cup and a quarter). Conversely, when your goal is weight loss, opt for filling, but still nutritious, Cheerios, which will satisfy you and your nutritional needs for half the calories.

Carbohydrates are a complex issue. Every human being, from the fetus to the senior citizen, benefits from a diet rich in high-nutrient, high-fiber complex carbohydrates, such as whole grains and dried legumes (peas and beans). They are rich in many vital vitamins and minerals, as well as in the trace metals we all need. If your diet contains adequate quantities of these carbohydrates, the milk you produce should contain adequate quantities of the right nutrients. If the Best-Odds Pregnancy Diet has put you in the habit of choosing whole grains over refined ones, stay in it—and not just while you're nursing, but for the rest of your life.

Sweet nothings—nothing but trouble. Calories that come from sugar are always empty. They offer nothing but trouble (obesity, tooth decay, and possibly an increased risk of diabetes and heart disease) to you and to any member of your family. If they regularly take the place of more nutritious foods, deficiencies in certain nutrients or even generalized malnutrition can result, which, of course, can affect the quality of your milk. That doesn't mean the nursing mother can't occasionally enjoy a sugar-sweetened treat, but it does mean she shouldn't partake of them frequently. (She can, of course, enjoy Best-Odds sweet treats any time.)

Eat foods that remember where they came from. This principle is also one you'd do well to carry over from pregnancy to lactation and then to the rest of your life. Processed foods generally lose much of their nutritive value during processing, which may leave your milk lacking, too. And they often contain excesses of sodium, sugar, fat, and additives, all of which are not good for you, and the last of which may contaminate your milk. So, whenever possible, select foods that are closest to their natural state.

Make good eating a family affair. If you stuck to this principle during pregnancy, it will be easy to continue during lactation and forever after. Do—for everyone's good health.

Don't sabotage your diet—or your milk. Absolute prohibition (of alcohol and caffeine) ends with delivery. Even if you are breastfeeding you can have an occasional cocktail, as well as your morning cup of coffee. But because alcohol and caffeine cross into your breast milk and can drug your baby, make moderation your motto. Have no more than two cups of coffee daily, alcohol only occasionally, and then no more than a drink or two. Avoid illicit drugs completely—they are bad for you both.

Any amount of tobacco is hazardous to both you and your baby. Nicotine enters the breast milk, the smoke you exhale fills your baby's lungs (as it does yours), putting him or her at greater risk for respiratory problems and, possibly, Sudden Infant Death Syndrome (also called "crib death"). If you gave up smoking during pregnancy, don't take it up again. If you didn't give it up, well, better now than never; see page 192 for tips on quitting. The longer you smoke, the more extensive the risk to you and your family.

THE BREASTFEEDING DAILY DOZEN

The Daily Dozen are a flexible bunch. They can adjust, with alterations in serving requirements, to anyone's nutritional needs: the pregnant or nursing woman, the toddler or preschooler, the child or teen, the adult of any sex or any age. The following alterations are specifically geared to the breastfeeding mother.

Calories

Even more calories are needed to nourish your baby outside the uterus than inside—baby is, after all, larger and needs more fuel for growth and activity. Instead of the 300 extra calories a day needed in pregnancy, you will need about 500 when you're breastfeeding. If you're not a calorie-counter, there's no need to start counting now. As long as you're eating all of the Breastfeeding Daily Dozen every day, you can feel fairly confident that you're getting enough calories

(you will certainly be getting enough nutrients) to produce your baby's six to twelve meals a day. To feel completely confident, watch your scale. Too rapid a weight loss, or none at all after delivery, means you're not on target.

While it's perfectly safe, even desirable, to lose excess pregnancy pounds during lactation, losing more than two pounds per week after the first three weeks can interfere with your milk production, as can dipping significantly below your ideal weight. Your milk production factory draws on your fat stores, and when you have none, or when your dieting body competes for these stores, production may be hampered. If you become too thin, increase your food intake (concentrating on calorie-dense foods as marked with a ↑ in the Food Selection Groups).

On the other hand, if you don't seem to be shedding pregnancy pounds at all, you're taking in too many calories, probably because of inefficient food selections. Satisfy your nutritional needs with the fewest calories by opting for the items in the Food Selection Groups marked with a ↓. Exercise (anything from a formal postpartum fitness program to daily brisk walks with the baby carriage) can help burn excess calories while not interfering with your utilizing the nutrients they come with. It'll also firm up the inevitable postpartum flab.

Since an infant's appetite increases with weight, you may find you need more calories when baby is 15 pounds than when he or she was eight. On the other hand, when your baby begins to take supplementary formula or significant amounts of solids, the quantity of milk he or she takes (and consequently, your caloric needs) is going to drop. As always, your scale is your guide to increasing or decreasing your caloric intake.

Protein—three servings daily

For meat-and-fish-loathers who spent nine months struggling to meet daily protein requirements, there is good news: You'll only need three servings of protein a day while you're nursing, not four (see page 44). This is still one more serving than you need ordinarily; though your milk is barely more than 1 percent protein, the extra protein is needed for its production.

Vitamin C Foods—two servings daily

Since your baby can't get a daily dose of C from a glass of orange juice (at least not for many months), your milk will have to provide all he or she needs of this essential vitamin. (Many pediatricians will also prescribe vitamin drops that contain vitamin C as added insurance.) Because your body can't store vitamin C, you'll need to take in two fresh servings of C foods a day to ensure that your milk is a good source of the vitamin for your baby (see page 55).

Calcium—five servings daily

If you became adroit at fitting calcium into your diet during pregnancy, you'll have to become even more skillful now (see page 46). During lactation, your calcium requirement increases by one serving daily over your pregnancy requirement, for a total of five servings. Of course, you don't have to drink milk to produce it. As during pregnancy, any source of calcium will do (see page 56), including a supplement if necessary (see footnote, page 104).

Green Leafy and Yellow Vegetables and Yellow Fruits—two to three servings daily

It may never again be so easy to ensure that your baby gets the nutrients in green leafy and yellow vegetables (as you will discover less than a year from now, when the spinach gets smeared on the high-chair tray and the carrots dropped neatly on the floor). Right now, all you have to do is take in enough of these vegetables yourself to guarantee the presence of the vitamin A and other essentials they contain in your milk. The requirement—three servings daily, preferably at least one green and one yellow—is the same as it is during pregnancy, as are the number of delicious ways you can satisfy it (see page 57).

Other Fruits and Vegetables—one to two servings daily

These less nutritionally glamorous foods (see page 58), though not dramatic in their vitamin and mineral contents, provide essential nutrients for both you and, through your milk, your baby. For you, there is the added benefit of fiber—particularly important in the early postpartum period, when constipation is common. (Your breastfed infant, incidentally, won't share your problem; a baby on mother's milk is virtually never constipated.)

Whole Grains and Other Concentrated Complex Carbohydrates—six or more servings daily

If you started your baby out on the goodness of whole grains and other complex carbohydrates while he or she was still in the uterus, don't stop now. (If you didn't, begin immediately.) Complex carbohydrates are one of the best sources of B vitamins and trace minerals, as essential to a growing baby as they are to a developing fetus. Make sure your milk contains ample supplies of these nutrients by making sure your diet contains ample amounts of these foods (see page 59). And don't undo all the nutritional good you began during breastfeeding by weaning your baby from your vitamin- and mineral-rich milk to white teething biscuits and refined bread; get junior's tastebuds acclimated to whole grains early and they'll become a lifetime eating habit.

Iron-Rich Foods—some daily

Menstruating women aren't the only ones who need iron. Baby girls, who are some dozen years away from the onset of menses, need it, too, as do baby boys, who will never menstruate. And so do nursing mothers, who aren't menstruating but need to replenish their blood stores after delivery. To ensure that you and your baby are getting all the iron you both need, eat some iron-rich foods daily. However, since it's almost impossible to meet iron requirements through diet alone, you will probably need to fill in the gap with an iron supplement. Take at least 30 to 60 milligrams daily, more if you're diagnosed as iron-deficient after delivery.[1]

High-Fat Foods—one to two servings daily

Contrary to what some diet purveyors would have you believe, fat is a necessary constituent of everyone's diet. It is also a necessary component of breast milk, about half of the calories of which come from fat. This fat not only supplies the baby with calories needed for the unparalleled growth spurt that occurs during the early months, but with essential fatty acids, too. Some of the fat in your breast milk will come from the fat stores you accumulated during pregnancy, and some from your diet—from both the added fat allowance and the ordinary foods that contain some fat. As in pregnancy, fat intake should be adjusted according to fluctuations in your weight. If you find you are losing too much, or losing too quickly, increase your fat

allowance to up to four servings daily. If you are not losing, or worse, are gaining unwanted weight, cut back to a minimum of one serving daily—but don't cut out added fat altogether. In general, most authorities recommend that no one take more than 30 percent of their total calories from fat in any form. Some recommend as little as 10 percent. Choose your fats wisely. The blanket protection against the undesirable effects of foods high in cholesterol or saturated fats that you had during pregnancy has now ended, though you will continue to have some, courtesy of the estrogens your body produces, until menopause.

Salty Foods—in moderate quantities

Though you no longer need the extra body fluids required during pregnancy, you don't want to lose what you need for milk production, either. So, use salt in moderation; pick up the shaker somewhat less frequently than you did during pregnancy. It is vital that the salt you shake be iodized; your baby needs iodine and the quantity in your milk depends on the quantity you take in. As always, stay away from processed and fast foods in quantity; they contain more salt than anyone needs.

---

1. Though your baby probably gets sufficient iron from your breast milk and from the iron stores built up during his or her stay in the uterus, your pediatrician may recommend iron supplementation after birth. Iron will certainly be prescribed when your baby is four to six months old, by which time stores are depleted and the introduction of solids into the diet means a reduced proportion of nourishment will come from breast milk.

Fluids—at least eight glasses daily

Though a woman can produce milk for a short time if she's not eating, she can't produce any at all if she's not drinking. Breast milk is nearly 90 percent water, and that water basically comes from the fluids in your diet. (Caffeinated tea, coffee, cola, and alcoholic beverages, however, don't count because their diuretic action draws fluids out of the body; see page 51.[2]) Drink eight glasses daily—more if it's very hot or if you lose a lot through perspiration or fever. (Thirst or a reduced urinary output, especially when the urine is darker than usual, is a clue to inadequate fluid intake.) Don't, however, overdo a good, and necessary, thing. Flooding yourself with fluids (more than 12 glasses a day) can actually decrease milk production.

Fluid intake should be spread throughout the day. Guzzling four glasses of water at a time will only prompt your body, which won't be able to hold it all, to excrete most of it. The best time to drink is while your baby's drinking, or just before, so that you can replace the fluids baby is getting. Since you will probably, at the beginning, be nursing at least eight times a day, drinking a glassful at each feeding will assure you your Daily Dozen in fluids.

Supplements—a pregnancy/lactation vitamin formula taken daily

Continuing to take your prenatal supplement while breastfeeding will ensure that you and your baby are getting enough of the major vitamins and minerals both of you need, even if your diet is sometimes less than best. Remember, however, that vitamin supplements should never take the place of a good diet.

THE BREASTFEEDING DIET IN SPECIAL SITUATIONS

Women who are nursing are not all alike, nor are their lifestyles alike. In most cases, breastfeeding women in special situations can follow the suggestions made for expectant mothers with special dietary needs (see page 102). There are two exceptions: the breastfeeding vegetarian and the breastfeeding mother of twins. The needs of these women during lactation will differ from their needs during pregnancy.

2. More than two caffeinated or alcoholic beverages a day may result in the excretion of necessary fluids. They may also reduce your capacity for necessary beverages.

The Breastfeeding Vegetarian

What does eating meat (and other animal products) have to do with making quality milk? Actually, quite a lot. The vitamins and minerals in a woman's breast milk are directly related to those in her diet. Some essential vitamins, particularly B_{12}, are found only, or primarily, in animal proteins (most predominantly in red meats, in smaller amounts in fish, eggs, milk, cottage cheese, and other cheeses). Since the effect of B_{12} deficiency on a baby can be devastating, all vegetarians and other non-meateaters (unless their diets are extremely rich in eggs and dairy products) should be sure that their prenatal supplement contains at least four micrograms of B_{12}. For women who do not drink milk (which is fortified with vitamin D), the supplement should also contain that vitamin. For women who eat neither eggs nor dairy products (and, as a precaution, for everyone else) folic acid supplementation is advisable.

In the competition for calcium, it's the nursing mother who is more likely to come out the loser. If she doesn't take in enough of this essential mineral, the additional that's needed to produce milk will be drawn from the body stores in her own bones. This could set her up for osteoporosis (a thinning of the bones that can result in collapse of the vertebrae and susceptibility to fracture) later in life. To make sure that there's enough calcium for both competitors, it's very important to fulfill the five Daily Dozen calcium servings faithfully. This is most difficult for the vegan, who does not drink milk or eat dairy products. As during pregnancy, she should consume as many of the nondairy calcium foods listed on page 56 as possible. Because it may be difficult to consistently consume five full servings daily, a calcium supplement may also be necessary.

Of the other Daily Dozen requirements, only protein may present a problem for the breastfeeding vegetarian. Inadequate protein may mean inadequate breast milk. So the nursing mother should be scrupulous in getting three servings daily if she is an ovolacto or lacto vegetarian, and four servings (because of the poorer quality of vegetable protein) if she's a vegan or strict vegetarian.

The Breastfeeding Mother of Twins (or More)

You don't need twice as many breasts to successfully breastfeed twins (though twice as many arms might come in handy). You don't even need twice as many nutrients in your diet. A breastfeeding mother of twins can safely follow the Breastfeeding Diet with only the following modifications:

More calories. To produce adequate amounts of milk without losing too much weight, a breastfeeding mother of twins needs to take in about 800 to 1,000 more calories than she would need to maintain her pre-pregnancy weight, or about 400 to 500 extra calories per baby (for the mother of triplets, that's a total of at least 1,200 extra calories). The amount may need to be increased as the babies get bigger and hungrier, or decreased as they begin to get more of their nourishment from other sources. Again, look to the bathroom scale for caloric guidance. If you're losing too much weight or losing it too quickly (see page 77), increase your intake. If you're not losing enough, or not losing at all, decrease it.

More protein. Have an extra serving of protein above the three recommended in the Breastfeeding Daily Dozen for each extra baby. With twins, that would mean four servings, triplets five.

More calcium. You will need one additional calcium serving for each additional baby: six for twins, seven for triplets. Since getting it all down in the form of dairy products may be difficult

or impossible, feel free to turn to a calcium supplement if necessary (see footnote, page 104). The new calcium-added milk may be helpful. Each glass contains 500 milligrams of calcium, 66 percent more than regular low-fat milk. Three glasses would supply your quota if you're feeding twins.

More fluids. Be prepared to drink a lot. With twins, you may need as many as 12 glasses of fluids a day, with triplets, even more. Use your urinary output as a gauge; if it seems scant and dark in color, increase your fluid intake.

GUIDE FOR A PURE MILK SUPPLY

One of the major benefits of breastfeeding for the busy new mother is that she doesn't have to worry about sterilizing bottles, safely storing formula, or being sure baby's food hasn't been contaminated by bacteria. Breast milk has its own safe storage containers, avoids contamination by airborne germs by going directly from mother's nipple to baby's mouth, and is unsullied by external matter. Or is it?

Not exactly. It's true that once the breast milk is produced, the process protects it from contamination. But unlike

THE BEST-ODDS NOT-BREASTFEEDING DIET

Just because you're not breastfeeding doesn't mean you don't have special dietary needs after childbirth. Your body has gone through nine months of physical and emotional stress culminating in the trauma of childbirth; good nutrition will not only speed your recovery, it will give you the energy to keep up with the extrauterine demands of your baby.

If, however, the vast amounts of food you had to eat during pregnancy have wearied your appetite, there's some relief in store. Unlike the breastfeeder, you won't have to continue eating for two—in fact, if you do, you'll soon end up looking like two. Cut back, but only to the sensible levels of the Prepregnancy Daily Dozen (page 146).

Use the Nine Basic Diet Principles for the Breastfeeding Mother as a dietary guide (it can serve as the foundation for a lifetime of healthy eating), ignoring the references to breastfeeding (since you will be eating to your health, and not to your baby's) and with just a couple of variations. Because what you eat and drink will no longer affect your baby (unless it affects your energy level and/or your temperament), you can be more liberal about the amounts of sugar, caffeinated beverages, diet soft drinks, and alcohol in your diet. Be aware, however, that: excesses in sugar can cause a litany of problems, including, once a sugar-high has ended, deep lows in energy; excesses in caffeine can lead to jitteriness, emotional instability, and, with doses of 10 cups or more, ringing in the ears, delirium, irregular heartbeat, muscle tension, and trembling; the effects of excesses in diet soft drinks are as yet unknown; excesses of alcohol can impair your ability to cope with your life and your baby and aggravate postpartum depression; and excesses of any or all of these empty foods can interfere with your intake of necessary nutrients.

Because you'll certainly want to return to your prepregnancy weight (unless you were too thin to begin with), or even to venture below it (if you were overweight), eat a little less than you'd need to maintain your prepregnancy weight (see page 70). But don't go on a diet severely restricted in calories and nutrients during the six-week postpartum period. Iron supplementation is particularly important, since pregnancy and childbirth may have left you anemic and because, if you're not breastfeeding, the monthly iron-depleting process of menstruation will soon resume.

formula, of which every single ingredient is (or should be) carefully measured and checked for purity and safety, breast milk can be contaminated during the production phase. Not by bacteria, but by a wide range of foods, drugs, and other chemicals.

Does everything that goes into a mother's mouth go into

her milk? Fortunately, no. But of those substances that do, which pose a threat to the nursing baby and which do not? Since thousands of new chemicals are produced each year in laboratories—some of which end up in our food, others in drugs we take, still others elsewhere in our environment—and years of study are required to test the effects of these chemicals on human life, very few definitive answers are available. Enough is known or suspected, however, to help a breastfeeding mother make sensible choices about what she should or shouldn't put in her mouth.

A few substances seem to be harmful to baby even if mother takes them in very small quantities—certain drugs, for example. Others are apparently harmful only in large doses—alcohol and caffeine, for example. Still others appear to be harmless in the doses the nurs-ing mother generally takes them, and some seem to have no ill effects at all. Like environmental threats in pregnancy, those that may contaminate breast milk need to be viewed in nonalarmist perspective. To learn which substances to avoid entirely when you're nursing, which to limit, and which you can cross off your worry list entirely, see page 189.

Exposure to large doses of some hazardous chemicals (such as DDT or PCBs) even before you begin nursing can affect your breast milk. These chemicals are stored in the body fat, which is drawn on for the production of milk. Such exposure is rare, but if you have reason to believe that you've had such an exposure, you can have your breast milk analyzed. Ask your physician or the local EPA office or department of health where such testing is available in your area.

SIX

Eating for the Next Baby

BABIES, UNLIKE WEDDINGS AND VACATIONS, AREN'T always planned. Often, they just happen—when we least expect it, when we're most unprepared. When our finances aren't what we'd like them to be (that "nest egg" hasn't been laid, never mind hatched). When the roof over our heads barely covers two. When our careers are at a critical juncture, or are just starting to take off. When we've been skipping breakfast, getting through the day on coffee, Danish, and Häagen-Dazs, overdoing the cocktails before dinner and the wine with.

Sometimes, however, babies are conceived according to plan. They're scheduled months, even years, in advance, at the most convenient, best-prepared time in our lives. When the nest egg is hatched and carefully invested, the new roof fits three (or more) comfortably, the careers have settled on a stable, less demanding plateau. And when we've had the advance warning we need to plot out and stick to a healthier life-style—one that includes a balanced breakfast and lunch, and doesn't include caffeine, alcohol, and junk food, at least not in large doses.

As this book stresses, it's never too late to start giving your baby the best nutritional odds possible—even a switch to the Best-Odds Diet in the eighth month ups the odds for both you and baby. But it's never too early, either. Your mother sowed the nutritional seeds when she carried you; during that gestation, your egg cells, one of which will develop into your baby, were formed, and her diet had an impact on them. (In the same way, your diet during pregnancy will affect the health, not only of your baby, but of your baby's babies.) What you've eaten since you left your mother's womb will also have some influence on your pregnancy and your offspring. The closer you get to conception, the more significant your diet becomes.

PLANNING AHEAD

For the woman who has the chance to plan ahead, the Best-Odds Prepregnancy Diet is the best preparation her body can have for her baby. It provides an opportunity to build nutritional reserves before baby starts tapping them, to fill in nutritional deficits before baby misses them, and to change dietary habits while the stakes aren't as high. It can start boosting your baby-to-be's odds a year before egg meets sperm, or a week before. Either way, it lays the foundation not only for a healthier pregnancy, but for a healthier rest-of-your-life.

Certain factors, because they have a direct affect on your nutritional status, require special prepregnancy attention. These include:

Spacing of pregnancies. Having a baby is a draining experience, one capable of depleting much of a woman's nutritional supplies. Having a baby, and then nursing him or her, can drain resources still further. Having a lot of babies, or having them in quick succession, can severely reduce body stores.

Staying on the Best-Odds Prepregnancy Diet between having or weaning one baby and conceiving the next is the ideal way to replenish those body stores and reduce the nutritional risk that comes with having a large or closely spaced family.

Weight. Being significantly under- or overweight is never in your body's best interest. During pregnancy, unless they are carefully monitored and compensated for (see pages 23 and 74), either can be responsible for a number of complications and nutritional risks.

If you are 10 percent or more under, or 20 percent or more over the weight that is ideal for your size, you should make a concerted effort to get closer to that ideal number before conception. (If you don't reach your goal, see page 70.) This will uncomplicate the issue of weight gain during pregnancy, assuring you won't be tempted to diet at your baby's expense (if you're overweight) or forced to force-feed yourself beyond capacity to be sure your baby is adequately nourished (if you're underweight).

Eating habits. Surveys show that most American women say they aren't satisfied with their eating habits and would like to improve them. The same surveys show that for all the talk, there's little action on the part of many of these women. So it's not good intentions that are lacking, it's the motivation to take the first step. Here, women who are planning to become pregnant have a distinct advantage. They have the best possible motivation: a safer pregnancy and a healthier baby.

Before conception—before morning sickness, food cravings and aversions, indigestion, and emotional instability begin to confuse and confound your appetite, and before the needs of a developing embryo make instantaneous (and probably helter-skelter) change necessary—is the most practical time to start changing any less-than-best eating habits. Go gradually or cold turkey, but do it so that by the time you're ready to be pregnant, you're ready to eat pregnant.

Cutting back on or cutting out caffeine and sugar, which are addictive for some people, is especially important prepregnancy if your transition to the Best-Odds Diet is to be a smooth one. Limit your consumption of caffeinated beverages to no more than two cups daily prepregnancy, cut down to one or none while you're trying to conceive. Try reducing all the sugar-sweetened foods in your diet (including such things as sodas, ice cream, pastries, candy) to one a day, and then to one a week prepregnancy. If you have an addiction to sugar-free soft drinks, try to break this, too, during the prepregnancy period; limit your consumption to one a day, then eliminate them completely once you begin your conception campaign. To help you make the Best-Odds Diet a habit (and break those bad ones), see the Prepregnancy Daily Dozen (page 146).

Put dad-to-be on the Best-Odds Diet. While a father-in-waiting's diet during his wife's term has no effect on the outcome of her pregnancy (except as it relates to her eating), what he eats and drinks before her pregnancy can. A prospective dad who drinks heavily, eats an unbalanced diet based on junk foods, and/or does drugs, can contribute less healthy sperm capable of making less healthy babies. So persuade your husband to join you on your Prepregnancy Diet (his requirements are listed on page 185) for the months before conception, avoiding drugs, excess alcohol, and too many empty calories. (It will, incidentally, make your own enlistment more enjoyable if you have company.)

Life-style habits. For some women, those who don't smoke and rarely toast an occasion with anything stronger than tomato juice, getting their life-style habits into shape for conception is an effortless undertaking. For those whose habits are less becoming an expectant mother, certain preconception alterations can prove a challenge. But because smoking and regular drinking pose direct threats to the fetus (and because the stress of quitting these habits is an extra stress you won't need during pregnancy), it's a challenge that should, when possible, be met in the prepregnancy period.

Smoking is an addiction. Though some smokers are able to kick their habits themselves— through sublimation, by substituting other occupations, by avoiding the settings and foods associated with their smoking, with relaxation and tension-reducing techniques and exercise, and with sheer willpower— many are not. If you feel you need help to stop smoking, get it now. Try a group program at a local hospital, or a private one, such as Smokenders, or see a physician who uses hypnosis to help patients break unwanted habits.

For some people, alcohol is an addiction. For others, it's just a casual social habit. The trick is discovering (or admitting) which category you fall into. The Best-Odds Prepregnancy Diet can help you do this.

The first step is to cut back to no more than one drink (one cocktail made with 1½ ounces of liquor, one 5-ounce glass of wine, one 16-ounce glass of beer) a day. When you are ready to conceive, stop altogether.

You don't have to quit the habit of "drinking," just the habit of having alcohol in your drinks. At the end of a long day, unwind with a Mock Daiquiri, a chilled Innocent Sangria, a glass of Sparkling Punch, or an orange juice or grapefruit juice spritzer (half juice, half seltzer, with a twist). Serve your drink at the accustomed cocktail hour, in your usual cocktail glasses (and don't forget a toast). If you're used to having wine with dinner, take your iced water, sparkling water, cider or grape juice, or nonalcoholic wines in attractive wine glasses. (Check labels to be sure the mock wines don't contain preservatives.)

If substitutes for alcohol don't satisfy you, and you find you can't cut back to one drink a day, much less none, your drinking is more than social; you will need help in breaking your habit. If your family doctor is trained in dealing with alcohol problems, he or she may be a good source of help. Many people also find Alcoholics Anonymous helpful (there are chapters in virtually every big city and small town in the U.S.). If you're not convinced you have an addiction, A.A. may seem like an extreme solution, but if it's the only way you can stop drinking entirely, then it's the only solution that makes sense.

Birth-control history. When a woman selects a method of birth control, she's not likely to consider the effect it might have on her nutritional status—particularly her nutritional status should conception occur. But two common methods, the IUD and the oral contraceptive, do have such an effect. Because the IUD frequently increases menstrual blood loss, it may deplete iron stores. Oral contraceptives appear, for uncertain reasons, to reduce body levels of several important nutrients—specifically, folic acid, B_2 (riboflavin), B_6, B_{12}, C, and some trace metals.

If you use either of these methods of birth control, you should compensate for the loss of nutrients, just in case you conceive accidentally. That means taking a vitamin supplement containing at least 60 milligrams of iron if you are using an IUD and one containing folic acid, the B vitamins, C, and such trace metals as zinc and magnesium if you are taking oral contraceptives.

Three months before you plan to conceive, stop using these methods of birth control and switch to a condom—without spermicide.[1] (This is wise for medical as well as nutritional reasons because the IUD has been linked to serious problems in pregnancy and oral contraceptives to a very slight increased risk of birth defects.) Continue with the supplements and begin making the Best-Odds diet a part of your life. If you are an IUD user, have your physician check you for iron deficiency so that a supplement can be prescribed if necessary. When you conceive, you should switch to a vitamin and mineral supplement specifically formulated for pregnancy (see page 336).

THE PREPREGNANCY DAILY DOZEN

Though the Daily Dozen were originally developed to fill the nutritional needs of expectant mothers, only the number of servings need change to make them appropriate for the not-yet expectant (or, since the Daily Dozen make nutritional sense at any stage of your life, for those not planning to be pregnant).

---

1. Spermicides have been accused of contributing to birth defects, but there is no solid evidence to support this contention. Those who conceive while using them appear to have nothing to worry about, but for those who have a choice, prudence suggests avoiding their use in the three months before trying to conceive.

Calories

Everyone needs calories; some people just need more (or less) than others. How much daily food energy you need prepregnancy will depend on your weight. If it's about where you want it to be, simply eat enough to maintain it.[2] If it's more than you'd like it to be, and especially if it's more than 20 percent over your ideal weight, eat less than you need to maintain it, and you'll lose weight. (But don't go on a very restrictive diet in the three months before you start trying to conceive.) If your weight is less than you'd like it to be, and especially if it's 10 percent or more below your ideal weight, eat more than you need to maintain it, and you'll gain weight. Be careful, however, to gain the weight on nutritious fare, not junk food.

Protein—two servings daily

Those Americans who begin their day with ham and eggs,

2. The scale is usually your best gauge of whether your calorie needs are being met, overfilled, or underfilled. But if you'd rather count calories, calculate your needs by multiplying your ideal weight by 12 if you are sedentary, 15 if you are moderately active, and up to 22 if you are very active. The product is a rough estimate of the calories you need to maintain or reach that ideal weight. Be aware, however, this formula is subject to the vagaries of metabolism and other factors. In the end, only your scale can tell you if your diet plan is working.

move on to lunchtime quarter-pounders, and wind up with 14-ounce sirloins eat far more protein than they need. Only during pregnancy, lactation, recovery from surgery, or in certain other medical conditions are large intakes of protein warranted. For the average adult female, the Food and Nutrition Board of the National Academy of Sciences National Research Council's Recommended Dietary Allowance (RDA) for protein is 46 grams, about two moderate servings daily (see page 53 for serving sizes). That's all you'll need during the prepregnancy period.

Vitamin-C Foods—one serving daily

As British seamen discovered back in the late 1700s, we can't survive without vitamin C. On every long fruit-and-vegetableless sea voyage, these sailors (later to be called limeys) risked dying of the debilitating disease called scurvy, characterized by bleeding gums and other tissues, muscular pain, and weakness in the beginning, and diarrhea and kidney or pulmonary failure at the end. The disease virtually disappeared among seamen in 1795 when the British navy mandated the use of lemon juice (later replaced, for economic reasons, by limes, thus the nickname). Thanks to citrus (fresh and frozen) in the markets year round, scurvy isn't a problem in the U.S. today. But because the body doesn't store vitamin C and we need a fresh dose daily, it's important not to skip a day, especially when you're getting into shape for pregnancy. Have at least one serving each day of any of the vitamin C foods on page 55.

Calcium—three-plus servings or the equivalent

Growing children and pregnant (or nursing) women are not the only ones who need calcium for strong bones. Scientists now know that we lose old bone and lay down new throughout our lives. Because the drop in estrogen levels as women approach and reach menopause increases the rate of bone loss, they need compensatory calcium to increase bone replacement. The more bone mass a woman builds up in her early years, the more she will bring with her to menopause, so it is now recommended that women of all ages increase their intake of calcium. The old U.S. RDA of 800 milligrams, or about 2⅔ servings of calcium foods (most American women don't even come close to that), is now considered insufficient by many experts. They suggest a safer minimum intake of at least 1,000 milligrams, or about 3⅓ calcium servings. If

you find it difficult to get this amount from diet itself without exceeding your prepregnancy calorie need (unless you are trying to gain weight), it's a good idea to consider getting 500 or 600 milligrams from a calcium supplement (see page 56) or to drink calcium-enriched milk.

Green Leafy and Yellow Vegetables and Yellow Fruits—two servings daily

The more that is learned about nutrition, the more the importance of deep yellow vegetables and fruits (rich in carotene, now believed to aid in inhibiting cancer) and green leafies (some of which may also aid in preventing cancer; see page 57) is recognized. Green leafy and yellow vegetables and yellow fruits have other virtues to recommend them: They're rich in many essential vitamins and minerals, high in fiber, usually low in calories, and always high in taste. Have two servings a day, preferably one green and one yellow.

Other Vegetables and Fruits—one or two servings daily

These aren't in the superproduce category, with whopping doses of vitamin A or C, but they are significant sources of fiber and many vitamins, minerals, and trace metals. They're also, for the most part, perfect fodder for the dieter, since they fill and satisfy but don't add a lot of calories. Have one to two servings daily (see page 58).

Whole Grains and Other Concentrated Complex Carbohydrates—four servings daily

Many authorities are now suggesting an increase in the consumption of complex carbohydrates, such as cereals, breads, other whole-grain products, and dried legumes (beans and peas). Contrary to the popular misconception, complex carbohydrates are not fattening (it's usually the butter on the bread, the sauce on the pasta, the pork in the beans that put on the pounds). What they are is very rich in vitamins (particularly those of the B complex), minerals (especially the trace minerals such as zinc, and fiber (see page 59).

Iron-Rich Foods—some daily

In general, women, because they lose menstrual blood each month, are the likeliest candidates for an iron deficiency (the risk is even greater if they have an IUD). Because pregnancy can be expected to put a serious

drain on iron stores, women who are planning to conceive should be sure these reserves are in good supply. That means eating iron-rich foods daily and taking a vitamin and mineral supplement that contains iron.

High-Fat Foods—one to two servings daily

Here's where the calories mount up, often without a parallel accumulation of other nutrients. The added calories, particularly because they come in such a concentrated, unfilling form, may be welcomed by the woman who is trying to gain weight during the prepregnancy phase. But for those who wish to maintain or lose weight during this or any time, an excess of fat in the diet can easily and quickly usher in unwelcome pounds. Have two servings daily if your weight is no problem, one serving if you're trying to lose weight, and up to four if you're trying to gain. Remember, you will be getting fat in other forms in your diet as well. Choosing your fats carefully in the prepregnancy phase is more important than when you're pregnant because you don't have the protection pregnancy seems to confer.

Salty Foods

Sodium chloride, also known as table salt, is a necessary nutrient

without which we couldn't survive. But while we can't live with
too little of it, many Americans
have trouble living with too
much of it. An excess of sodium
in the diet is closely connected to
the development of hypertension, one of the major killers of
American adults, and is also related to some kidney problems.
The excess doesn't usually come
naturally (though there is sodium in virtually every food, including milk, fruits, and vegetables) or even when we salt at the
table; its primary sources are
processed and fast foods Americans favor. These can often contain more than one gram of sodium (the limit some authorities
recommend for an entire day) in
a single serving. Though healthy
pregnant women don't need to
rigidly restrict their salt intake,
women who are planning to become pregnant, like everyone
else, should try to pare excess
sodium from their diets.

Fluids—six to eight glasses daily

Water is the most necessary ele-
ment in the human diet, needed
for every cell in our bodies, yet
many of us get too little of it.
Prepregnancy is the time to start
getting into the habit of
drinking—plain or sparkling water, juices, soups. Milk can also
provide fluid, but remember that
a glass of milk is only two-thirds

water. Foods with a high water
content (such as salad greens,
melons, citrus fruits) can also
contribute to your daily quota,
but don't count alcohol or caffeinated beverages in your fluid
intake, because they tend to de-
hydrate you. Be sure to increase
your intake in hot weather or
when you are exercising or running a fever.

Supplements—a vitamin and mineral formula taken daily

Whether or not the average person should take a vitamin and
mineral supplement daily as nutritional "insurance" is controversial. What isn't controversial,
however, is the advisability of a
woman beginning to take a multiple vitamin and mineral supplement that contains folic acid
three months before her target
conception date. Such supplementation, continued through at
least the first eight weeks of
pregnancy, has been linked to a
dramatic reduction in neural
tube and possibly other birth defects[3]. It also reduces the possibility that you'll start pregnancy
with nutritional deficiencies. But
be sure your supplement does
not contain more than 4 or 5,000
IU of vitamin A.

---

3. This is not to say that women who don't
take a supplement before pregnancy are at
great risk of having a child with a neural tube
defect. The general risk is slight.

PART TWO

Getting Practical

SEVEN

Preparing for the Best-Odds Diet

S TARTING ONE OF THE LOSE-SEVEN-POUNDS-IN-SIX-days diets that regularly make the covers of the major women's magazines and weekly tabloids takes relatively little preparation: clip the menus and tape them to the refrigerator door, invest in the requisite crate of grapefruit, and wait for Monday morning.

Starting a diet that is designed to last at least nine months—and hopefully, in a modified form, a lifetime—takes a good deal more time, effort, and dedication. But its results (unlike the usually short-lived effects of most quickie diets) can pay off for a lifetime, in fact, several lifetimes: yours, your baby-to-be's, your husband's, and that of any other children, present or future.

While starting the Best-Odds Diet won't be easy, sticking with it eventually will be. Also unlike those diets-of-the-week, in which Monday-morning bang dissolves into Wednesday-morning fizzle after grapefruit number six, you'll find the Best-Odds Diet will require less willpower with each passing day. Gradually, but inevitably, your new eating habits will become as ingrained as those they replace.

First things, however, must come first. Preparation for starting the Best-Odds Diet is vital to following it successfully. Though you shouldn't wait until the preparations are complete to begin eating to the best odds of your ability (today, after all, is the first day of the rest of your baby's prenatal life), you shouldn't continue the Best-Odds Diet too long without making some fundamental alterations in your kitchen, your shopping and cooking techniques, and, possibly most important, in your family's eating habits.

BLUEPRINT FOR A BEST-ODDS KITCHEN

The average American kitchen: More diets have fallen victim to it than to all the cream sauces on the Left Bank of Paris. Glance around yours. As innocent as it may look, chances are that therein lurk enough insidious, diet-destroying demons to way-lay the best laid of Best-Odds Diet plans.

Even the better-than-average American kitchen probably needs some remodeling before it can measure up to Best-Odds specifications. But before you call in an architect, start pulling down your wallpaper, pulling up your formica, and deciding between hi-tech and country French cabinets, you should know that you can't judge a Best-Odds kitchen by its decor. You have to look beyond the colors and patterns to find what will make or break your Best-Odds Diet. The demons are hidden behind pantry and refrigerator doors, in cookie jars, deep within the icy recesses of the freezer compartment. And they've got to go.

Still, it's not enough to exorcise the demons. To transform an ordinary kitchen into a Best-Odds kitchen, you've got to replace the bad with the best, so that all that's good for you and your baby is ready to pull out for healthy snacking and cooking.

Out with the Old

Why bother baring your shelves? After all, you have self-control. But is your self-control a match for the pair of Twinkies that winks seductively at you every time you open the cupboard? Or for the quart of Swiss Chocolate Almond that tempts you when you open the freezer door? Probably not. If you're like most mere mortals, you'll have ripped the cellophane off the Twinkies before you remember you were saving them for the baby sitter, have the lid off the ice cream before you remember it was the frozen juice you went to the freezer for.

Keeping temptation out of immediate sight won't necessarily keep it out of your mouth either. Freeze the leftover coffee cake, and some rainy afternoon you'll discover it tastes great frozen. Put the caramel corn on the pantry shelf you can't reach without a stepstool, and it won't be long before an urgent craving sends you up on that stool to "clean out" that very shelf. Bury the Mars bars in the farthest regions of the fridge, behind the apple juice, the mayonnaise, and the baking soda you haven't changed in three years, and you'll suddenly find the need to

VARIETY: THE KEY TO HEALTHY EATING

Variety has long been known to add spice to dining. But now we know it can do a lot more. Because not all nutrients come in the same packages, and varying the foods you eat gives you the best odds of getting all the nutrients you need, variety can make your diet more nutritious. It can also make your diet safer.

There is no food in the supermarket that is hazardous if eaten only occasionally (unless you are allergic to it); yet even the foods we consider harmless and wholesome can be toxic if consumed consistently and in huge quantities. A very occasional nitrated hot dog or glass of wine won't harm you or your baby, but daily doses of spinach can interfere with calcium absorption, and a massive overdose of milk can be fatal.

For safe and healthy eating:

❖Vary your choices of grains and other kinds of complex carbohydrates (oatmeal for breakfast one day, shredded wheat the next; brown rice as a side dish at lunch, chick-peas in your salad at dinner).

❖Vary your choices of protein foods (chicken one night, fish the next, and ground veal the third). If you only eat fish, or eat it often, vary the variety (halibut one night, sole the next, sea trout the third).

❖Vary your choices of vegetables and fruits (alternate selections from the Green Leafy and Yellow list, such as broccoli and carrots one day, kale and sweet potatoes the next, chicory and cantaloupe the third day; also alternate from the Other Vegetables and Fruit list, green beans and apples one day, Brussels sprouts and raisins the next).

❖Vary your vitamin C choices (orange juice and green peppers one day, mango and tomatoes the next, cantaloupe and cauliflower the third).

❖Rarely eat those foods that contain a lot of additives; vary them when you do. Try not to get the same additives (BHT, for example) repeatedly. (See page 313 for a list of additives of which you should be particularly wary.)

change the baking soda.

That's the reason for this first phase of the Best-Odds kitchen alteration, the object of which is to identify and remove all the ready-to-eat foods that won't yield nutritionally high returns for you and your baby. Some, like Twinkies, will be easy to spot; others may deceive you. The "all natural," "no sugar added" granola, for instance, which appears as wholesome and as healthy as a hike through the Rocky Mountains, may be of little more value than an artificially flavored, sugar-sweetened "kids" cereal. High in fat, low in protein for the calories it supplies, and containing hives-full of honey or sacks-full of sugar, it belongs among the discards. To screen for such deceptive products on your shelves, and to avoid restocking with similar mistakes, memorize Reading Labels (page 160). In general, toss out foods that are high in sugar (and all of its aliases; see page 168), contain mostly refined flours (even those that are enriched; see page 49), or whose ingredients list reads like the formula for a chemical cocktail. Good candidates for tossing are those on the Forbidden Fruit and Less-Than-Best Foods lists (page 32).

Of course, you wouldn't down a handful of uncooked white rice, devour a raw hot dog, or guzzle a can of sweetened condensed milk in a moment of weakened willpower. But you might open your cupboard one evening and, finding it otherwise bare, boil up a white rice dish, slice hot dogs into a casserole, or stir condensed milk into a pudding that, odds are, would not give your baby a Best-Odds meal. So to eliminate desperation, as well as temptation, as a motivation for nutritional shortchanging, weed off your shelves and out of your refrigerator and freezer even the seemingly harmless box of white rice or stuffing mix.

It's not necessary to sweep your cupboards completely clean. Though baking and cooking staples that are not beneficial to you, your baby, and your family (such as sugar, corn syrup, and white flour) should not be used for the duration of your pregnancy, they needn't be discarded. Since they aren't perishable, they can be stored away for occasional postpartum use. Sugar substitutes, such as aspartame (Equal, NutraSweet) and saccharine, while not appropriate for pregnant or very young Best-Odds dieters, can be kept for table use by resident or visiting nonpregnant adults. So can soft drinks and other products containing sugar substitutes—assuming you won't have any trouble resisting them.

Once you've assembled your discards, you need to determine their fate. Here there are two choices. The first is to pile them into a sturdy plastic bag, say your goodbyes, and let the sanitation department take care of the rest. (This is less wasteful than it sounds. Considering that empty-calorie foods are wasteful to begin with, everyone in your family—particularly baby—will benefit more from their being thrown out than eaten.) The second choice is for those in whose ears mother's admonitions about wasting food, even poor-quality food, still ring: unload the undesirable on others. Send some over to a neighbor. Donate to a bake sale. Give some to neighborhood kids to sell alongside their lemonade. Use them to cater a party at the office (but don't forget to bring something *you* can eat). A few items (such as rice and pasta) may be suitable for donating to a pantry for the hungry, but in general, such food collections will not accept cookies, cakes, and other junk foods.

BEST-ODDS KITCHEN TOOLS

If a poor workman blames his tools, a Best-Odds eater who is getting poor results could blame her kitchen utensils. But there's no blaming a kitchen stocked with the following:

Steamer. For crisp-tender vegetables that are still loaded with the vitamins and minerals they had when they were picked, a steamer is almost essential (a waterless pot, microwave, or pressure cooker can be used, but with less reliable results). Use it in a pot that has a tight-fitting lid to retain the steam.

Nonstick skillet. Low-fat or no-fat frying, sautéing, and pancake making can be a sticky business without a nonstick skillet. Silverstone is a better choice than Teflon, which is thinner and less durable. Have them in several sizes, if possible.

Nylon spatulas, spoons, and pancake turners. To keep your nonstick skillet from scratching and wearing out before its time, invest in a set of quality nylon utensils.

An accurate meat thermometer. Since too rare meat can present a potential hazard in pregnancy (see page 207), an accurate meat thermometer is essential for the meat-eating expectant mother.

Small scale. For the Best-Odds novice, a postage or kitchen scale is handy for weighing out portions of meat, fish, and poultry. Once you've learned to eyeball it (approximations are fine for Best-Odds purposes), you can put your scale away.

Measuring cups and spoons. You don't have to be fanatical about measuring out your yogurt, milk, cottage cheese, and wheat germ. But until you become an adroit estimator of portion sizes, it's a good idea to regulate them with measuring cups and spoons to make sure you don't shortchange yourself or your baby.

Acrylic chopping board. If you're not lucky enough to have a food processor to do your chopping and slicing for you, your chopping board will be an important tool in preparing Best-Odds meals. Opt for acrylic over the wooden variety. Wood boards may harbor germs that can cause food poisoning, and one of the last things you need during pregnancy is an attack of bacteria-triggered nausea, vomiting, and diarrhea.

Best-Odds Nice-to-Have Extras

Nonstick bakeware. Making your own Best-Odds goodies will seem less of an effort if you eliminate the chore of scrubbing muffin tins and cookie sheets. If you can, buy nonstick (Teflon will do for these pans, since the surface won't take quite the beating the skillet surface will) muffin and cake tins, cookie sheets, bread pans. If you can't, use a vegetable cooking spray on your old pans to minimize sticking and cleanup.

Waterless pot and/or pressure cooker. Both of these old standby cooking tools can yield crisp-tender vegetables that retain their vitamin and mineral content. Just be sure to read the instructions before using them and to time cooking carefully.

Salad spinner. For most people, it's not the salad-eating that's unappealing, it's the salad-making. Two of the least appealing phases of salad preparation—washing and drying—will be a lot less onrous if they're done with the help of a salad spinner. An added bonus: well-dried greens will need less dressing.

Blender. Purée vegetables with evaporated milk to make a "creamed" soup. Blend cottage cheese to make a Best-Odds Cheesecake. Double your calcium intake with a Double-the-Milk Shake. When you've a blender to work kitchen magic, it's easy to get your Daily Dozen.

Food processor. Almost anything a knife can do (and some things your hands or blender can do), a processor can do faster. By chopping, slicing, and shredding the endless vegetables of Best-Odds eating; making puréed fruit or vegetable soups; mixing and kneading whole-grain doughs; and grating cheese, a food processor can, in short order, eliminate one of the popular excuses for not eating well: "I don't have the time."

Juicer. Feeding the vegetables and/or fruits you don't find appealing in pregnancy to the juicer before feeding them to yourself may make them more palatable. Juicers extract for your nutritional benefit many of the important vitamins and minerals from plant foods—but don't

BEST-ODDS PRODUCTS ON THE SUPERMARKET OR HEALTH FOOD STORE SHELVES

This is only a partial list of products which are particularly appropriate for use in the Best-Odds Diet. Since new products are appearing on the shelves almost daily, many others will doubtless be available by the time this list is in print. Others which are not available nationally may be distributed in your area. Carefully screen your supermarket or health food store shelves to uncover them.

Fruit-only jams and preserves	Sorrel Ridge, Polaner, Poiret (LifeTime)
Fruit-sweetened cranberry sauce	Sorrel Ridge; RW Knudsen Family
Syrups and toppings	RW Knudsen Family; Sorrel Ridge
Natural whole-grain breads	Matthews, Pritikin, many local brands
Natural whole-wheat english muffins, dinner rolls, and burger buns	Matthews
Salad dressing (no additives, sugar, oil)	Pritikin, Nasoya
Peanut butter (sugar free)	Smuckers, many health food brands*

*If you find the peanuts-only peanut butter not to your liking, you can use Skippy, which has less sugar than other popular brands.

make juices your prime source of fruits and vegetables or you won't get enough of the fiber you need.

Frozen-pop molds. The long hot summer you're carrying through may seem a lot shorter when you've got an assortment of frozen juice pops waiting in your freezer. Buy plastic pop molds; fill them with unsweetened apple, apple-berry, orange, grape, pear, or any other favorite unsweetened juice or juice blend; freeze; and enjoy. Or just use paper cups and insert the popsicle sticks when the juice is partly frozen.

Ice-cream maker. Those who yearn for something sweet and

Fruit juice-sweetened baked goods	Barbara's (most items), Health Valley (some items)
Unsweetened applesauce	Very Fine (our favorite), Motts, store brands
Canned fruit in juice	Dole's, many store brands
Blended pure fruit juices (unsweetened)	Apple and Eve, Snapple, After the Fall, Juice Works (frozen)
Brown rice	River Brand, Uncle Ben's
Whole-wheat flour	Hecker's, Pillsbury, King Arthur
Whole-grain flours	Arrowhead, Elam, Shiloh
Wheat germ	Kretchmer
Ready-to-eat cereals (no sugar added)	Shredded wheats (all brands), Nutri-Grain, Grape Nuts, No-sugar-added Familia, Barbara's Toasted O's and Raisin Bran, other health-food brands
Whole-wheat pasta	De Bole's
High-protein pasta	Buitoni, Prince's Superoni
Textured vegetable protein (meat analogs)	Worthington, Loma Linda, Sovex
Frozen vegetarian main courses (tofu-based)	Legume

cold that's also creamy will be well satisfied with the naturally sweet ice-milk and sorbet creations that can be turned out with a home ice-cream maker (and with the recipes beginning on page 289). If you can afford one, the self-contained, electrically operated kind—which needs no ice, no salt, no people power, and makes no mess—is ideal. If not, any ice-cream maker will do. (In a pinch, you can even use a freezer and an ice-cube tray.)

Microwave oven. For busy mothers-to-be, the microwave can provide full meals in half an hour from market bag to table. Microwave cooking is also nutritious, since little or no water is used in preparation and quick-cooking saves nutrients. (Just don't stand in front of the microwave when it's in operation.)

BEST-ODDS SHOPPING

A trip to the supermarket used to be a fairly undemanding venture. Shopping list in hand, commercial jingles running through our heads, the most pressing decisions we had to make were between brand names of the same product ("new and improved" usually swung the tide, as did a more appealing "serving suggestion" photo). We filled our carts effortlessly, the methodical among us basing selections on carefully drawn weekly menus, the free-spirited shoppers letting whim, fancy, and appetite guide them. We knew vaguely that it was important to eat nutritiously, but were even vaguer on what constituted nutritious eating. Subliminally, Madison Avenue's four-color ads and TV extravaganzas combined with the seductive packaging and displays on grocer's shelves to send the message that everything from our friendly food manufacturer was "wholesome," and therefore "healthy." It was a comforting thought, one most of us, expectant mothers included, accepted.

Then came the consumer revolution. All of a sudden we're told that we shouldn't be so accepting. We shouldn't fall prey to catchy slogans. We shouldn't judge a product by its flashy cover. We ought to know—especially if we're pregnant—what's inside the foods we bring home. We are warned of the dangers of everything from hidden sugar to unpronounceable chemicals.

Have these admonitions made us better shoppers? Maybe. But more often, it seems, they've made us confused and frustrated shoppers. The questions are endless and seemingly unanswerable. Is sugar by any other name (there are at least a dozen) as dirty a word? Does low cholesterol mean low fat? Is "natural" a guarantee of healthfulness? Do you, as an expectant mother, need a combined degree in nutrition and chemistry to cut through the confusion and answer the questions? Not quite. All you need to master the market is a mini-course in Best-Odds Shopping.

Reading Labels

What would shopping be like without labels? Wandering blindly down aisles lined with naked aluminum cans and faceless cardboard boxes, we'd have no way of telling the green beans from the peaches, the raisin bran from the elbow macaroni. And if, by shaking or sniffing, we were able to track down the item we were looking for, we'd still have no way of discerning its ingredients, its style of preparation, its nutritional content.

But how helpful are labels? Are they always our allies? Do manufacturers place them on food packages solely as a public service, to aid consumers in their efforts to discern the "good" foods from the "bad"? Unfortunately, not always. Since most are in the business of selling the bad with the good, they would like you to believe that all their products are good for you. They hope to convince you of that by putting what they want you to believe in big type, in effect as mini-billboards, and what they hope you won't notice, the ingredients lists and nutrition labels, in tiny print. We, the consumers, have to learn to distinguish the fact of the small type from the fancy of the large.

The Big-Type Hype

Surveying your supermarket's shelves—where label after label calls out: "No preservatives," "all natural," "no sugar added," "wholesome," "no cholesterol"—you might get the impression that manufacturers are as concerned with our nutrition as we increasingly are. What they are concerned with, however, is getting us to buy their products. And the easiest way to do that, they feel, is to meet or appear to meet consumer demand—in this case for healthful foods.

Unfortunately, the profusion of "healthy" foods is often no more than label deep. Some manufacturers have indeed altered their products: reduced salt, eliminated sugar, eradicated additives, trimmed cholesterol. Others, whose products were natural and nutritious to begin with—apple juice or oatmeal, for example—had only to alter their labels to emphasize their newly fashionable old-fashioned virtues. But many in the food industry, unwilling to alter formulas, simply altered their labels to make it seem as if they had.

Labels are intended to entice, not inform; their seductive large print is meant to lure you into buying without reading the fine print. But you needn't be an easy mark for such label libel. By understanding the rules of the game the manufacturers are playing, you can become as accomplished at seeing through their labeling ploys as they are at perpetrating them.

Find the natural ingredient. It's in there somewhere between the artificial color and the polysorbate 80. All a manufacturer needs to do is track it down on his ingredient list and spotlight it on the label. It doesn't matter if it's the only "natural" ingredient in an otherwise synthetic, nutritionally vacant product. It doesn't matter if it has been added in infinitesimal amounts. It's natural, and it *sells*. Just ask one hot dog maker, who proudly emblazons his chicken franks, "Made only with ground natural spices." Never mind that there's no such thing as an unnatural spice, and that any spice that ends up in a hot dog is bound to be ground—it *sounds* good. So good that maybe nobody will notice the package body copy, which quietly lists less impressive ingredients, including nitrates and corn syrup, a sugar. Similarly, the six chemicals listed in small print on the side of a popular macaroni dinner are more likely to go unread when the shopper's attention is diverted by the easier to read banner: "Cheddar and Other Natural Flavors." (It's anybody's guess what "natural flavors," found increasingly in food products, are. Only the manufacturer knows for sure, and he isn't required to tell. And though the origin of natural flavor is always a food, the result is usually a chemical extract, which may or may not be safe. At least two "natural" flavors have been taken off the market after being relabeled by the FDA as carcinogenic.)

Highlight what's not in there. If you tell consumers what isn't in the product, maybe they won't notice what *is*. The manufacturer of a pancake mix is betting you won't notice the artificial colors and other chemical additives listed on the side of the box when the front of the package proudly proclaims "no preservatives." And the maker of "health food" cookies is sure you won't bother to read past the "no sugar added" banner to find out that honey *has* been added—and in vast quantities. Don't be fooled; bypass declarations about what isn't in a product, and read on about what is.

Fortify the weak. Today's consumer can't get enough vitamins. At least, that's what today's savvy manufacturers are banking on when they "fortify" otherwise nutritionally weak products with "essential vitamins and minerals." Dozens of glaring examples line the shelves of your market's breakfast food section: sugar-coated cereals, vibrant in artificially colored shades of purple, orange, and hot pink and intense with laboratory-created flavors of chocolate, vanilla, strawberry, and grape chorus "100% U.S. RDA of vitamins." By their side are toaster pastries, sugar-filled and -iced, that trumpet "fortified with six vitamins and iron." Around the corner on the beverage aisle are jars of "breakfast drink" with a "full day's supply of vitamin C." Long advertised as the space program's drink of choice, they also contain enough sugar to send a seven year old into a hyperactive orbit. (A glass of sugar-free orange juice contains as much C, in its naturally occurring form, plus other vitamins and minerals.)

Not every product that's fortified is a poor food to begin with. But fortification is often unnecessary and usually costly for the consumer. An already nutritious whole-grain cereal becomes significantly more expensive at the checkout counter when fortified, though the added vitamins cost the manufacturer no more than a few pennies. Buying a cereal that comes by its vitamins naturally, and taking a daily vitamin supplement, is a much more economical approach to guaranteeing your RDAs.

The exception to the forgo-the-fortification rule is milk. Since vitamins A and D are essential to the proper utilization of calcium by the body, all milk you buy should be fortified with both.

Enrich the poor. The manufacturers of "enriched" white breads and other baked goods do their best to convince consumers that replacing the germ and bran they've removed in the refining process with a few vitamins and minerals is an even swap. It isn't. Only Mother Nature knows the original formula for whole-grain goodness, and don't let a label tell you otherwise.

Reapportion portions. Those discovering the sudden doubling of the protein content in a serving of canned tuna may have wondered whether a new breed of high-protein fish had been netted. A more thorough reading of the fine print demonstrates that what has actually doubled is the portion size: from two 3¼-ounce servings to one 6½-ounce serving per can. Preferring division to multiplication, another tuna canner dramatically "lowered" the sodium and calorie content of its tuna by cutting its suggested serving to a scanty 2 ounces (or 3¼ servings per can). A major soup company also reduced calories and sodium by changing the typesetting on its labels and redefining its traditional serving size of 10-ounce portion (two servings to a can) to 8 ounces (two and one-half to a can). They changed the label, but not the fact that most of the soups are still unnecessarily high in sodium. So be sure to factor in portion size when comparing nutritional contents of potential purchases.

Play the name game. The rules of this game would seem quite clear. FDA regulations require that a product name (not the brand name) must identify or describe the basic nature of the food or its characterizing properties or ingredients in accurate, simple, and direct terms, such as "diluted orange juice drink" for a partial juice product.

But rules and regulations notwithstanding, many product names turn out to be misleading. "Wheat bread," for example, conjures up for the average consumer a picture of a healthful whole-grain loaf. But the majority of breads (and crackers and muffins) with the appellation "wheat" are composed mostly (sometimes entirely) of white refined-wheat flour. Because "wheat" refers to the type of grain (wheat as opposed to rye or barley) and not to whether the grain is refined or whole, manufacturers can use the term freely without protest from the FDA.

The name game can be played another way, too. Take the most nutritionally appealing ingredient in an otherwise valueless product—bran, for instance, in a largely refined muffin—and headline it in the product name. How much bran need be present in a "bran" muffin? A pinch will do.

To beat manufacturers at this game, look past the product name to the ingredients list when making your selections. You may find that there's even less in a name than Romeo thought.

Play with words. Because some product-describing words defy definition in the FDA and Federal Trade Commission (FTC) dictionaries, manufacturers use (some would say abuse) literary license to create meanings that suit their marketing needs.

Natural. Since surveys show that most consumers believe that "natural foods are more nutritious than other foods," and many regularly buy products because they're "natural" even if they have to pay a premium for them, it would be unnatural if profit-motivated manufacturers didn't seize every opportunity to label their products "natural." No regulations define the word, so only imagination—and a sly sales promotion director—is needed to use it. One company proclaims "100% Natural Lemon Flavor" for its chemically concocted lemonade on the grounds that the lemon flavor is natural, even if nothing else in it is. Another's chemical-rich instant dinner boasts "natural chicken flavor"—hardly what mother would have simmered in her stew. The company that takes the granola cake, however, is the one that rationalizes an unfounded claim of naturalness by philosophizing existentially, "Our products exist, therefore they are natural. After all, they aren't supernatural!"

Wholesome. Before there was "natural," there was "wholesome." There still is—and it still doesn't mean anything. Certainly not when it's used to describe a "peanut butter oatmeal fudge jumble" cookie mix, whose list of ingredients is headed by sugar and followed by bleached flour, hydrogenated shortening, artificial flavors, and artificial colors. Or a "wholesome" serving of mini doughnut-shaped breakfast cereal that contains 11 grams of sugars for its 1 gram of protein, and an allstar cast of chemical additives.

Organic. Earthier than "natural" or "wholesome," "organic" is equally meaningless under the law. Any manufacturer can claim that a product is organic—that is, grown without chemical fertilizers or pesticides. Why, then, should the buyer beware? Studies demonstrate that organic foods are neither more nutritious nor freer of chemical residues than other foods— except possibly in Oregon, where they are checked for pesticides. The only thing you can be sure of is that they're more expensive. Products designated "health foods" are in the same gray category. The term has been dubbed by the FTC as "undefined, undefinable, and inherently deceptive."

Hi-energy. To a pregnant woman trudging sluggishly through the supermarket, "hienergy" on a label might sound like the product is the perfect antidote to her ever-present fatigue. It isn't. "Hi-energy" is nothing but a code word for the less marketable "high calorie." No technical deception here: Food energy *is* calories, after all. Just enough doublespeak to mislead the weary into an inappropriate purchase.

Lite/Light. From peaches to potato chips, there's a "light" (or "lite") at the end, beginning, and middle of every supermarket aisle. Though manufacturers using this increasingly popular product modifier hint at the lightening of calories and fat, they often follow through with neither. Makers of fried fish filets and sticks dubbed a new variety "Light and Crispy," though it contains almost 50 percent more calories and 16 percent more calories from fat than original varieties. A "light dough" ravioli is lighter on dough, but heavier on filling, therefore yielding more fat and calories than its thick-doughed counterparts. Be forewarned: With no federal standard for use of the word, many consumers who think they've seen the "lite" may really be in the dark.

The word *dietetic* can also lead you astray. It doesn't, as many of us may assume, automatically mean low in calories; it means the food has been adjusted for a special diet. According to the FDA, when the word appears on a label, the type of diet the product is appropriate for (low calorie, low salt, low sugar, or whatever) must be specified. Look for this information; if it doesn't appear, don't buy the product—the manufacturer is intentionally trying to mislead you.

For a more reliable guide to foods that will lighten your diet, look for the phrases "low calorie" or "reduced calorie." Both are FDA regulated. "Low-calorie" food may contain no more than 40 calories per serving and no more than 0.4 calories per gram. "Reduced-calorie" items must have at least one-third fewer calories than normally prepared equivalent foods.

The Fine Points of Fine Print

While the bold type can help to camouflage the contents of a food package, the fine print can help to reveal them. But as with a legal contract, you need to know how to decipher the fine print before you can use it to your advantage. So polish your magnifying glass (if your eyes aren't up to the job), and read on to find out how the small print can be a big help in determining what you get in the packaged foods you buy.

The ingredients list. The most valuable guide to what's behind a label, the ingredients list is required by the FDA on almost all food packages. The exceptions are certain staple products (such as mayonnaise, ketchup, canned vegetables, milk, ice cream, margarines, and some breads prepared from standard recipes stipulated by the FDA) and alcoholic beverages. Today, the ingredients are usually listed even when not required. Consumer advocates are pressuring the FDA to require ingredients information listed on the labels of alcoholic beverages.

Not only do ingredients lists tell you what's in a product, they tell you the relative abundance of each item. Ingredients appear in order of predominance, with the first ingredient the most plentiful and the last the least. So if you'd like to keep your sugar intake low, bypass products that have sugar (or any of its aliases; see page 168) at or near the top of the list. If you expect to get some protein from the meat sauce you're buying for your pasta, be sure that meat (not meat flavor) is among the first ingredients and not buried at the bottom of the list after salt and modified food starch. If you want to be wholly sure of your whole-wheat bread, check to see that whole wheat (not wheat or spring wheat) tops the ingredient list, and that no refined flours dilute the formula.

Also scan ingredients lists for additions food processors are not likely to brag about elsewhere on the label, such as hydrogenated or animal fats, and artificial preservatives, colorings, and flavorings.

The nutrition information label. A relative newcomer to the packaging scene, nutrition information labels are proliferating on supermarket shelves faster than health food stores in southern California, thanks to pressure from consumers and the FDA. More than 50 percent of the products that aren't required to carry this information do so anyway, with the cooperation of their manufacturers.

Nutrition information is offered in a standard form and must include: serving or portion size; number of calories per serving; grams of protein, carbohydrates, and fat, and milligrams of sodium per serving; and the percentage per serving of the United States Recommended Daily Allowance (U.S. RDA) for protein, five vitamins, and two minerals. Though the RDA for most nutrients is greater for pregnant and nursing women (see page 320), these tables can still be useful to you in evaluating the nutritional merits of a food. One that supplies high percentages of several nutrients for the average adult is a good candidate for your shopping basket. So is one that supplies a substantial number of grams of protein (remember, you will need four 20- to 25-gram servings daily) compared to calories (more than 300 calories per 25 grams of protein is high).

Optionally, a manufacturer may also include such information for multiple servings of food eaten more than once a day, such as bread or milk; the quantities (in commonly used units) of the listed nutrients; nutrition information for servings prepared as directed (cereal with milk added, pancake mix with egg added); ratio of polyunsaturated to saturated fats; amount of cholesterol; percentages of the U.S. RDA for 12 additional vitamins and minerals; and a breakdown of carbohydrates into starches, sugars, and fiber.

Warnings. Unlike warnings on over-the-counter drug labels, warnings on food labels aren't aimed directly at pregnant or nursing women. For example, the small type on saccharin products warns of the risk of cancer, but makes no mention of the possible effects of the artificial sweetener on the unborn child. When in doubt about whether or not a product warning extends to use in pregnancy, check with your practitioner or the March of Dimes. (For saccharin, see page 195.)

How to Not Get What You Don't Want

For the pregnant woman surrounded by a marketplace full of over-sugared, over-salted, and over-processed foods, knowing how to screen product labels for ingredients she doesn't want is almost as important as knowing how to identify those she does. The following ingredients are among those you will want to limit or to omit from your diet entirely through judicious label reading.

Sugars. To many shoppers, bypassing sugar seems as easy as passing by the cake, cookie, ice-cream, and candy aisles without stopping (see page 39 for why you *should* bypass sugars). It isn't. In fact, there is probably no aisle—besides household and beauty aids—in the entire supermarket that is sugar-free. Sugar is everywhere, including where you'd least expect to find it. It's a major ingredient in many popular condiments (most ketchups, barbecue sauces, and salad dressings, including some found in health food stores, are at least one-third sugar). It fills more than half of many cereal boxes and jars of nondairy creamer, and as much as a quarter of some packages of chicken coating mixes. Though not detectable by the untrained tongue, sugar also makes unexpected, but significant appearances in such "savories" as hot dogs, luncheon meats, gravies, soups, and spaghetti sauces.

And you can't banish sugar from your table simply by loading your shopping cart with products marked "No sugar added," or those that don't have "sugar" listed as an ingredient. "Sugar," when listed on a package label, usually means sucrose, or ordinary table sugar. But there are many other forms of sugar with less familiar names. All of the following not only taste as sweet, but are equally high in calories and generally devoid of nutrients: honey, brown sugar, turbinado sugar, raw sugar, corn syrup, high-fructose corn syrup, corn sweeteners, maple syrup, molasses, fructose, dextrose, dextrin, and sucrose.[1] Check ingredients listings for all of these.

It's crystal clear that a product is high in sugar when any of these sweeteners tops the ingredients list. It's less clear when a product contains two (or more) sugars, neither of which alone is a major ingredient but when added together, exceed any other single item on the list.

Occasionally, you may be

---

1. Honey, molasses, and maple syrup have insignificant traces of nutrients. Of all sugars, only blackstrap molasses can be considered to have nutritional value. It is notably high in calcium and iron.

lucky enough to find a product label that includes "carbohydrate information," which lists the total number of grams of sugar in a serving (most cereals labels do), both added sugars or naturally occurring ones. More than two grams of added sugar per serving (about one-half of a teaspoon) indicates a relatively high sugar content.

Artificial sweeteners. Ever since cancer scares (sparked by animal research) caused cyclamates to be removed from the market completely and saccharin products to carry a warning label nearly as threatening as those on cigarettes, sugar substitutes have provoked consumer uneasiness. This wariness toward non-caloric sweeteners slackened somewhat with the introduction of aspartame (NutraSweet, Equal), which is composed of two amino acids (proteins) and has not been shown to cause problems in normal healthy people, including women who are expecting a baby.[2] Still, occasional worrisome comments from skeptical researchers have prevented complete eradication of concern.

Because of this concern among consumers, some founded, some not, manufacturers

tend to try to sweet-talk their way into our shopping carts, carefully keeping the words we don't want to see ("sugar," "artificially sweetened," "saccharin") out of the big print, and instead boasting, "No sugar," or "No artificial sweeteners," or "Naturally sweetened," making products of dubious nutritive value sound desirable. To be sure no unwanted sweetener is lurking in the foods you buy, check the ingredients list. Check the list, too, to be sure the product is otherwise nutritious, which isn't always the case.

Salt or sodium. If sugar is found in every aisle, sodium is found in virtually every food in every aisle in your market. Unprocessed, some foods contain only a trace, while others (particularly dairy foods and some vegetables) are naturally high in sodium. Most processed foods (even those that don't taste salty, such as desserts, pastries, and cereals) have considerable amounts of salt (sodium chloride) added. (To find out how much salt is enough and how much is too much during pregnancy, see page 50.)

To help consumers keep the salt in their diets to acceptable levels (which may mean less than 1,000 milligrams per day for a person with high blood pressure), the federal government now specifies standards for the

---

2. Individuals with phenylketonuria (PKU) are unable to metabolize phenylalanine, one of the amino acids, and should not use aspartame. Nor should children under two.

STOCKING THE KITCHEN

Bare cupboards were fine for Mother Hubbard, but she wasn't pregnant. You are—or will be soon. So once you've stripped your kitchen of all the things babies don't need for growing and thriving, it's time to restock with all the things they do need (including those items that, though not necessarily nutritious on their own, are invaluable in the preparation of delicious and nutritious meals and snacks). Any or all of the following make Best-Odds shelf liners.

In the Cupboard

Brown rice, wild rice*
Whole-grain or high-protein pastas
Kasha (buckwheat groats), bulgur, triticale
Whole-grain unsweetened hot cereals such as old-fashioned oatmeal or rolled oats, Wheatena, Ralston's
Whole-grain unsweetened or lightly sweetened dry cereals such as shredded wheat, Nutri-Grain, Grape Nuts, Cheerios or its health-food store equivalent, Special K (or others containing no more than 2 grams of sugar per 1-ounce serving)
Raw whole-grain flakes such as wheat, oat, barley, available in health food stores
Flours*, including whole wheat, whole rye, whole cornmeal, soy flour, and unbleached all-purpose flour
Unprocessed bran*, for cooking or adding to cold cereal
Corn for popping

Canned foods

Evaporated skim milk
Tuna and mackerel packed in water, sardines, salmon
Beans and peas such as kidney, garbanzo, lentils, Northern, black-eyed
Unsweetened applesauce
Fruits packed in juice (for use when fresh is unavailable)
Unsweetened solid-pack pumpkin and squash
Tomato paste
Tomatoes, tomatoes in purée
Tomato sauce
Artichokes, pimientos, black olives
Vegetable protein meat and poultry analogs

Miscellaneous

Vegetable cooking spray
Vinegars (try a variety)
Natural flavorings (such as vanilla extract)
Carob powder (for use as a chocolate substitute)
Unsweetened cocoa
Nonfat dry milk
Dried fruits, including raisins, apricots, figs, prunes
Unsalted nuts*, seeds*
Decaffeinated tea and coffee

Baking powder, baking soda
Unflavored, unsweetened
  gelatin

Dehydrated meat analogs
Herbs and spices
Best-Odds cookies*

Produce

Sweet and white potatoes
Onions, garlic, shallots

Bananas
Tomatoes

In the bread box

Whole-grain baked goods such
  as breads, bagels, rolls, pita,
  English muffins, sour dough*

Whole-grain crackers, bread-
  sticks, matzoh

In the refrigerator

Skim, low-fat, or nonfat milk
Low-fat buttermilk
Low-fat cottage cheese and pot
  cheese
Low-fat plain yogurt
Hard cheeses (preferably low-
  cholesterol and/or low-fat)
Tofu
Fresh fish, poultry, meat
Mustard (have a variety on
  hand), horseradish
Mayonnaise
Butter, margarine, polyunsatu-
  rated oil
Yeast (for baking bread)

Eggs (including some ready-to-
  eat hard-cooked)
Wheat germ
Fruit butters and preserves
  made with fruit only
Peanut and other nut butters
Fresh seasonal vegetables
Salad greens
Fresh seasonal fruits
Tomato or vegetable juice
Natural fruit juices (including
  unsweetened blends)
Seltzer
Ice water
Wine for cooking

In the freezer

Apple, pineapple, grapefruit,
  orange juice, and unsweetened juice blend concentrates
Unsweetened fruit popsicles
Ripe bananas (peeled and
  wrapped before freezing)
Unsweetened berries for milk-
  shakes or snacking
Grapes for snacking

Frozen vegetables (for use
  when fresh is unavailable)
Frozen unsweetened fruits
Best-Odds or juice-sweetened
  commercial baked goods
Soup stocks
Nuts*
Whole-grain breads (for longer
  storage)*

*Asterisked items should be kept in the refrigerator (for medium-term) or the freezer (for long-term) storage. Bread should be frozen if not used on the day of purchase.

use of such claims as "low salt" or "unsalted." "Low sodium" means 140 milligrams or less per serving, "very low sodium" to 35 milligrams or less per serving, and "sodium free" to less than 5 milligrams per serving. "Reduced sodium" indicates that the salt content has been cut by at least 75 percent as compared to similar products, while "unsalted" means that no salt was used in processing a food that is usually salted.

The number of milligrams of sodium per serving is included as part of the nutrition information label. What it means to the pregnant consumer is relative. Three hundred milligrams of sodium in a main course is fine; 300 in a dessert or cereal is high. Keep in mind that authorities have set a safe outside limit of 3,300 milligrams of sodium daily for those not on salt-restricted diets, and many experts believe a much lower intake is desirable. If you're drinking four glasses of milk a day, you're already taking in about 500 milligrams of sodium; if you're tapping cheeses as a major calcium source, your sodium tally will be even higher. So calculate your other purchases accordingly.

Fat. A pregnant woman can easily overdo the fat before she's finished breakfast if she isn't familiar with the many disguises of this high-calorie nutrient. To avoid excess fat, don't buy foods with any of the following high on the ingredients list, or with two or more anywhere on the list: shortening; lard; salad, vegetable, partially hydrogenated, hydrogenated, sesame, cottonseed or other oil; animal, vegetable, chicken, beef, or other fat. "Low-fat" on a product does not necessarily mean it is low in fat. Low-fat and skim milk cheeses, for example, are often as high in fat as regular cheeses. Check the grams of fat per serving. They will range from only a quarter of a gram per ounce of low-fat cottage cheese to nine or more grams per ounce of Cheddar. The fewer grams of fat, the better off you are.

Don't be confused by labels that specify "no cholesterol." This doesn't mean a product is low in fat. Peanut butter, for example, has no cholesterol but is 50 percent fat; each tablespoon provides half a Best-Odds fat serving.

Cholesterol. Pregnant women (and to some extent, all women in their childbearing years) are thought to be naturally protected against the artery-clogging effects of cholesterol. Still, high intakes of cholesterol don't do anyone's body any good, particularly the body of any adult male in the family. Since "cholesterol" won't be found in an ingredients list, the only way to spot it if it isn't noted with the nutrition information is to look for the following high-cholesterol ingredients: eggs or egg yolks; whole milk or cream (sweet or sour) and dairy products (cheeses, yogurts) made with them; and animal fats (butter; suet; lard; chicken, beef, and other meat and poultry fats and drippings). Also high in cholesterol are fatty beef, lamb, and pork; organ meats; specialty meats (salt pork, sausages, frankfurters, cold cuts and luncheon meats); some shellfish (shrimp, scallops, lobster); some poultry (duck and goose); and all poultry skins. If a cholesterol count is listed on the nutrition label, remember that the American Heart Association recommends a cap on cholesterol of 300 milligrams a day for most people, as little as 150 milligrams for those with atherosclerosis or high cholesterol levels.

But cholesterol isn't the only culprit, and labels that boast "contains no cholesterol" or "contains no animal fats" do not automatically give the product a clean bill of health. Saturated fats from vegetable sources (such as those found in coconut oil, palm oil, cocoa butter, and hydrogenated fats), also raise blood cholesterol levels, increasing the risk of heart disease. Somewhat less hazardous, but still undesirable for the cholesterol-conscious, are foods that contain partially hydrogenated shortenings.

You needn't cut out all cholesterol during pregnancy. Moderate amounts from eggs, cheese, fish, lean meats, and poultry should be okay. When cooking, stick to the "good" oils, the ones that don't raise blood cholesterol levels and that may actually lower them. Particularly good are olive and canola, with safflower, sunflower, corn, and soybean next best. The margarine-butter controversy is a little less clear. Neither is especially good for the heart, so using them in minimal quantities is probably best. Stick to vegetable oils for cooking and baking.

Additives. Very few consumers buy a product for the additives it contains. Manufacturers recognize this. And though they're not always willing to omit additives from the insides of food packages, they are often more than willing to leave them off the outsides. They accentuate the negatives consumers see as positive: "no preservatives," "no artificial flavors." Unfortunately, these claims are no guarantee that the product is completely additive-free; the absence of one type of additive does not in any instance ensure the absence of all others. The only real insurance is their absence from the ingredients list.

All additives in a product

must be included in the ingredients list (although some, such as flavorings, colors, and stabilizers need not be identified by name, making it impossible for a consumer to know exactly which chemicals they're splashing on their pancakes, serving with tea, or guzzling after tennis). Not all are potentially harmful, however, and some are actually healthful (such as ascorbic acid, which is vitamin C). See page 313 for a list of safe, unsafe, and questionable additives.

BEST-ODDS COOKING

Your kitchen cupboards are now stripped of all traces of dietary indiscretion and laden with only the best food selections discriminately chosen from supermarket shelves. Your odds of making a success of the Best-Odds Diet are already quite good. By following through from the store to the stove, with the final phase of Best-Odds food preparation—Best-Odds Cooking—you can turn those good odds to excellent ones.

The demise of most dietary regimens is caused by tastebud ennui. That's why Best-Odds Cooking concentrates not just on turning out food that satisfies the baby's needs for nourishment, but also the mother's—and the rest of the family's—need for gastronomic pleasure.

That sounds like a tall order, but it's no mystery to master if you pull these ten Best-Odds cooking tricks from your chef's hat. Apply them to any of your favorite recipes.

Trimming the Fat

Keeping to your limit of one or two tablespoons of added fat daily can be extremely difficult or relatively easy depending on the cooking techniques you use. These can make it almost effortless.

Low- or no-fat sautéing. Do all your sautéing in a nonstick pan coated with a vegetable cooking spray. For no-fat sautéing, add small amounts of stock, wine,[3] or water, as necessary, and stir frequently to keep food from sticking. For low-fat sautéing, use ½ to 1 full teaspoon of oil or butter spread evenly on the bottom of the pan.

No-fat browning. Brown chicken and meats without fat in a preheated nonstick pan coated with a vegetable cooking spray. Pour off any fat that accumulates in the pan before cooking meats further.

---

3. Simmering wine or other spirits for five minutes during the cooking process evaporates their alcohol content, making them safe for pregnancy use.

Low- or no-fat egg and pancake cooking. Fry, scramble, omelet your eggs or prepare pancakes or French toast in a nonstick pan coated with a vegetable cooking spray. For a buttery flavor, add just ½ teaspoon of butter or margarine before cooking.

Low-fat baking. Substitute another liquid (such as apple juice concentrate, apple juice, or milk) for half (or even more) of the oil or melted shortening called for in cake, cookie, and muffin recipes. The final result will be less oily or buttery, with a somewhat different texture than when made with more fat, but very acceptable—and often better than the original.

Fat-reduced salad dressing and dipping. Reduce the oil in a salad dressing recipe to ½ to 1 tablespoon per serving; substitute other liquids, such as stocks or juices (apple, orange, pineapple, tomato, depending on the desired flavor), yogurt, or buttermilk. When using mild-tasting vinegars, such as balsamic, the proportion of vinegar to oil can also be significantly increased to taste. Puréed raw vegetables (such as cucumber, zucchini, watercress, and arugula), tofu, cottage cheese, yogurt, and buttermilk (instead of sour cream and mayonnaise) can also give flavor to dressings and dips without adding fat.

Low- or no-fat broiling or barbecuing. For no-fat broiling or barbecuing of fish and poultry, rub with complementary herbs, garlic, and/or spices, and baste with wine (see footnote, page 174), lemon, stocks, or a combination. For low-fat grilling, brush lightly with oil, melted butter, margarine, or mayonnaise before seasoning and basting. (For all low- or no-fat barbecuing, be sure the grill is well coated with a vegetable cooking spray before heating in order to prevent sticking; a "grilling rack"—again, sprayed—makes turning easier, especially when grilling fish.) When using marinade recipes, decrease oil to one tablespoon per cup marinade; replace with wine or stock.

Reduced-fat roasting. Roast meats and poultry on a rack that will allow fat to drip off. Add one inch of water and a few pieces of celery, carrot, and onion to the pan before cooking, adding additional water as needed to prevent burning. When cooking is completed, remove vegetables (they can be discarded or puréed in gravy), drain accumulated liquid into a bowl, and chill. Remove fat when congealed, and use remaining drippings for gravy.

Fat and skin trimming. Trim all visible fat from meats and remove all skin and fat from poultry before cooking.

Fat skimming. When possible, prepare soups, stews, potted meats, and gravies ahead of time and allow to chill (in the freezer for fastest cooling) so that fat can be easily skimmed off the top. When this isn't possible, allow a few minutes for the fat to rise after the soup (or other dish) is removed from the heat. When the fat has collected on the top, skim with a spoon or skimmer. If the mixture is at room temperature, an ice cube or a paper towel brushed over the surface may also lift off some of the fat. For separating fat from pan drippings, invest in an inexpensive gravy separator.

Low-fat thickening. Instead of thickening sauces, soups, and gravies with egg yolks or the traditional roux of flour and butter, try cooking them down and/or thickening with puréed cooked vegetables (particularly tasty in soups), tofu (adds a creaminess), mashed potato (gives a very smooth texture), or a combination. In some dishes, corn or potato starch may do the trick. If you do use a roux, use a minimum amount of fat to flour. In pâtés and desserts that usually depend on melted fats such as butter or pork fat, which harden later for firmness, substitute unflavored gelatin (dilute 1 tablespoon in each 2 cups of liquid or semi-liquid) for perfect form without the fat.

Striking the Sugar

Though most cooks are accustomed to using sugar in everything from soup to nut tortes, it is one of the easiest ingredients to strike from recipes. Here's how.

No-sugar baking. When baking cakes, cookies, and muffins, omit the sugar and use instead thawed and undiluted frozen juice concentrates (apple, orange, pineapple, or a combination, depending on the desired taste), unsweetened fruit juices (apple, orange, prune, pear), and puréed banana for all or part of the liquid (milk, water, oil, melted shortening, juice, or egg yolks) in the recipe. In general, if approximately equal amounts of juice concentrates replace the sugar, the result will be equally sweet. (Omitting the sugar will change the texture of baked goods somewhat; however, what is lost in texture is gained in richer flavor.) Raisins, dates, or other dried fruits can also be added to batters; chopping and/ or simmering them in juice concentrates can increase their sweetening power further. Stepping up the spices somewhat (particularly cinnamon) and the vanilla will also add sweetness.

No-sugar cooking. Impart extra sweetness to milk shakes, fruit soups, puddings, ice cream, and sorbets with mashed or puréed *very ripe* bananas (for convenience, peel and freeze ripe bananas whenever you have a bunch on hand, and process frozen as needed), fresh or un-sweetened frozen fruit or ber-ries, fruit juices, or fruit juice concentrates (depending on sweetness desired). Substitute apple juice concentrate, mixed with orange or pineapple juice concentrate when tanginess is desired, for sugar-water syrups in sorbets, fruit soups, and poached fruits. Add fruit-only preserves for extra fruit flavor, sweetness, and thickness. Use these, too, with or in place of fresh fruit in plain low-fat yo-gurt. Cook apples for applesauce in small amounts of apple juice or cider.

Sugar-free savory seasoning. Where a pinch or so of sugar is called for in salad dressings, soups, sauces, biscuits, and other nonsweet foods, an equal amount of apple juice concen-trate will do the job as well. Sweet and savory dishes (stuffed cabbage, borscht, carrot-sweet potato tzimmes, Cumberland sauce, oriental sweet-and-sour dishes) are not only as good sweetened with fruit juice, they are usually more flavorful.

Watching the Salt

Salt, for most pregnant women,

is a necessary dietary staple (see page 50). But recipes often call for an unnecessarily heavy hand with the salt shaker, and using excess salt in cooking isn't a good habit to get into. Learning to use other seasonings that can replace salt wholly or partially is a skill that can have lifelong ben-efits. If anyone in your family is on a salt-restricted diet, cook without salt using the following tips and let yourself and those who are on normal diets salt at the table. If you are only trying to reduce your family's intake of salt as a precaution, salt lightly in cooking and use these tips to enhance flavors.

Low- or no-salt seasoning. Lightly salted or unsalted dishes can be made rich in flavor if taste compensation is made in the form of garlic, onions, shallots, herbs, and spices. In these cases, excess is best; heady amounts of garlic or biting amounts of hot spices will leave diners blissfully unaware of salt reduction or elimination.

Salt substituting. Lemon juice added to a bubbling pot of pasta will have almost the same effect as salt. You can also substitute a slightly acidic taste for a slightly salty one by using lemon juice, wine, or vinegar in salads and vegetable, fish, and poultry dishes. Lemon chicken, for ex-ample, does very nicely without salt. Do not use potassium chloride, sold as a salt substitute, without medical advice. It can be hazardous.

Sweet seasoning. A pinch of sweetness (juice concentrate, not sugar, please) can often substitute for salt in bringing out the flavor of foods. Sweet dishes, or sweet-and-sour ones, can go salt-free more easily than savory ones, so serve them often if you must restrict salt.

Low-salt baking. Although it's not commonly recognized, we get a lot of our sodium intake from sweet baked goods. To reduce this source of salt, use low-sodium baking powder, substituting 1½ teaspoons for each teaspoon of regular baking powder.

Sneaking in the Milk

Expectant mothers needn't drink a single glass of milk during their entire pregnancies in order to supply their growing babies with adequate amounts of calcium. For those who don't have a milk intolerance but just can't tolerate drinking milk, the taste can be disguised.

Nonfat dry milk fortifying. A third of a cup of dry milk is equivalent to a cup of liquid milk. Stir it into hot or cold cereals; include it in pancake, cake, and muffin batter; use it in milk shakes, decaffeinated coffee (for café au lait), and in puddings and other desserts. In baking, reduce the dry ingredients by the amount of unreconstituted dry milk you add.

Evaporated skimmed milk "creaming." A half cup of evaporated skimmed milk is equal to one cup of regular skim milk in both calories and nutrients. Though it has no fat, it adds richness as well as calcium and protein to soups, homemade ice "cream," puddings, and sauces.

Yogurt enriching. Nonfat or low-fat yogurt in soup, salad dressing, or topping for poached fruit provides cup-for-cup more calcium and protein than milk. It offers the same benefits when turned into a frozen dessert or a predinner vegetable dip, added to a sauce or gravy, mixed with fresh or frozen fruit, or topping a bowl of cereal and fruit.

Saving the Vitamins

Even the fruits and vegetables that are richest in vitamins and minerals stand to lose a lot of what they have to offer if stored and prepared incorrectly. Here's how to best reap the benefits of their just-picked goodness.

Separating the greens. The greens on root vegetables, such as carrots, continue to thrive on nutrients drawn from the roots. So buy such root vegetables with the greens already removed, or remove them immediately on purchasing.

Cutting the cooking. Eat fruits and vegetables raw at least part of the time. Since heat destroys some vitamins, particularly vitamin C, the availability of nutrients in all fruits and most vegetables is greatest when they are uncooked. (Carrots are an exception; though unquestionably nutritious and high in fiber when raw, their carotene is more easily absorbed by the body when cooked.) When cooking is called for, lightly does it. Vegetables cooked to a crisp-tenderness retain their nutrition best.

Storing the vitamins. Cold temperatures help keep vitamins from getting away, so store ripe fruits and vegetables in the fridge. To further avoid unnecessary vitamin loss, don't wash and cut them before storing. And definitely don't store them soaking in cold or ice water to stay crisp; the water will end up with more of the nutrients than the vegetables.

Vitamin-preserving preparation. Air, light, and water speed vitamin loss. So the less peeling, cutting, and soaking vegetables and fruits undergo, the more vitamins are saved. Prepare just before cooking, so there is less time for nutrients to migrate (don't shell those peas until you're ready to throw them in the pot). Peel and cut only when necessary (keep zucchini unpeeled, potatoes unpeeled and whole, for instance, during cooking; but be sure unpeeled produce is scrubbed well first, see page 204). Puréeing allows the escape of many nutrients, so limit the use of this preparation process and when you do use it, purée just before serving.

Vitamin-retaining cooking. Fruits and vegetables don't need to be watered once they've been harvested. Cook them in water, and you'll throw out the vitamins with the cooking water. Instead, steam vegetables, cook them in a "waterless" pot with only a drop of water, pressure cook, or stir-fry them—again, to the just-tender stage. (Cooking in water is fine for soups and stews, as long as you'll be consuming the liquid into which the vitamins have escaped, but even then, don't overcook vegetables. Add them at a point that will have them tender when the rest of the dish is cooked.) Poach or bake fruits and serve them in their juices. Never retain the color of produce by adding baking soda during cooking; your vegetables will be sprightly in hue, but sluggish in nutrition. A bit of salt added to vegetables just after they begin to steam can help retain color without depleting nutrition.

Pouring on the Protein

With your protein requirement doubled during pregnancy, you'll have to be doubly as inventive to meet your daily quota. These additions to your diet will barely intrude on your caloric intake, yet will help push your protein count to the recommended 100 grams.

Wheat germ. Not just an esoteric health food to be stirred into your carrot juice, protein-rich wheat germ is one of the most valuable and versatile items in your refrigerator. Each quarter-cup of wheat germ added to your hot or cold cereal; sprinkled on your yogurt, fruit, salads, puddings, pasta, or pizza; or baked into your cakes, breads, cookies, casseroles, or meat loaves provides 9 grams of protein plus a bevy of essential B vitamins almost unequaled in any other food.

Egg whites. The two parts of the egg are not created equal. Slightly more than half of the egg's protein, and none of its fat, is stored in the white. What's more, egg-white protein is the best-quality protein, and is available at only about 15 calories per medium white. Add hard-cooked egg whites to all kinds of salads, including egg salad, extra egg whites to pancakes, loaves, and fritters.

Nonfat dry and evaporated skimmed milk. Milk isn't just an excellent source of calcium, it's a potent source of protein, too: each full cup of dry milk is a full protein serving, and so is each cup and a quarter of evaporated skim milk. Add them in all the ways suggested on page 178.

Cottage cheese. For a mere 180 calories, a cup of low-fat cottage cheese yields more than a full serving of protein. Enjoy its yield in fruit and vegetable salads, in soups and oatmeal (serve à la mode, then stir in for rich creaminess), as a cream cheese substitute in desserts (such as our Cheesecake), as a ricotta substitute in casseroles and pasta dishes, and as a sour cream substitute (puréed with buttermilk to the desired consistency) in dips (see page 294). And, of course, enjoy it as a ready-to-eat main course whenever you're short of time.

Tofu. Because it has little taste of its own and a texture that allows it to be creamed, crumbled, sliced, or chunked, this chameleonlike soybean derivative can add protein to almost any dish. Puréed, it can become a dip or the creamy base for a soup or dessert. Frozen for a few days, thawed, and crumbled, it makes an excellent base for chili or "meat" sauce for pasta. Breaded, seasoned, and sautéed or baked, it becomes a crunchy hors d'oeuvre; sliced, layered with cheese and tomato sauce, it's a lasagna. Add it to salads, to stews, to soups—each five or six ounces, depending on the variety, is a full protein serving.

Fitting in the Fiber

The growing evidence that high-fiber diets may prevent some kinds of cancer and even heart attacks may be of less interest to the expectant woman than the long proven fact that it prevents constipation. Though most plant foods start out high in fiber, preparation and cooking can have an impact on whether they are still high in fiber when eaten.[4]

High-fiber food selection. Choose foods high in fiber (see page 83) when you market.

High-fiber food preparation. The closer to its original form a plant food is when you serve it, the higher its fiber content. A raw apple, for example, is higher in fiber than a baked apple, which in turn has more fiber than applesauce; apple juice is fiberless. So keep peeling, cut-

ting, and puréeing to a minimum, and use edible stems and leaves whenever you can.

High-fiber baking. Use only whole grains, which have far more fiber than refined flours, in all your baked goods (see page 107 for flour equivalents). Add extra fiber by substituting 2 tablespoons bran for 2 tablespoons flour in each cup called for in your favorite recipes. Adding nuts, dried fruit, or wheat germ will increase fiber, too. Bran can also be added to meat, fish, and vegetable loaves, but should first be soaked in broth, juice, or other liquid until softened.[5]

High-fiber cooking. Cooking breaks down the fibers that constitute roughage, so the less cooking of most plant foods, the better. Eat vegetables and fruits raw or cooked just-tender. Grains and legumes (beans and peas), of course, are rarely eaten raw or even lightly cooked. Fortunately, they retain most of their fibrous structure even after long cooking.

Going for the Whole Grain

Banishing refined grains from your kitchen and replacing them

---

4. Try to avoid serving foods high in fiber, such as bran, at the same meal as foods high in calcium because fiber interferes with the absorption of calcium by the body. Don't add bran to your cereal if you are getting a major part of your calcium requirement from the milk in your bowl; don't wash your bran muffins down with a glass of milk. If you do mix bran and milk, count only half of the milk in your calcium allowance.

5. If your diet includes your Daily Dozen requirements for complex carbohydrates and fruits and vegetables, you needn't add additional bran unless constipation is a problem. Excess fiber in the diet is both unnecessary and unwise, since it can interfere with the absorption of several nutrients.

with whole grains is relatively easy. But for those who've never tackled whole-grain cooking before, just what to do with these unfamiliar, if nutritious, ingredients may be a major barrier to using them.

Whole-grain selection. Start with whole-grain ingredients; see the Food Selection Group, page 59.

Whole-grain baking. Whole grains can be used successfully in virtually every type of baked good—from cookies to pie crusts—providing more flavor and a heartier texture. Substitute the appropriate whole-grain flour or meal for the refined using the chart on page 107. Since the whole grains are heavier, more rising power will be needed; add an extra half teaspoon of baking powder for every teaspoon called for.

Whole-grain coating and stuffing. Whole-grain bread-crumb mixtures and stuffing mixes aren't widely available in the market, but they are readily made at home. To make dry bread crumbs for coating poultry and fish, process in the blender whole-wheat matzoh or whole-wheat bread that has been toasted until dry, but not browned. (For fresh bread crumbs, process fresh or frozen bread.) Or use one part wheat germ to one part whole-wheat flour. To either coating mixture, add desired seasonings, such as salt, pepper, Parmesan cheese, paprika, garlic and onion powders, and appropriate herbs to taste. For stuffings, substitute whole-wheat bread cubes, corn bread made with whole-grain cornmeal, and brown or wild rice for the refined products you usually use.

Whole-grain filling. Cut the cost of meat loaves, hamburgers, and meatballs without cutting the nutrition by using wheat germ, soft whole-grain bread crumbs, and/or rolled oats or other raw flaked grains as fillers.

Splitting the Eggs

Though you can safely have a whole egg every day when you're expecting, your husband (or any adult male) probably shouldn't. So when cooking for the two of you, keep in mind that his total, according to American Heart Association standards, should not exceed three whole eggs a week. In most recipes, you can easily substitute whites only for whole eggs, generally two whites to one whole egg.

Egg-white binding. You can use egg whites alone to bind meat, fish, and vegetable loaves, burgers, pancakes, croquettes, and quiches. French toast can also be prepared with egg whites only, or with a mixture of whole eggs and egg whites.

Egg-white baking. In baked goods that call for whole eggs, egg whites can be successfully substituted as above. When a recipe calls for separating eggs, substitute liquid, such as apple juice concentrate, for the yolks (measure yolks before discarding[6] and substitute an equal amount of liquid). Other liquids will not beat until "thick and yellow," but in most cases, this will not significantly affect the results.

Egg-white coating. Substitute lightly beaten egg whites (plus milk or water) for whole eggs when breading fish or chicken.

Adding protein and volume with egg whites. Adding extra egg whites to scrambled eggs, omelets, and egg salads will increase protein content and volume with very little increase in calories and virtually no alteration in taste and texture. Use hard-cooked egg whites as a salad garnish.

ENLISTING FAMILY SUPPORT

You've read about remodeling your kitchen, changing your

---

6. Ask your veterinarian about feeding unused egg yolks to your pet. Discarding yolks may be difficult at first, but after a while it will be as easy as dumping the shell.

shopping ways, and revamping your style of cooking. All of which sounds sensible—and, unless you live alone, impossible. Your husband will never consent to a freezer that doesn't contain a half gallon of rum-raisin ice cream. Your three year old will doubtless balk at your unloading his chocolate chip cookies at the office. And both will surely protest the sudden appearance of unfamiliar breads in their lunch bags and unfamiliar cereals at breakfast.

Even if you did manage to sneak the Best-Odds Diet into your house, how long could it hold out in the face of such hostility? How long would it be before your husband refilled the freezer to his satisfaction, before your three year old started spending his afternoons at the better-stocked homes of friends whose mothers understood a kid's need for chocolate, before they both began demanding the return of familiar foodstuffs? And how long would your self-control last should their demands be won and your Best-Odds kitchen be refurnished in an irresistible array of worst-odds foods?

The answer? Not very long at all. Which is why your preparations for the Best-Odds Diet cannot be complete without a very important fourth step: the enlistment of your family as allies in your endeavor.

What's In It for Them?

It's obvious what's in it for you and the expected new family member if the rest of the family takes on the Best-Odds Diet. But what's in it for them?

For Father. A father-to-be whose wife gorges on doughnuts and heavenly hash (and all the other caloric rationalizations she's heard pregnant women are entitled to) is likely to put on almost as many extra pounds during her pregnancy as she is. Unlike those gained by his wife, none will be dropped at delivery. His wife's no-holds-barred eating is also likely to reinforce the worst in his eating habits, setting him up for a lifetime struggle against creeping obesity, making him a candidate for all the ailments of middle and old age—and a poor example for his unborn child (and those who preceded or will follow).

A father-to-be whose wife is on the Best-Odds Diet, however, has a much rosier prognosis, particularly if he goes on the regimen with her. While the Best-Odds Diet is designed to produce the healthiest possible baby, it can also yield a healthier, fitter father. Though it is intended to put between 20 and 30 pounds on you, it can, in its modified form (see following page), keep—and even take—

pounds off your husband. And should his new Best-Odds eating habits stick with him after delivery, the benefits multiply. Because it is low in cholesterol, saturated and total fats, free of refined sugars, and high in whole grains and fiber, the Best-Odds Diet can also help him ward off heart disease, certain types of cancer, and, possibly, diabetes.

For siblings. The ploys that your mother's generation used to get their children to eat better ("Popeye eats his spinach," "There are children starving in Africa," "No dinner, no dessert") may have changed slightly, but the goal of today's mother is the same: a healthier child through healthier eating. It's ideal, of course, to start your offspring off on Best-Odds nutrition in the uterus, as you're planning to do with the one you're presently expecting, but it's never too late for children to reap the benefits of improved diet.

The Best-Odds Diet has plenty to offer your already born. It can keep their resistance to illness and tooth and gum disease high, help them avoid the increasingly common problem of childhood obesity, and perhaps control hyperactivity (which has been linked in some children to the consumption of sugar and/or certain food additives). And, as another plus: Well-nourished children tend to do better in school. In the teen years, good diet can also reduce the possibility of acne. If the good eating habits stay with your children into adulthood, your children will, like their father, increase their chance of living a longer, healthier, and more productive life by lowering their risks of heart disease, cancer, and possibly other chronic illnesses. And, because good nutrition in childhood sets the stage for making healthy babies, they are likely to give you healthy grandchildren.

THE DAILY DOZEN FOR THE BEST-ODDS FAMILY

The Daily Dozen (see page 42) are as essential for fathers- and siblings-to-be as for mothers-to-be. But some alterations in quantities are necessary:

Calories. Father's calorie intake should be based on his needs. If he's gaining weight and doesn't want to, he's eating too many calories. If he's losing weight and doesn't want to, he's eating too few. And if he's maintaining a weight he's satisfied with, he's eating just the right number.

For children, the principles are the same, but the details are somewhat different. You know a youngster is getting the right number of calories when growth and weight gain continue on approximately the same curve from month to month and year to year. If there is a sudden jump in weight without a concurrent jump in height, he or she is probably consuming too many calories. On the other hand, if the weight gain doesn't keep up with height, then probably too few calories are being consumed. In either case, a consultation with your pediatrician should be made before making any drastic change in diet.

Protein. Everyone needs protein, but under normal circumstances no one needs as much protein as an expectant mother—and many non-pregnant Americans eat too much protein. Your husband probably needs about half your intake, or about two servings daily, and the children will need even less, depending on their ages. For toddlers ages one to three, the equivalent of about one adult serving or 25 grams is right (perhaps 1 ounce of hard cheese, 1½ cups milk, and 1½ ounces meat, fish, or poultry). For four to six year olds, increase that to about 30 grams (add an egg or ⅓ cup of cottage cheese or another ounce of meat). The requirement goes up another five or six grams for the seven to ten year olds (which means, perhaps, another cup of milk). By the early teens, the protein requirement is about two Best-Odds servings.

Vitamin C foods. The importance of vitamin C to health is becoming more and more apparent. Everyone in the family will benefit from at least 2 servings daily.

Calcium. If you've got teenagers at home, their calcium needs are just about the same as yours: 4 calcium servings a day (see page 56). For your husband and younger children, the requirement is lower, about 2⅔ calcium servings a day.

Green leafy and yellow vegetables and yellow fruits. Two or more servings a day will benefit all family members (see page 57). For toddlers, portions will be smaller.

Other vegetables and fruits. Two or more servings of these will provide vital fiber and added vitamins and minerals for husbands and children (see page 58).

Whole grains and other concentrated complex carbohydrates. Like you, the rest of the family should have six or more servings of bread, cereal, or other complex carbohydrates daily (see page 59). And like you, they should emphasize whole-grains. Again, portions for young children will be smaller.

Iron-rich foods. Though the iron requirement is always higher in women of childbearing age, and is higher still in pregnant women, all the members of your family should eat some iron-rich foods every day (see page 60).

High-fat foods. Everyone in the family over two years old should limit fat intake to 30 percent of calories. And no more than one-third of that should come from saturated animal or hardened vegetable fats. For the typical active 150 pound male, that means about 85 grams of fat (6 full servings). For a small child,[7] 6 to 7 half-servings are about right. Best fats to use in cooking: olive and canola oil. Next best, safflower, corn, and other polyunsaturated oils.

Salty foods. Too much salt isn't healthy for pregnant women, or other living things, including children and husbands. While a salt-restricted diet isn't necessary (unless your husband has been put on one by his doctor), salt should be used lightly in cooking and at the table, and high-salt foods (see page 169) should be avoided most of the time. This will keep your children from developing a taste for overly salted foods. To insure iodine intake, use iodized salt.

---

7. Babies and children under the age of two should drink whole milk.

Fluids. Now is a good time to get other members of your family used to drinking more healthy liquids, too. This is particularly important in hot weather and/or when they are exercising. Drink six to eight cups minimum daily.

Supplements. Though vitamin supplementation isn't as vital for your family as it is for you, it does make good dietary sense. Particularly for children, who may eat sporadically, a daily vitamin (in tablet or liquid form) is insurance that nutritional requirements will be filled even when appetite isn't up to par.

Winning the Family Over

Don't expect your family to jump on the Best-Odds bandwagon just because it's "good for them" (although your husband may thank you eventually). They are much more likely to participate if they know this is one way they can directly help both you and the baby. Some persuasive arguments for Best-Odds family dieting include:

It's hard to go it alone. Having to eat differently from everyone else in the family is a strain and, since it's everybody's baby you're eating carefully for, inherently unfair. For the father-to-be, sharing your Best-Odds regimen, supporting you through those moments of weakness, is possibly more important than coaching you through childbirth. It's a job that lasts nine months, instead of nine (or so) hours, and has far more impact on the outcome of pregnancy. For siblings-to-be, who in most cases won't even be able to take part in the birth, joining dietary forces with you is one of the few concrete ways they can contribute to the development of their brother- or sister-to-be.

Explain to your family how their eating habits can affect yours. How that box of cookies or that carton of ice cream meant for them calls out to you when your resistance is low. How their ordering your favorite pie à la mode in a restaurant can make you resentful, and ultimately rebellious. How a call for fast-food burgers every night is going to strain family unity.

Also explain that preparing special meals for one can be tiresome; preparing them for all, especially when everyone chips in, can be a treat.

It can be fun to go it together. There isn't only strength in numbers for you. A team effort, as any Little Leaguer can tell you, is rewarding for all its members. If other kids in the family are old enough to read, put them in charge of checking labels at the store and foods that come into the house for Best-Odds suitability. Have the kids help plan menus and bake Best-Odds treats to share with friends.

It tastes good. A prime point to push and to remember yourself: Healthy eating can be just as delicious, if not more delicious, than unhealthy eating. A batch of Fruity Oatmeal Cookies, a dish of Brown Rice Pudding, or a celebratory Nut Torte will state the case eloquently. Though a little adjustment is usually necessary for palates accustomed to a highly sugared or refined-flour taste, once it's been made, those palates may come to reject their former favorites.

Their efforts can pay off. By helping you stick to a better diet, they'll be helping you toward an easier pregnancy, a healthier baby, and a safer delivery (see pages 16 to 21 for explanations). For a concerned father, all of these can be prime motivations, as can the incentive of a slimmer postpartum wife (see page 23). For siblings, knowing that they're helping to "make" the baby can give them a sense of pride and accomplishment.

EIGHT

What's Safe to Eat—and What's Not

O PEN A NEWSPAPER TODAY TO A VARIETY OF ALARM-ing reports on the dangers of foods and other ingestibles, and you may wonder if it's safe to open your mouth—especially if you're pregnant or nursing. Is oral gratification as hazardous to expectant and nursing mothers and their babies as we read and hear it is? The answer, happily, is rarely. True, a few things that we can put in our mouths are completely unsafe and should be avoided. Some things are questionable and should be limited. Others are risky but can be made safe. But most, your taste buds will be happy to know, appear to be harmless—at least when consumed in moderation as part of a sensible diet, and when you're observing one of the cardinal principles of a safe diet: variety (see page 154).

WHAT TO AVOID WHEN YOU'RE EXPECTING

The only substance known to be damaging to the fetus in every instance of use is the drug thalidomide, and even this drug is teratogenic (capable of causing birth defects) only during certain stages of development. Most items that have been labeled hazardous to a developing fetus only increase the risk of birth defects or of pregnancy or birth complications, they don't guarantee them. Still, with some substances (alcohol, for example) the increased risk is significant enough for the Food and Drug Administration (FDA), the

March of Dimes, and most obstetricians to suggest total or near total abstention from them during pregnancy, and limitation during nursing. Some—tobacco, for example—should be avoided during pregnancy *and* lactation.

Alcohol. The signs posted in bars and liquor stores in New York City reading "Warning: Drinking alcoholic beverages during pregnancy can cause birth defects" may be new, but the message they're carrying isn't.[1] Though many expectant women and their health-care providers chose to ignore it, the writing was on the wall long before the signs went up. In fact, the theory that the use of alcohol in pregnancy presents hazards to the fetus has been around since ancient times. And as far back as 1759, the London College of Surgeons attempted to persuade lawmakers to raise taxes on gin to make it less available to expectant mothers.

Today, the United States Surgeon General recommends that women who are pregnant or who are considering pregnancy abstain from alcoholic beverages. And the evidence that supports this recommendation continues to grow. Studies show that women who drink heavily (usually considered to be five or six cocktails, glasses of wine, or bottles of beer a day) during pregnancy have a 30 percent to 50 percent chance of having children with Fetal Alcohol Syndrome, a set of signs and symptoms that includes mental retardation, central nervous system disorders, growth deficiencies, facial abnormalities, and other malformations, particularly of the skeleton, urogenital tract, and heart. It's been estimated that alcohol may be responsible for five out of every 200 congenital anomalies and is the most frequent substance-related cause of mental retardation in the Western world. Though the evidence is less clear, more moderate drinking has been linked to such negative pregnancy outcomes as low birth weight (at levels of as low as one to two drinks a day) and miscarriage (at levels of two drinks two to six times a week). Some studies show that alcohol use increases the chance of premature delivery, others do not.[2]

The truth is, the facts are confusing. Just what level of alcohol consumption at what point

1. An increasing number of communities are posting similar warnings to pregnant women.

2. Since tests on the effects of alcohol on human pregnancy cannot be scientifically regulated, evidence is based on animal studies or on epidemiological evidence, in which women are asked to report on how much alcohol they drank (or are drinking) in pregnancy. Their answers are correlated with the rate of birth defects or birth effects in their pregnancies. This is not an extremely accurate methodology, since many people tend to under-report their drinking.

during pregnancy is risky is not at all certain. The issue is further confused because other factors can influence the effect of alcohol on the fetus: genetic predisposition (one of a pair of fraternal twins may be affected by the mother's drinking, while the other is not); smoking (smoking *plus* alcohol poses a greater risk than either alone); and poor nutrition (not only does inadequate nutrition compound the effects of alcohol, but women who drink tend not to eat properly).

Since even light drinking throughout pregnancy hasn't been cleared, and since no "safe" upper limit has been determined, abstinence is the only completely risk-free position an expectant mother can take toward alcohol. Every drink taken during pregnancy is shared with the unborn baby. The alcohol crosses the placenta in concentrations almost identical to those in the mother, having immediate impact on the fetus' central nervous system and interfering with its breathing movements.

This doesn't mean the expectant mother should worry about the drinks she had before she found out she was pregnant. Even a couple of episodes of binge drinking during early pregnancy haven't been proven to be harmful—many women have unwittingly indulged before they discovered they were pregnant without there being

any ill effect. And it also doesn't mean the woman should despair if she's already drunk herself halfway into her pregnancy; an expectant mother's chances of bearing a healthy child are significantly increased *whenever* she gives alcohol up (whereas they are significantly decreased if she continues to drink in the third trimester).[3]

What it does mean is that a pregnant woman should give up alcohol completely. Don't even use wines or other alcoholic beverages in cooking, since recent research shows the alcohol does not fully evaporate. If you decide to take a very occasional celebratory sip or two, do so with food, which slows the absorption of alcohol into the system. Even a sip, of course, is risky if you have a history of uncontrolled drinking. If you are a heavy drinker and do not intend to take steps to become sober, you should discuss this fact with your doctor. (For tips on giving up alcohol, see page 145.)

That alcohol might also present a problem for nursing mothers is a more recent discovery. A generation ago, the prescription for a copious milk supply was a daily glass of beer. Today we know that it takes a

---

3. It appears that damage done by alcohol during the formation of organs may often be repaired, and inadequate growth compensated for, by abstention in the latter half of pregnancy.

good overall diet and not fermented hops and barley malt to produce adequate milk for an infant. In fact, although an occasional cocktail or glass of wine or beer won't interfere with milk production or be harmful to baby, daily or heavier drinking may.

First of all, alcohol is dehydrating, causing valuable fluids to be excreted rather than utilized in making milk. Second, like most drugs, alcohol passes into the breast milk. In large doses, this depressant is capable of making a baby sleepy (and thus unable to suck), sluggish, and unresponsive, and in very large doses can interfere with breathing. And as little as one drink a day has been linked to slower motor development. Third, excessive quantities of alcohol can impair your functioning as well as your baby's. It can make you a less effective mother, more susceptible to depression, fatigue, and lapses in judgment, as well as a less effective source of milk since it weakens the let-down reflex. Finally, like any nutritionally empty food or beverage, alcohol can either add excess calories (and thus pounds) or divert your appetite from taking in the necessary nutrients.

So go ahead and enjoy an occasional drink. Many women find that after a particularly hectic day, a drink can relax a tense let-down reflex. But limit yourself to no more than one drink at any one time (one drink equals 12 ounces of beer, 5 ounces of wine, or a 1½-ounce shot of distilled liquor). Take it with food, or at least not on an empty stomach, and be sure to rehydrate yourself with a glass of water or other nonalcoholic fluid for each drink you have.[4]

Other socially used drugs. Like alcohol, marijuana, cocaine, PCP, heroin, methadone, and other "recreational" drugs can cause catastrophic problems in the fetus and newborn, including addiction, low birth weight, premature delivery, placental problems, behavior disorders, and birth defects. Don't put any drug in your mouth (or anywhere else) if you care about your baby-to-be. Or, in fact, if you care about yourself.

Tobacco. Smoking has always been hazardous to human health; it's just that we haven't always known it. However, since 1964, when the U.S. Surgeon General's report on the hazards of smoking came out, officially implicating cigarettes in the development of lung cancer, millions of Americans have been knowingly risking their lives to

---

4. Some brands of beer and Scotch have high levels of a form of nitrosamines, which are believed to be carcinogenic. Look for brands that say "no preservatives."

smoke. Expectant and nursing mothers continue to risk their own lives when they smoke, but studies now show they also risk the lives and well-being of their babies.

It's not lung cancer or heart disease that is a risk for your baby if you smoke when you're pregnant, but a myriad of other, often no less devastating, medical problems, including low birth weight (the major cause of newborn death), placenta previa (a placenta located dangerously low in the uterus), placenta abruptio (a placenta that separates prematurely), miscarriage, major congenital malformations, Sudden Infant Death Syndrome (crib death), and, possibly, long-term intellectual deficiencies and behavioral difficulties. The effects of tobacco on pregnancy are serious enough to warrant a warning from the surgeon-general on cigarette packages.

Why talk about smoking in a book on nutrition? First, because cigarettes, like food, are a form of oral gratification, one which often serves to replace food and thus interfere with nutrition. And second, because much of the good you can do with the Best-Odds Diet can be undone with smoking. Smokers are notoriously poor eaters (many consciously choose to smoke rather than eat, a habit that is particularly dangerous during pregnancy). This is one of the rea-sons why smokers are much more likely than nonsmokers to have low-birth-weight babies. On the other hand, an expectant mom who smokes can partially compensate for this deleterious effect by eating a great deal. This, of course, presents her with another problem: although she may have a normal weight baby, she risks the many hazards of excessive weight gain in pregnancy.

But a compensatory weight gain will not prevent or reverse the other complications related to maternal smoking. The by-products of smoking, such as nicotine and carbon monoxide, cross the placenta. They, plus alterations in the mother, such as increased blood pressure and reduced blood flow to the uterus, caused by smoking, are believed responsible for a deprivation of oxygen, which interferes with growth and development—both of the fetus and the placenta. If you don't believe that your baby is smoking with you, smoke a cigarette in your practitioner's office (with permission, of course), and ask to have the fetal heartbeat monitored as you do. You'll find that your baby's heartbeat speeds up abnormally during the first 7½ minutes or so after the first puff and continues rising for another 10 minutes.

Though cutting back is better than continuing to smoke at your usual rate, it is rarely a successful ploy. The smoker who cuts back usually compensates unconsciously by taking more puffs and smoking more of each cigarette in an attempt to get his or her usual quota of nicotine. It won't help to switch to low tar and nicotine cigarettes, either. Not only will your body, craving its nicotine fix, prompt you to smoke more, you (and your baby) will still be taking in many of the other hazardous constituents of tobacco that are not reduced in such cigarettes. Quitting is the only safe route for both you and baby. Quitting as soon as possible in pregnancy is ideal, but even quitting two days before delivery can reduce the risk of oxygen deprivation to the fetus during childbirth. For tips on quitting, see page 145.[5]

A woman who gives up tobacco during pregnancy but plans to start lighting up again after delivery should know that smoking when breastfeeding is no more salubrious for her or her baby than when she's pregnant. Nicotine and other toxic substances in the tobacco smoke inhaled by the mother pass from her bloodstream into her milk. The baby gets additional doses of these substances by breathing in the smoke the mother exhales. All of the long-term health effects of these toxic carcinogenic

substances aren't known, but we can assume they aren't positive. Short term, we know that a baby whose parents smoke is much more likely to suffer from respiratory illnesses than one who isn't exposed to secondhand smoke ("passive smoking"). Presumably, you wouldn't stick a lighted cigarette in your baby's mouth. Don't give him one indirectly by sticking one in your own.

Smoked or cured meat and fish. Cigarette smoking isn't the only smoking that's potentially hazardous during pregnancy and lactation. Smoked and cured meat and fish can present a risk, too, if they contain sodium nitrite, which can be converted in our stomachs to nitrosamines, powerful carcinogens and possible teratogens. Bacon, ham, cured pork, sausage, smoked salmon and other smoked fish, dried beef, luncheon meats, salami, and frankfurters usually do. Eat them, or other foods containing sodium nitrite, only rarely or not at all during pregnancy and while you're breastfeeding. (Beer and Scotch can also contain high levels of nitrosamines, and since manufacturers aren't required to list the ingredients of alcoholic beverages, you won't be able to find out by checking a label—unless the label specifies "no preservatives." Avoid beer or liquor that may

---

5. A more complete program for tobacco cessation appears in *What to Expect When You're Expecting* (New York: Workman, 1985).

contain this chemical when you're breastfeeding, and all alcoholic beverages when you're pregnant.)

Sugar Substitutes. Whether they fear for their weight, their teeth, or their general health, Americans today are shying away (or at least talking about shying away) from sugar. They are turning instead to a mixed bag of other sweeteners—which, depending on the sweetener, may be wise, or not so wise. Though no fetal damage in humans has been linked to saccharin use, it has not been proven safe for use in pregnancy, and so using it would fall in the not-so-wise category. Also unwise would be using products sweetened with cyclamates (presently banned but under review in the U.S. and available abroad), which has been linked to birth defects. Aspartame (NutraSweet, Equal), on the other hand, appears to be safe for pregnant women who do not have a problem metabolizing phenylalanine (see page 169), so moderate use should pose no problem. Be wary, however, of ingesting a lot of aspartame-sweetened foods that are otherwise nutritionally empty or filled with questionable chemicals. And consider fruit-juice sweetened products, when they are available, a wiser option.

There appear to be no deleterious health effects from sorbitol and mannitol, two relatives of sugar that are absorbed more slowly by the body than sugar, though large doses can have a laxative effect. Sorbitol is not of any benefit to the weight watcher since it has as many calories for its sweetening power as sugar. Mannitol can be used for calorie-reduced diets because it is not completely absorbed by the body. Both appear safe to use during pregnancy, though, like sugar, they offer only empty calories.

Caution in using sugar substitutes is necessary, too, when breastfeeding. Since saccharin crosses into the breast milk, don't have more than an occasional product sweetened with it while you are breastfeeding. Aspartame (Equal, NutraSweet) seems to pass into the breast milk in only small quantities, so its moderate use, as well as the use of sorbitol and mannitol, in otherwise nutritious foods shouldn't pose a problem while you're nursing.

Caffeine. When your mother was pregnant, she may have given up coffee because she developed an early first trimester aversion to it. Today, pregnant women are giving up (or cutting down on) coffee and other caffeinated beverages (teas, colas, chocolate drinks) even when

KICKING THE CAFFEINE HABIT

For the casual coffee drinker, giving up the occasional cup won't take any special effort. But even for the one-cup-a-morning drinker, and, especially, for the heavy caffeine user, the habit won't be so easy to kick. There will be both physical and emotional withdrawal symptoms (including headache, fatigue, and lethargy), which can range from minor to temporarily debilitating. With the following decaffeinating program, they can all be minimized or eliminated, and even the most ingrained habit kicked.

Identify your motivation for quitting. In all kinds of habit-kicking, this is the first step. And in your case, it should be clear-cut: to give your baby the best odds of being born healthy.

Determine what needs the caffeine (or the beverage it's in) fills. If it's the need for a hot start to your day or end to your meal, switch to a naturally decaffeinated coffee or tea. If it's the taste of coffee or tea you crave, a good-quality, brewed decaffeinated variety is likely to satisfy even the most particular palate. (Decaffeinated espressos are as dark and rich as the caffeinated kind.) Unfortunately, if it's a caffeinated cola your taste buds are hankering for (or that your thirst is thirsting for) you can't opt for a decaffeinated variety, since all soft drinks are taboo in pregnancy. You can, however, substitute a refreshing glass of club soda or seltzer, flavored with lime or lemon or mixed half-and-half with any unsweetened fruit juice. If you pour a cup of coffee, tea, or cola for lack of something better to do with your hands or your time, do something else. Work out on your stationary bicycle. Clean out the closet you're planning to use for baby. Make a baby layette list or a list of prospective baby names. Bake up a batch of Best-Odds Banana Muffins, or scrub and cut a selection of vegetables for snack-time crudités. If your habit is more of a ritual—you take your coffee with the morning paper, your tea with the late-night news, a cola after your

they don't develop an aversion—and for good reason. While caffeine was not suspected of being harmful to the unborn a generation ago, recent studies have raised some questions about the safety of this stimulant drug during pregnancy.

The questions have yet to be fully answered. Although animal studies have shown a connection between caffeine intake and birth defects (particularly delayed skeletal development), human studies have not. Still, until more conclusive evidence is available, the Food and Drug Administration and many experts recommend that women run—change the time and place of the ritual and the beverage that goes with it. Read the paper on the way to work, watch the late news in bed, end your run at a juice bar.

For most caffeine abusers, it will be the caffeine lift that's most missed. Though there is no pregnancy-approved direct substitute for this drug-induced high, there are roads to reaching a more natural one. Orange juice may do the trick, particularly for that midmorning or late-afternoon droop. Once the fatigue of caffeine withdrawal has worn off (see below), you'll be able to get more long-lasting lifts from exercise (dancing, walking, jogging, tennis doubles, swimming, making love) and good food (particularly protein).

Taper off if you're a heavy drinker. If you're accustomed to six cups of coffee a day, cold turkey quitting will be too great a shock to your system, which is used to several caffeine fixes daily. Let your body down easy; cut back by a cup every day until you're off the stuff.

Keep your energy up. A dipped-down blood sugar level will only aggravate your withdrawal fatigue and headache. Eat frequently (either snacking between three large meals or eating six small meals a day), concentrating on high protein and complex carbohydrate foods, and don't skip your vitamin supplement. Exercising in moderation (particularly in the fresh air) can also pick up a sagging energy level, though overdoing it will only compound your fatigue. Getting enough sleep is necessary if you're trying to combat fatigue; let your body be your guide in filling your shut-eye requirement. (Nap, if need be, to get through the worst of the withdrawal drag.)

The caffeine-withdrawal droop should last only a few days after you've had your last dose of the drug. It should not be confused with the fatigue of pregnancy, which is most pronounced in the first and third trimesters, but which some women find stretches unabated throughout their nine months.

should discontinue or, at least, reduce their intake of caffeinated beverages while pregnant.

For the nursing mother, caffeine in large doses presents other problems. Newborns don't need caffeine to keep them up at night; they usually do a good job of that on their own. But pump a baby up with too much caffeine (through the coffee, strong tea, or caffeinated sodas you drink) and you may find him or her having trouble sleeping, day or night, and being jittery and irritable. One or two cups of caffeinated beverages a day will probably not affect your baby; more probably will. (More may also affect your ability to cope calmly with the stresses of new motherhood. And because your body becomes dependent on the caffeine "lift," you will feel more tired when the caffeine wears off than you would feel if you'd had no caffeine.) Supplement the real thing with the decaffeinated varieties, if necessary.

There are other reasons for avoiding caffeine during pregnancy and lactation. It's a diuretic that draws out of your body the fluids you and your baby need during pregnancy and that you need in order to make milk when you're breastfeeding. In addition, caffeinated beverages offer poor nutrition; they fill you up without filling a single requirement for nutrients. And they are often loaded with either sugar or the still questionable sweetener aspartame.

Monosodium glutamate. Since 1908, when a Tokyo researcher discovered that this sodium salt of glutamic acid, an amino acid, could greatly enhance the flavor of protein foods, MSG has been popular both in oriental cookery and in processed foods. It can cause what has been dubbed Chinese Restaurant Syndrome, usually characterized by a burning sensation in the back of the neck and forearms, tightness in the chest, and headaches. The symptoms are temporary and believed harmless. More serious is the brain damage it has caused

in studies on infant animals. Because it could presumably do damage to human infants as well, it has been removed from baby foods. Whether it can also damage a developing fetus is not certain, and so expectant mothers are wise not to consume MSG in large quantities. Do not use it in cooking, ask that it be omitted from your meal at oriental eateries, and avoid processed foods that list it as an ingredient. If, however, you occasionally ingest some MSG accidentally, there doesn't appear to be any cause for concern.

WHAT TO USE WITH CARE

Though the list of potential prenatal and postnatal perils you may have heard or read about may be a supermarket-aisle long, you can still eat, drink, and enjoy—if you take a few precautions when shopping for, preparing, or using the following.[6]

---

6. Reducing your intake of unwanted chemicals now is important, but previous ingestion may cause a problem, too. Potentially harmful substances you may have been exposed to prior to becoming pregnant are stored in your body's fat tissue. To avoid their being released suddenly into your bloodstream (and thus into your fetus') when you're pregnant, or into your milk when you're breastfeeding, do not diet strenuously between conception and weaning. You should avoid losing weight entirely during pregnancy, and should lose only gradually while breastfeeding your baby.

Processed foods. The chemical revolution that took American kitchens by storm in the 1950s was cheered on wholeheartedly by an entire generation of convenience-craving home-makers. As preservatives, artificial colors, artificial flavors, and stabilizers multiplied faster than laboratory mice across the nation, Americans marveled at the miraculous properties of additives. They heightened the intensity of flavor and color in foods, they kept salt and spices from caking, bread from molding, ice cream from melting too fast. Because of them, commercial sauces and gravies could stir up as thick as home-simmered in seconds; hot cereals, potatoes, even whole dinners could appear cooked and ready at the first pang of hunger.

After scarcely two decades of celebration in the home and marketplace, however, these heroes of the fifties became the villains of the seventies and eighties. Today's health-conscious consumers look askance at additives, consider them unnatural, and thus, unhealthy. They view "natural," on the other hand, as synonymous with "good" and "safe." This generalization, however, is a false one. Sugar and eggs are natural, but sugar is nutritionally bankrupt and causes tooth decay, and eggs are implicated in heart disease. Natural farm-fresh spinach contains oxalic acid, which can be toxic in large doses. Natural aflatoxins, sometimes found on spoiled peanuts and grains, are the most potent carcinogens known.

And just as everything natural isn't naturally good for you and your baby, everything that is "chemical"—formulated in a laboratory—isn't naturally bad. All foods, from the garden variety tomato to the laboratory variety tomato-flavored sauce, are made of chemicals. A just-picked, organically grown strawberry, for instance, is composed of acetone, acetaldehyde, methyl butrate, ethyl caproate, hexyl acetate, methanol, acrolein, and crotmaldehyde. Chemical additives found in processed foods are synthesized in the lab from a wide variety of organic and inorganic materials, or extracted from completely natural sources (sodium caseinate from milk, lecithin from soybeans). Some are suspected of being harmful (those that are indisputably proven to be harmful are taken off the market), more are believed to be harmless (though testing is often inadequate), others are necessary and even beneficial (for example, ascorbic acid). None that are currently being used have, to this date, been proven teratogenic or toxic to a nursing baby. Most, however, have not been conclusively cleared.

Under these circumstances,

KNOW MORE ABOUT FOOD SAFETY

The Center for Science in the Public Interest is a nonprofit public interest organization that produces an excellent newsletter *(Nutrition Action Health Letter)* and a variety of other materials, books, even software for the nutrition-conscious consumer. If you want to know more about the safety of a particular food, write CSPI, 1501 16th Street, NW, Washington, DC 20036.

a bit of caution is advisable. Read labels carefully and avoid frequent, repeated use of the additives on page 313 that are considered suspect or are not recommended during pregnancy and/or nursing.

Even when they aren't on the "least-wanted" list, additives should signal "think again" when you are considering a product. A long list of additives on a label is a clue that the item doesn't contain top-grade ingredients and may be less nutritious than a similar food without additives. Using a few tomatoes plus tomato flavoring and thickening agents and water in a tomato sauce, for example, is a lot cheaper and quicker for a manufacturer than using a lot of tomatoes and cooking them down. Adding inexpensive red color to the sauce gives it the appearance of a homemade sauce without the costly ingredients in Mama's recipe. (Sometimes, a coloring is added to make a food look even more vibrant than its homemade cousin. The result is often unnaturally vivid in hue, something those reared on processed foods are unlikely to discern.) Heavy doses of salt and sugar are also used in processed foods to compensate for the lack of quality ingredients, another reason to avoid such foods. Preservatives, on the other hand, are sometimes used for the opposite reason: to preserve the freshness of a quality ingredient (such as whole-wheat flour) that might otherwise spoil on the shelf.

Herbal tea. Some of the greatest oral perils for pregnant and nursing women are not manufactured in laboratories, but in fields and forests by Mother Nature herself. They are marketed not with warning labels, but as natural and healthy, and they line the shelves not of pharmacies but health food stores. They are herbal teas. Though touted by their proponents as "natural tonics" or "remedies," many have been condemned by medical experts as unsafe, even deadly. Some are capable, particularly in large doses, of causing a variety of alarming symptoms, including diarrhea, vomiting, and heart palpitations. In Mexico, tea brewed from the zoapatle leaf is used to induce abortions, and ergot alkaloids have also been used to terminate pregnancies. Slippery elm, cohosh, pennyroyal, mugwart, and tansy have been linked to miscarriage.[7]

Herbs are often such powerful drugs that many are used in purified form in pharmaceuticals. Foxglove, for example, is refined into digitalis, used to treat heart ailments. Because no drug, no matter how "natural" its origins, should be used during pregnancy and lactation unless under the advice of a physician, stay away from unprescribed herbs or herbal teas that contain any ingredient not ordinarily found in your diet (orange rind and dried apples would be okay, but hibiscus and chamomile might not be). If you enjoy herbal-type teas, make your own using juices, orange or lemon rinds, fresh mint, cinnamon, cloves, or other familiar ingredients, and, if you like, decaffeinated tea.

Vitamin supplements. Because vitamins cross the placenta during pregnancy and are excreted in the breast milk during lactation, when you take vitamins your baby is taking them, too. This can be good—and bad. Good if the vitamins you are taking are specially formulated for use during pregnancy and lactation (see page 32)—this guarantees that your baby will get, either through the placenta or your milk, many of the major vitamins he or she needs. Bad if you take additional vitamins, especially in megadoses (large doses far in excess of the RDA) without your physician's approval. Those vitamins that present the most danger are A and D, both of which can be toxic in doses not very much higher than the RDA. Vitamin C is also suspect. A small-scale 1960s study showed that vitamin C in megadoses could make a fetus or baby dependent on the vitamin. Further studies have not substantiated this, but it's unwise, nevertheless, to take large doses of vitamin C without your doctor's approval. More recently, animal studies have fingered lecithin, a phospholipid, frequently found in supplements. The research showed that even slightly higher than normal intakes of lecithin could cause brain abnormalities in rats. The message for expectant mothers: Don't supplement your diet with lecithin.

Random use of megadoses of any nutrient is risky because vitamins work synergistically in

7. Raspbery tea is frequently touted as a surefire way of inducing a lazy uterus into labor. Do not experiment with it without your practioner's permission.

the body. A very high dose of one may increase the need for another, and thus may set up a deficiency that didn't exist before. Very high doses of zinc, for example, may lead to iron deficiency.

Also avoid unpurified sources of nutrients. Calcium from bone meal or dolomite, for instance, has been found contaminated with lead, arsenic, mercury, and other potentially toxic metals. "Herbal health pills" have been found to be contaminated with lead.

Drugs and medications. The warnings plastered on most over-the-counter medications and on the package inserts of prescription drugs would suggest that drugs and pregnancy and drugs and breastfeeding don't mix. In most cases, this is a wise suggestion. The vast majority of drugs do pass through the placenta or into the breast milk, with a variety of effects at varying concentrations.

During pregnancy, some drugs appear not to affect the fetus at all; others definitely do, some slightly, some significantly. (Except for the infamous thalidomide, no drug taken by the expectant mother has been found to invariably cause damage to the fetus, and even thalidomide did its damage only at specific stages of fetal development. Like thalidomide, most,

but not all, drugs are more dangerous early in pregnancy; these drugs are often safe to take when prescribed in the final trimesters. In general, taking a potentially harmful drug increases the risk of birth defects, but it doesn't guarantee a negative effect on the fetus. In fact, the increase in risk is often very small—doubling, for example, as in from 1 in 1,000 to 2 in 1,000.) Many drugs, however, are in a gray area at present—the centers listed on page 206 will provide the most up-to-date information).

During lactation, some drugs taken by the mother appear to have no effect on her baby at all; others have a mild transient effect, while still others are capable of having a significant detrimental effect.

Before the decision to use a drug during pregnancy or lactation is made, the potential effect of the drug on the fetus or baby should be weighed against the potential therapeutic benefits of the drug to the mother. Since our knowledge and understanding of these effects is constantly growing (and lists for lay people of drugs safe or unsafe for use during pregnancy or lactation are usually out of date before they're in print), the best source for guidance in making such a decision is a physician who is knowledgeable on the subject and has access to the most current reports on drug safety in pregnancy and lactation. If you're pregnant, your obstetrician should be most helpful, even if it's your family doctor or internist who is treating you for an illness (any doctor seeing you for any condition should be aware that you're pregnant). If you're nursing, your child's pediatrician will probably be the most useful consultant. Check with the appropriate physician before taking any drug (even an aspirin, acetaminophen, or ibuprofen tablet, an antacid, or a laxative). For additional information on drug safety, call the local chapter of the March of Dimes Birth Defects Foundation.

Sometimes, taking a medication can be postponed until after delivery (or until a later stage of pregnancy, when the development of vulnerable organs is complete) or weaning; sometimes a safer medication, or even a nondrug regimen, can be substituted for a risky one.[8]

When you're breastfeeding, there may be other ways of reducing the risk of drug therapy. One is to time the taking of the medication and the breastfeedings so that the lowest possible concentration of the drug is in your breast milk when your baby suckles. (Ask your doctor

to help you determine the best schedule.) Another is a temporary halt to breastfeeding. When you're pregnant you can't take your baby off placental feedings while you're taking a medication, but when you're nursing you can switch temporarily from breast to bottle if you're put on a potentially hazardous medication for a brief period. Pump your breasts to keep them from "drying up," and discard the milk. When drug treatment is completed, switch back to breastfeeding (your physician will be able to tell you when your milk will be drug free). Don't be discouraged if baby doesn't seem to want to resume nursing; it's easier to extract milk from a bottle than your breast. But if you persist (and don't give in to the bottle), the odds are good that baby will eventually pick up where he or she left off.

WHAT YOU CAN SAFELY EAT

Produce. Media reports on the presence of pesticides and other chemical contaminants in produce may have you wondering whether you have more to fear if you do eat your vegetables (and fruits) than if you don't. Since such chemicals can reach your baby, either through the placenta or through your breast

---

8. A variety of nondrug treatments for most common illnesses are described in *What to Expect When You're Expecting* (New York: Workman, 1991).

milk, it's a reasonable fear during pregnancy and lactation. It's a fear, however, that needn't keep you and your produce apart.

First of all, it's important to keep in mind that fetal damage linked to pesticides has shown up in the babies of women who were accidentally exposed to large quantities of the chemicals, not to those who ate too many apples. There is no hard evidence at this point that the small quantities of chemical residues found on produce can have a damaging effect on unborn children. Second, you can reduce any possible risk by being careful to follow the three principles of fruit and vegetable safety. *One*, always wash all non-organic produce with water and dish (*not* dishwasher) detergent or a product especially designed for washing produce. (A water rinse will suffice on produce you will be peeling). Scrub with a vegetable brush when possible; don't try scrubbing lettuce, mushrooms, or grapes, of course, but do scrub such produce as zucchini, bell peppers, apples, and potatoes. Then rinse thoroughly before eating or cooking (don't rely on cooking to inactivate the chemicals; it often doesn't). *Two*, vary the produce you eat; the types and quantities of residues differ from item to item, so the more variety, the less risk of a buildup of any one chemical. *Three*, when in doubt, peel. It's true that in the ideal world, where pesticides and other chemical residues don't contaminate our fruit and vegetables, we would never peel most vegetables and fruits (the peel retains nutrients and provides fiber), but in this imperfect world, peeling is sometimes necessary. Peel cucumbers, for example, when they seem coated with wax, or apples if the skin still has a film after scrubbing. Unfortunately, peeling removes only external residues; it does not remove those chemicals that have been absorbed by the fruit or vegetable.[9]

During the well-publicized Alar-apple scare several years ago, it was charged that the chemical daminozide (tradename Alar)—which was used to prevent preharvest fruit drop, increase storage life, and promote red color in apples—might cause cancer. Parents who were feeding their children gallons of apple juice each week were, not surprisingly, particularly worried. Because of heavy consumer concern and major press coverage most food processors quickly stopped using produce sprayed with Alar and the use of the chemical on produce was subsequently banned. Most significantly, the episode raised a number of questions about the safety of our food supply, many of which remain unanswered.

9. Always peel parsnips, which have naturally high levels of the chemical psoralen.

(There are even more questions about imported produce, which sometimes doesn't meet U.S. standards; pesticides banned here may still be in use abroad.) Though it's wise to be consumer concerned and to press both the government and farmers for a reduction in the use of pesticides on produce, it's important to keep in mind that to stop eating vegetables and fruits because of fear of chemical contamination is unwise. Not only do fruits and vegetables provide vital nutrients (nutrients that are particularly important in pregnancy), but many also contain natural substances that *protect us* from many of the very chemicals we fear.

Ideally, of course, all the produce we consume would be grown without hazardous chemicals—and someday that ideal may be realized. More and more supermarkets and health food stores are stocking organically grown produce these days. As demand for organics goes up, prices are coming down, though they are still usually higher than those charged for conventional produce. If you can find and afford organics (check to be sure those you buy are certified), by all means, buy them. Not only will you be giving yourself and your baby-to-be the benefits of pesticide-free food, you will be helping to protect the soil and water of this earth from further chemical contamination. If you can't, continue to take the above precautions—and don't worry.

Meat and poultry. Things aren't quite as wholesome down on the farm and back at the ranch as they used to be. There's an antibiotic, we hear, in pig feed to prevent outbreaks of swine dysentary and in chicken feed to control necrotic enteritis. There are traces of pentachlorophenol, a wood preservative and herbicide, in cattle feed and in the wood of the holding pens on which the animals like to chew. There are organophosphate insecticides on the crops grown for animal consumption, and on the animals themselves—applied to keep them free of grubs and flies. And there may even be steroid pellets (though they are illegal, their effectiveness in promoting weight gain and feed efficiency makes use tempting to the unscrupulous) implanted in the ears of cattle and sheep and in the necks of chickens.

Since all of these chemicals are believed to pose potential health hazards to all humans—particularly developing fetuses and nursing infants—the U.S. Department of Agriculture and the FDA have designed rigid inspection programs to help prevent significant residues from ending up in the meat we eat. However, with millions of animals slaughtered annually, only

TERATOLOGY INFORMATION CENTERS
IN THE U.S.

Through the following sources, your physician can obtain up-to-date information on current environmental hazards.

For computerized bibliographic searches

Environmental Mutagen, Carcinogen and Teratogen Information
   Department
Department of Pediatrics
T0083
University of California School of Medicine
La Jolla, CA 92093 (619-294-3584)

For interpretation of literature of specific agents

Teratology Service Program
Department of Pediatrics
Division of Medical Genetics
UMDNJ-Rutgers Medical School
CN-19
Academic Health Science Center
New Brunswick, NJ 08903 (201-937-7889)

March of Dimes Birth Defects Foundations
Community Services Division
1275 Mamaroneck Avenue
White Plains, NY 10705
(914) 428-7100 or your local chapter

a small percentage can be checked. So there's always the possibility that meat and poultry containing illegal levels of chemical contaminants await our purchase at our local butcher or supermarket.

Does this threat necessitate a switch—at least during pregnancy and lactation—to a meat-free diet? No. First of all, the risks are mostly theoretical. Very rarely has any ill effect been traced to chemical contamina-tion of meat, usually only when massive, accidental exposure occurred. Second, by being selective in the parts of the meat we eat (as recommended on the Best-Odds Diet), we can avoid most of the contaminants that might have ended up in the cow, chicken, pig, or sheep we're having for dinner. Most chemicals tend to congregate and linger in the fat and fatty organs, such as the liver, kidneys, and brains of all animals. To avoid their entry into your system and thus your baby's, stick to lean meats, always carefully trim any visible fat from meat and poultry, and eat organ meats infrequently (in spite of their high vitamin content). Because poultry skins also harbor unwanted chemicals, don't eat them (it's best to remove them before cooking, so their fat doesn't melt down into the flesh). Finally, remember the importance of variety in eating safely and well. Don't have chicken (or lamb, or veal, or anything) every night of the week. Alternate protein choices and you're less likely to take in significant amounts of any one chemical.

Chemicals aren't the only hazards in the meat eater's diet—at least for the expectant meat eater. Ordering lamb (or other meats) well done may be frowned on by gourmets, but for a pregnant woman, it should be a way of life. Raw and undercooked meats can harbor a parasite that causes toxoplasmosis, a disease so mild (its symptoms include a slight rash, some achiness, swollen glands, a low-grade fever) in an adult that it often passes unnoticed. In the fetus who contracts it, however (some 40 percent of exposed fetuses do), there is a one in three chance that serious illness, lasting damage, or even death may result.[10]

If you favor your meat rare or raw (as in steak tartare)—or if you have a cat at home—it's very possible that you have already been exposed to toxoplasmosis, and are thus immune to it. A simple blood test will reveal if this is the case. And if it is, you can feel free to order your meat to your taste (with the exception of pork, which should always be cooked to at least 137 degrees, and should be ordered "well done" in restaurants to prevent the possibility of trichinosis). If you turn out not to be immune, play it safe by ordering your meat well done in restaurants, and by cooking it at home to a temperature of at least 140 degrees (rare)—the temperature at which the parasite is killed—on an accurate meat thermometer. (Since the infection is much more threatening to the fetus in the second half of pregnancy than earlier on, don't worry if you've eaten raw or rare meat in the first months. Do, however, ask your practitioner to test you, and take precautions for the rest of your pregnancy if you are not immune.)

Dairy products. The same problems with chemical contamination exist on dairy farms as on

---

10. Toxoplasmosis can also be transmitted in the feces of cats (who can contract the disease from other cats or from mice they hunt), so a pregnant woman who is not immune should avoid caring for cats or having a cat in her home unless the cat is free of infection and is not allowed out of doors. And she should not garden in soil cats frequent.

cattle and chicken farms, which means that some residues end up in the dairy case as well. These, too, are easily avoided with a little informed picking and choosing. As with meat and poultry, fat is the storehouse for chemicals that end up in a cow's milk. Dairy products that are high in fat, such as butter, cream, whole milk, high butter-fat and cream-cheeses, and whole-milk cottage cheese and yogurt, are more likely to contain chemical residues than low-fat ones. For this reason (as well as the fact that they are inefficiently high in calories and dangerously high in cholesterol), high- or full-fat dairy products are not recommended on the Best-Odds Diet. Use low- or nonfat products instead.

Fish and seafood. Like other items in the food chain, fish (at least those that swim or spawn in inland waters that have been used as receptacles for chemical wastes) have not escaped the scourge of industrial society: pollution. The most serious hazard in such fish presently are polychlorinated biphenyls (PCBs). Because of the potential risk to the unborn (and to the already born, through contaminated breast milk), it's recommended that all women of childbearing age avoid fish that swim or spawn in lakes and rivers (including trout, perch, whitefish,

carp, salmon, and striped bass), unless the waters these fish have frequented are known to be unpolluted. Fish raised on "farms," for instance, won't be contaminated; salmon from the East Coast aren't safe, but those from Scandinavian or Pacific waters (as are most canned salmons) probably are.

To find out which fish sold in your area are risky and which aren't, contact your local Environmental Protection Agency (EPA) or health department. For the most part, the other fish in the sea (flounder, sole, snapper, tuna, sea bass, and sea trout, for instance) are your best Best-Odds bets. The exception is swordfish, which can contain high levels of methylmercury. Though the FDA sets limits on permissible amounts in swordfish for human consumption, it's probably a good idea not to have this fish on your menu frequently.[11]

Remember, of course, that as with most environmental risks, occasional exposure is unlikely to be hazardous to your fetus. Don't worry if you unwittingly tucked away a few lake trout dinners early in your pregnancy, just refrain from ordering it in the future.

---

11. If you believe you have had extensive exposure to PCBs, either through your work, through eating a lot of contaminated fish, or through other means, have your breast milk assayed before nursing your baby. High levels may mean you should not breastfeed.

All raw fish and seafood, such as sushi and oysters, should be strictly avoided during pregnancy and lactation. The parasitic organisms that fish and seafood sometimes contain can be dangerous, and will be killed with cooking.

Decaffeinated coffee. Just when caffeine refrainers thought they'd discovered a way to have their coffee and drink it without guilt, too, researchers began to find fault with decaffeinated coffee. They fingered the solvent used in the decaffeinating process, trichloroethylene, as a carcinogen. When the FDA threatened to pull it from the market, coffee companies switched to natural solvents, to a water process or other processes that employ no chemicals, or to another chemical solvent, methylene chloride. Though one 1981 study linked this new solvent to cancer, further studies found no such link. In addition, many contend that the chemical is rinsed away in processing and very little residue is left. According to the National Coffee Association, it would take 25 million cups of chemically decaffeinated coffee a day to cause any ill effects to the drinker. This may be an exaggeration, considering the associations' vested interests, but even if the danger level is much lower, it's pretty certain the most confirmed coffee addict isn't likely to get an overdose of methylene chloride by drinking decafs.

Faithfully adhering to the under 25 million cups a day limit, however, doesn't mean you're automatically safe. Because decaffeinated beverages (even those that are "safely" water processed) are no more nutritious than their caffeinated counterparts, both pregnant and nursing women should limit their consumption to no more than two or three cups a day. Decaffeinated soft drinks containing saccharine or sugar should generally be avoided during pregnancy and lactation; those sweetened with aspartame can be used in moderation (see page 195). Replace these questionable chemical cocktails with seltzer or mineral waters when you want calorie-free thirst quenching. If it's a sweet drink you crave, the sugar-free juices available are virtually limitless; they refresh best if mixed with seltzer.

Tap water. Water, water, everywhere, but is there a drop that's safe for expectant mothers to drink? In most cities across the country the answer is yes. Water is, in general, a lot safer today than it was a century ago when typhoid and other deadly diseases were spread through contaminated water. With the advent of chemical purification

FOOD POISONING: THE ALL-NATURAL PERIL

Though the risks from chemical contamination and chemical processing are largely theoretical (only in cases of accidental overexposure have there been proven significant ill effects on the population), these synthetic perils capture a great deal more public concern than the all-natural peril of food poisoning. But the risks from tainted food are not theoretical. An estimated 10 million cases of food poisoning occur each year in the United States; most are mild, but some are severe and a few even fatal.

For the pregnant or nursing mother, even a mild case of food poisoning can interfere with her nourishing her baby, so taking preventive steps is particularly important. To keep undesirable microorganisms from multiplying in the food you eat at home and to avoid tainted food when eating out, observe the following:

❖Wash your hands with soap and water before touching food and after handling raw meat, poultry, fish, or eggs, all of which harbor bacteria.

❖Cover any exposed cuts on your hands and arms before handling food to avoid germs from the wound contaminating the food. If you have a cold or other infection, wash your hands thoroughly before beginning, and again if you touch your nose or mouth.

❖Use a fresh, clean spoon for tasting (every time you taste) and serving food. Don't leave a perishable residue of yogurt in your mustard jar by using the same spoon in each. Wash can openers after using so particles from the food in one can won't stick to the blade and fall into the next.

❖Keep hot foods *hot*. Reheat leftovers thoroughly; bring gravies and soups to a rolling boil.

❖Keep cold foods *cold*. Food spoils fastest at between 60° and 120°F; do not keep at these temperatures more than two hours. Refrigerate foods that won't be served or cooked immediately. Don't stack food in the refrigerator or overload the shelves with warm foods; refrigerator air must circulate to preserve food.

processes, outbreaks of such diseases became nearly nonexistent. Do frequent water drinkers have as much to fear, as some environmentalists claim, from the chemicals that have wiped out these illnesses as from the illnesses themselves? If the answer was yes, then we would be seeing epidemic levels of birth

❖Never cool foods at room temperature. Quick-cool before refrigerating by dipping sealed containers in cold water.

❖When in doubt, throw it out—or send it back. If the odor or color of any food is poor or questionable it may be dangerous. Get rid of it, or, if you're in a restaurant, send it back to the kitchen. *Don't taste it first;* even one bite of contaminated food can be harmful. Also, discard cans that are swollen or leaking, jars that are cracked or have loose or swollen lids, and liquids that should be clear but are cloudy or milky.

❖Defrost meats and poultry in the refrigerator, in cold water (changing the water every 10 minutes), or in a microwave oven, rather than at room temperature.

❖Don't stuff meats and poultry until they are ready to go into the oven; cook stuffing to at least 165 degrees F. Store cooked stuffing and meat separately.

❖Clean all dishes, utensils, and work surfaces thoroughly with soap or detergent and water after each use, giving special attention to dirt-harboring cracks and corners. Don't use wooden chopping boards or butcher blocks for food preparation; their many natural and knife-created crevices collect potentially hazardous bacteria. For the same reason, discard chipped or scratched wooden bowls. Wash cutting boards with a soft sponge instead of an abrasive pad or cleanser, which can cause germ-harboring scratches.

❖Refreeze only those foods that are still cold or contain ice crystals and have been held no longer than one or two days in the refrigerator since thawing. *Do not* refreeze ice cream, or any food that is either off color or has a bad odor.

❖When selecting a restaurant, pass by those that have unrefrigerated perishable foods on display on the counter or in the window, and those that appear dirty and/or are fly-infested. Buy only from licensed street vendors; check to see if the food is kept properly heated or refrigerated, covered, and not handled with dirty hands.

defects today. The truth is, more healthy babies are being born than ever before.

That's not to say, however, that all tap water everywhere in the U.S. is uniformly safe for pregnant, or nonpregnant, people to drink. Because of variations in natural chemicals and run-off from industrial sites and in the modes of purification, water safety varies from community to community. To find out about the water that flows from your tap, check with your local health department, the Environmental Protection Agency (EPA), or a consumer advocacy group. Some questions you might want to raise are: Is the water chlorinated or filtered? (Filtering water is the safest way to purify; chlorinating risks the possibility of too high levels of chemicals, though in most cities levels are below the danger point.[12]) Is there run-off from farms or industries, or possible seepage from underground gas storage tanks, into reservoirs or other water sources? (These can raise the level of hazardous chemicals in the water.) Is there leaching of lead or other metals from pipes in the water supply? (This may be the case in your own home if lead has been used to solder the plumbing pipes.)

If you have any serious doubts about the safety of your water supply, don't just sit back with a glass of bottled water and worry about it. Check your Yellow Pages or ask the EPA to recommend a lab that does water analysis. Have the analysis done for the particular chemicals you are worried about. If your water does turn out to be questionable, there is much you can do. You can get a filter (what kind depends on the offending substance; check with your local EPA or the National Sanitation Foundation, P.O. Box 1468, Ann Arbor, MI 48106). Or, if chlorine or germs are a problem, you can boil your water before using for drinking or cooking. Or you can use bottled water that has NSF certification. (Avoid distilled water, which has been so purified that even the health-giving elements have been removed.)

If the problem is lead solder on your pipes, and replacement is out of the question (it's an expensive proposition), the solution may be as simple as letting the water run for five minutes first thing in the morning, or whenever it hasn't been used for six or eight hours, to clear out any standing water that has accumulated the poisonous metal. (If water is in short supply in your community, draw water in the evening and refrigerate for morning coffee, cereal, and drinking.) And don't use hot water from the tap for cooking; it leaches more lead from the pipes than cold.

12. Though high levels of chlorine compounds in water have been linked to cancer, they have not been linked to birth defects. And, in fact, in an animal study, rats drinking chlorinated tap water had no more birth defects than those drinking distilled water with minerals removed.

PART THREE

The Best-Odds Recipes

NINE

The Best-Odds Recipes

MOST COOKBOOKS FALL NEATLY INTO ONE OF TWO categories. Either they're a general collection, fairly evenly divided between appetizers, soups, salads, main courses, and desserts, or they concentrate on a single food or course, for example, all cheese dishes or all desserts. The Best-Odds recipes falls into neither category, and at first glance may seem oddly balanced, heavy on the desserts and baked goods and light on the main courses.

But there is a sound reason behind this selection. While most of your favorite main course recipes can be used as is or with a few Best-Odds adjustments (see below), most desserts and baked goods cannot. These recipes are intended to fill in the gaps left by your other cookbooks and in your own recipe repertoire. They concentrate on naturally sweetened sweets, whole grains, dishes rich in calcium and low in fat, nonmeat main courses that are high enough in protein to meet the needs of the pregnant or nursing vegetarian, and nutritious party foods, including festive nonalcoholic and sugarless beverages. Unless otherwise specified, the nutrition information accompanying each recipe is for one serving.

A COOKING PRIMER

Put down your spatula and pull up a chair. Like most recipe collections, this one repeats certain words, phrases, and ingredients over and over. Because even the most accomplished cooks may be unfamiliar with some of the following, acquaint yourself thoroughly with them before you begin cooking.

Juice concentrate. Instead of sugar, ubiquitous in most recipe books, you will find juice concentrate—most often, apple juice concentrate—in the Best-Odds recipes. This is the frozen juice concentrate found in your supermarket freezer. Use it completely undiluted, but, to measure it accurately, defrost it first.

Unsweetened juices, fruits, etc. To make sure that no sugars or artificial sweeteners have been added to your juices and prepared fruits, read labels carefully. Use canned fruits that come packed in unsweetened fruit juice or juice concentrates.

Fruit-only preserves. These are increasingly available in health food stores and supermarkets. They have both the sweetness and the texture of sugar-sweetened preserves but are sweetened only with fruit and fruit juices.

Eggs and egg whites[1] We generally used extra large eggs in testing these recipes, so this size will work best for you, too. Egg whites are on the ingredients lists much more often than whole eggs, not because you are at risk from the cholesterol-laden yolks (during pregnancy you probably are not), but for two other significant reasons. First, we assume you are cooking for

more than one and that the others who will be enjoying your culinary efforts are not expecting. They should be cautious about cholesterol. Second, the Best-Odds Diet, though designed primarily for use by pregnant women, is intended to steer you onto a dietary path you can stay on for life.

Vegetable oil. Any vegetable oil will work in Best-Odds recipes, but canola and olive are best, followed by such polyunsaturated oils as safflower and corn.

Margarine. Though margarines generally contain no cholesterol, they are very high in fat (as high as butter) and much of that fat is saturated or partially saturated. Look for a high ratio of polyunsaturates to saturates. Best margarines are health food store brands made without additives.

If you prefer butter, and spread it very lightly (no more than half a pat or teaspoon on a slice of bread), by all means, enjoy. A pat of butter has only 11 milligrams of cholesterol, and one a day shouldn't be a problem.

Skim milk. Our recipes specify "skim milk," but in many parts of the country milk from which the fat has been skimmed is called "nonfat milk" or "skimmed milk." Skim, skimmed, and nonfat milks are identical and interchangeable in recipes.

---

1. Recently, raw or undercooked eggs have been the source of serious salmonella infection. If the eggs you buy are suspect (ask your health department), shun recipes that use them raw.

Low-fat yogurt and other dairy products. We always recommend low-fat, skim, or nonfat dairy products because generally they are higher in protein as well as lower in fat, cholesterol, and possibly, chemical residues.

Rolled oats. This is the slow-cooking variety of oatmeal, which works better in cooking and baking than the instant. It is used raw.

Unflavored gelatin. This can be from animal or vegetable sources, but it must be unsweetened as well as unflavored. Check the label.

Stock. Stocks and broths give flavor to gravies, soups, and other dishes. Make a batch of vegetable and/or chicken stock to keep in the freezer, if possible. Or use bouillon cubes that contain no or few additives, no MSG, and preferably no sugar; thay are most likely available in the health food store.

The garlic core. How does one enjoy the garlic both while eating it and hours later when the indigestion usually sets in? By removing the slender core (or heart or germ) at the center of the clove when using the garlic raw or almost raw. The core slips out easily with a nudge from the tip of a knife when the clove is cut in half lengthwise.

Salt to taste. Each of us develops a different "salt palate." What tastes like just the right amount of salt to us may taste like too little or too much to you, so we suggest salting to taste. But, remember, although you needn't limit salt in pregnancy, a heavy salt habit is not good for anyone in your family.

Nonstick. Because nonstick surfaces require less fat in cooking, we recommend using them whenever possible (see page 156). We like to enhance their efficiency with a quick coating of a vegetable cooking spray (such as Pam). This spray can also turn an ordinary pan into a nonstick surface to some extent, and is perfect for "greasing" baking tins; so keep a can on your shelf.

Daily Dozen Servings. Following most recipes is information on how many Daily Dozen servings each provides per portion. This information is approximate, but you can safely use it as a guide in planning your day's food intake. When no listing appears, there is no preponderance of one single ingredient to make a Daily Dozen serving, but you can be sure that there is plenty of good nutrition.

Cereals

It's not news that cereals make excellent breakfast, but if you shut your cereal cabinet after 9 A.M. you're missing the opportunity to add snap, crackle, and nutrition to lunch, snacks, and even dinner. So, don't hesitate to enjoy cereal all day long, particularly when your stomach can't seem to tolerate anything else. Use ready-to-eat varieties with no or little added sugar (no more than 2 grams per serving). Cook up whole grains—there's everything from the old-fashioned oats and Wheatena your mother used to serve to seven-grain concoctions your mother never heard of. Whichever cereal you use, add calcium by stirring extra nonfat dry milk into the milk you pour over your cold cereal or into the pot when you've finished cooking your hot cereal (⅓ cup dry milk equals 1 Calcium serving). Add extra nutrition by stirring in 2 to 4 tablespoons wheat germ (2 tablespoons equal 1 Whole-Grain serving). And if constipation is a problem, add a tablespoon or two of wheat bran.

If you can't tolerate milk, don't forgo the pleasures of cereal. Use fruit juices instead, and enjoy.

ORANGE MUESLI

If you can't tolerate milk or don't consume dairy products, that doesn't mean you can't enjoy a good bowl of cereal in the morning. This muesli is one of the best. Prepare it the night before for easy morning eating.

Serves 2

1 cup rolled oats
¼ cup wheat germ
2 tablespoons raisins or currants
2 dates or figs, chopped
2 cups orange juice
1 tablespoon orange juice
   concentrate
1 cup diced seasonal fruits
¼ cup sliced almonds

1. Combine the oats, wheat germ, raisins, dates or figs, orange juice, and juice concentrate in a glass or stainless bowl. Refrigerate, covered, and soak at least 1 hour or over night.

2. Add the seasonal fruits and the almonds. Stir and serve.

3 Whole-Grain servings; 2 Vitamin C servings; 1 Fruit serving (depending on fruit used); ¾ protein serving.

GREAT GRANOLA

A versatile, crunchy treat to eat by the handful or bowlful, mixed with other cereals, and topped with milk or yogurt.

Makes about 5 cups

3 cups rolled oats
½ cup raisins
¾ cup plus 2 tablespoons apple juice concentrate
¾ cup wheat germ
¼ cup unsalted soy nuts
¼ cup unsalted sliced almonds or chopped walnuts
2 tablespoons raw sesame seeds
1 teaspoon ground cinnamon, or to taste

1. Preheat the oven to 350°F.

2. Spread the oats in a non-stick baking pan, 11 x 9 inches or larger. Toast in the oven for 10 minutes. Remove from the oven and reduce heat to 300°F.

3. Meanwhile, combine the raisins and ½ cup of the juice concentrate in a small saucepan. Bring to a boil. Reduce the heat, and simmer for 5 minutes. Drain, reserving the liquid and the raisins separately.

4. Add the raisin liquid and remaining ingredients except the raisins to the oats; combine well with a wooden spoon. Return the pan to the oven and toast for 20 minutes, stirring twice during baking.

5. Stir in the raisins well and press the mixture firmly into the pan. Bake another 5 minutes. Let cool to room temperature. Break up the granola and store it in a tightly covered container.

½ cup = 1½ Whole-Grain servings; ½ Protein serving; ½ Other Fruit serving.

CORNMEAL MUSH

Not only will your queasy tummy appreciate this dish, your taste buds will, too. Leftover mush can be chilled, sliced, then browned in a nonstick skillet for a tasty accompaniment to eggs.

Serves 2

½ cup whole-grain cornmeal (preferably yellow)
½ cup cold water
¼ teaspoon salt, or to taste
1½ cups boiling water

½ cup nonfat dry milk
½ cup low-fat buttermilk or yogurt
¼ cup wheat germ
¾ cup low-fat cottage cheese
White pepper to taste

1. Mix the cornmeal and cold

water together until smooth.

2. Stir the salt into the boiling water. Gradually add the cornmeal mixture to the boiling water, stirring constantly, and heat until the mixture comes to a boil again. Partially cover the pan and cook over low heat for 7 minutes, stirring frequently.

3. Stir in the dry milk, buttermilk, and wheat germ. Continue stirring over low heat until the mixture is hot. Stir in the cottage cheese, season to taste with white pepper and more salt, if necessary, and serve hot.

1½ Whole-Grain servings; 1 Protein serving; 1 Calcium serving.

Variation: For Cheesy Cornmeal Mush, substitute 3 ounces grated low-fat Cheddar or Swiss cheese for the cottage cheese and buttermilk. Serves 2

1½ Whole-Grain servings; 1²/₃ Calcium servings; 1 Protein serving.

MIXED-MEAL MEDLEY

A chunky, nutty blend of cereals that's worth the extra cooking time. Prepare it the night before if your mornings are hectic and reheat with a little extra water or milk on top of the stove or in the microwave. The wheat and barley flakes are available in health food stores and some supermarkets.

Serves 2

3 cups water
½ teaspoon salt, or to taste
¼ cup rolled oats
¼ cup wheat flakes
¼ cup barley flakes
⅔ cup nonfat dry milk
¼ cup wheat germ

1. Bring the water and salt to a boil in a small nonstick saucepan. Gradually stir in the cereals. Cover and cook for 30 minutes, stirring occasionally.

2. Remove the pan from the heat and blend in the dry milk and wheat germ thoroughly.

Serve immediately, with skim milk if desired.

2 Whole-Grain servings; 1 Calcium serving; ²/₃ Protein serving.

Variation: For a Mixed-Meal Medley for a Sweet Tooth, omit the salt, substitute ⅓ cup apple juice concentrate for ⅓ cup of the water, and stir ¼ cup raisins or currants into the cereal after 15 minutes of cooking.

2 Whole-Grain servings; 1 Calcium serving; 1 Other Fruit serving; ²/₃ Protein serving.

FRUITED OATMEAL

If you can't finish a bowlful of this at breakfast, don't toss out the leftovers. Instead serve it cold topped with yogurt and sprinkled with nuts as a dinnertime dessert.

Serves 2

1¾ cups water
¼ cup apple juice concentrate
⅔ cup rolled oats
1 apple, pear, or peach, peeled and diced; or 1 small banana, peeled and sliced; or ½ cup berries, hulled; or ¼ cup chopped dried fruit
⅔ cup nonfat dry milk
¼ cup wheat germ
Dash of ground cinnamon, or to taste (optional)

1. Bring the water and juice concentrate to a boil in a non-stick saucepan. Stir in the oats and cook covered over low heat for 5 minutes.

2. Add the fruit and cook for 5 minutes more. Add the dry milk, wheat germ, and the cinnamon, if desired, stirring until the milk is dissolved.

3. Serve hot with skim milk and/or chopped nuts or seeds, if desired.

2 Whole-Grain servings; 1 Calcium serving; ½ Other Fruit serving; ¾ Protein serving.

CHEESY HOT CEREAL

A savory breakfast that packs half a day's calcium and whole-grain requirements into every bowl.

Serves 2

1 recipe Mixed-Meal Medley (page 219) or your favorite cereal prepared according to package directions with 2 tablespoons wheat germ and ⅓ cup nonfat dry milk added per serving
3 ounces Swiss or Cheddar cheese, preferably low fat

1. Make the hot cereal. Meanwhile, grate the cheese.

2. When the cereal is ready, add the grated cheese and stir over low heat until the cheese is partly melted. Serve immediately.

2 Whole-Grain servings; 2 Calcium servings; 1 Protein serving.

CEREAL A LA MODE

For those who find plain old oatmeal uninspiring to the palate, try a little à la mode excitement.

Serves 2

1 recipe Mixed-Meal Medley (page 219) or your favorite cereal prepared according to package directions with 2 tablespoons wheat germ and ⅓ cup nonfat dry milk added per serving

1 cup low-fat cottage cheese or 1 cup low-fat yogurt

½ cup unsweetened applesauce or ¼ cup fruit-only preserves or jam

1 tablespoon chopped nuts (optional)

Make the hot cereal and divide between two bowls. Top each portion with half the cottage cheese or yogurt and half the applesauce or preserves. Sprinkle with nuts, if desired. Serve hot.

2 Whole-Grain servings; 1⅓ Calcium servings; 1¼ Protein servings (with cottage cheese); ¾ Protein serving (with yogurt); ½ Other Fruit serving.

Eggs and Pancakes

You don't have to cut out your favorite breakfast, brunch, and light meal egg dishes to cut down on cholesterol. Half an egg is better than none, particularly when it's the white half, which is a source of quality protein. Cholesterol-free, and virtually as versatile as a whole egg, the white can be used in omelets, pancakes, waffles, and more.

ONE-YOLK OMELET

All the taste of a whole egg omelet without all the cholesterol.

Serves 1

1 whole egg
2 egg whites
1 tablespoon milk
½ teaspoon margarine or butter
1 to 1½ ounces low-cholesterol cheese, thinly sliced

1. Beat the egg, egg whites, and milk together.

2. Melt the margarine in a nonstick skillet over medium heat. Add the egg mixture and cook until set, lifting the edges to allow the raw egg to flow un-

derneath. When the omelet is almost set, place the cheese over half of it. Fold the other half over the cheese and cook until the cheese melts, about 2 minutes. Serve hot.

1 Protein serving; 1 Calcium serving.

Optional Fillings: Lightly sauté any of the following in ½ teaspoon vegetable oil and add to the omelet when you add the cheese:

½ cup sliced or diced apple or pear
¼ cup thinly sliced mushrooms
½ small red or green bell pepper, thinly sliced

No-Yolk Omelet

This omelet will provide plenty of protein for your baby-to-be and help keep your husband's arteries plaque-free.

Serves 1

½ teaspoon margarine or oil
4 egg whites, lightly beaten
1 to 1½ ounces low-cholesterol cheese, thinly sliced

Melt the margarine in a nonstick omelet pan over medium heat. Add the egg whites and cook until almost set. Place the cheese over half the omelet. Fold the other half over the cheese and cook for a minute or two until the cheese melts. Serve immediately.

1 Protein serving; 1 Calcium serving.

Optional Fillings: See One-Yolk Omelet (recipe precedes).

Tofu Hash

Stripped of the high fat, salt, and nitrate content of corned beef, can hash still be flavorful? Yes—and it packs plenty of protein, too.

Serves 2

2 tablespoons vegetable oil
1 large onion, diced
1 medium potato, cooked and diced
8 ounces tofu, diced
¼ teaspoon dried thyme (optional)
Salt and pepper to taste
4 egg whites, lightly beaten

1. Heat 1 tablespoon of the oil in a heavy nonstick skillet over medium-low heat. Add the onion and sauté until softened. Add the remaining oil, the potato, tofu, thyme, and salt and pepper. Cook, turning frequently, until mixture browns.

2. Pour the egg whites over the hash and cook until the are set and browned. Serve hot.

1 Protein serving; ½ Other Vegetable serving; 1 Fat serving.

SWEET COTTAGE-CHEESE PANCAKES

Quick, delicious, nourishing—for breakfast, brunch, lunch, or a light supper.

Serves 3

1 cup low-fat cottage cheese, preferably salt-reduced
1 whole egg
3 egg whites
3 tablespoons apple juice concentrate
¼ cup skim milk
1 tablespoon melted butter or margarine, or oil
¾ cup whole-wheat flour
¼ cup wheat germ
Vegetable cooking spray

Toppings (optional)
Fruit-only preserves
Unsweetened applesauce
Unsweetened apple butter
Unsweetened frozen strawberries, thawed
Fruited Yogurt (page 224)

1. Place all ingredients (except the cooking spray) in a blender or food processor and blend thoroughly. Let the batter stand 5 minutes.

2. Heat a nonstick skillet or griddle coated with vegetable cooking spray over medium-high heat. Drop large spoonfuls of the batter on the hot surface and cook pancakes until the bottom side is nicely browned. Turn and brown the second side. Serve immediately with one or more of the toppings.

1½ Whole-Grain serving; 1 Protein serving.

Variations: For Blueberry–Cottage-Cheese Pancakes, stir ½ cup blueberries into the pancake batter after blending.

For Savory Cottage-Cheese Pancakes, substitute regular low-fat cottage cheese for the salt-reduced variety and an additional 3 tablespoons skim milk for the apple juice concentrate. Add salt and pepper to taste. Serve with plain low-fat yogurt.

WHOLE-WHEAT BUTTERMILK PANCAKES

Fluffy and golden, with a nutty whole-grain taste that puts them stacks ahead of the refined competition. Allow the batter to settle for 1 hour before making the pancakes.

Serves 3

1 cup low-fat buttermilk
1 teaspoon apple juice concentrate
¾ cup whole-wheat flour
5 tablespoons wheat germ
⅓ cup instant nonfat dry milk
Pinch of salt
Dash of ground cinnamon, or to taste (optional)
2 teaspoons baking powder
2 large egg whites
Vegetable cooking spray
Margarine or butter
Unsweetened applesauce or fruit-only preserves or apple butter
Plain low-fat yogurt

1. Combine the buttermilk, juice concentrate, flour, wheat germ, milk, salt, and cinnamon in a blender jar, and process until smooth. Add the baking powder and blend briefly on low speed.

2. Beat the egg whites in a large mixer bowl until stiff. Quickly beat in the buttermilk mixture, and let the batter stand for 1 hour.

3. Coat a nonstick skillet or griddle with vegetable cooking spray. Heat over medium-high heat to very hot. Brush lightly with margarine or butter. Lower the heat slightly, stir the batter, and spoon it onto the skillet to make pancakes of desired size. When the surface of the pancakes begins to bubble and the undersides are nicely browned, turn and brown the other side. Continue until the batter is used up. Respray the pan as needed (more margarine is optional).

4. Serve pancakes immediately with unsweetened applesauce or fruit-only preserves, and/or plain low-fat yogurt.

2 Whole-Grain servings; ⅔ Calcium serving; ½ Protein serving.

Variation: Add ¼ cup raisins to the batter.

FRUITED YOGURT

A sweet-and-tangy topping for pancakes, waffles, French toast, fruit salad, or cottage cheese. Or eat it by the bowlful.

Makes about 1 cup

¾ cup plain low-fat yogurt
½ cup fresh or frozen (thawed)
  unsweetened strawberries,
  blueberries, or raspberries
5 teaspoons apple juice concentrate
1 tablespoon orange juice
  concentrate
½ teaspoon freshly grated orange
  peel

½ teaspoon ground cinnamon, or to
  taste (optional)

Combine all the ingredients in a blender jar. Purée until mixture reaches desired texture.

1 cup = 1 Vitamin C serving (with strawberries) or 1 Other Fruit serving (with other berries); ¾ Calcium serving.

CRUNCHY OATMEAL-PECAN WAFFLES

The nuts and oats add texture and taste, as well as nourishment.

Serves 4 to 6

Waffles
2 tablespoons butter or margarine,
  melted
¼ cup apple juice concentrate
1 whole egg
3 egg whites
2 cups skim milk
⅔ cup nonfat dry milk
1⅓ cups whole-wheat flour
⅓ cup rolled oats
½ cup wheat germ
4 teaspoons baking powder
2 teaspoons vanilla
¼ cup coarsely chopped pecans

Toppings (optional)
Cottage cheese or yogurt
Fruit-only preserves
Fresh berries cooked in apple juice
  concentrate
Unsweetened frozen berries, thawed
Unsweetened applesauce
Fruited Yogurt

1. Preheat a waffle iron.

2. Beat the butter, juice concentrate, egg, egg whites, and skim milk together in a bowl. Combine the dry ingredients in another bowl, stirring to blend thoroughly. Add them to the egg mixture and stir just until blended. Fold in the vanilla and pecans.

3. Pour batter in batches onto a hot waffle iron and bake until nicely browned. Serve immediately with any of the toppings.

¼ recipe = 2 Whole-Grain servings; 1 Protein serving; 1 Calcium serving.

Variation: For Orange Pecan Waffles, substitute orange juice concentrate for apple juice concentrate. Add 1 tablespoon finely grated orange peel.

Breads and Muffins

Those wishing to keep trim often trim grains from their diets, turning their "daily bread" into a rare treat. This is unfortunate, unnecessary, and unhealthy, particularly for the expectant mother. Breads should be eaten four or five times daily. Fill your basket with these whole grain, no-sugar temptations.

BOSTON BROWN BREAD

A good old standard made even better. Spread it lightly with cream cheese or butter or unsweetened apple butter.

Makes 1 cylindrical loaf

Margarine
½ cup whole-wheat flour
¼ cup wheat germ
1 cup whole-grain cornmeal,
  preferably yellow
1½ teaspoons baking soda
¼ teaspoon salt
½ cup evaporated skim milk
⅔ cup low-fat buttermilk
½ cup apple juice concentrate
1 cup raisins
Vegetable cooking spray

1. Grease a 1-pound coffee can lightly with margarine and set aside.

2. Combine the flour, wheat germ, cornmeal, baking soda, and salt in a medium bowl.

3. Stir together the milks, juice concentrate, and raisins in another bowl. Stir the flour mixture gradually into the milk mixture, blending well.

4. Pour the batter into the prepared coffee can. Cover tightly with a piece of aluminum foil coated with vegetable cooking spray. Place the can in a pot large enough to hold it. Fill the pot to halfway up the side of the can with boiling water. Cover the pot and steam the bread for 2½ to 3 hours, adding additional boiling water as necessary.

5. Cool the bread in the can before unmolding. Open the bottom of the can with a can opener. Push the bread through about ½ inch at a time and cut off with a serrated knife or a strong thread using a sawing motion. Continue cutting until the entire loaf is sliced.

¹/₉ loaf = 1 Whole-Grain serving; ⅔ Other Fruit serving.

CHEESY SPOON BREAD

Eat your milk and get additional grain and protein servings in the delicious bargain. Add a salad and you've got a complete Best-Odds brunch or lunch.

Serves 6

3½ *cups evaporated skim milk or
2⅓ cups nonfat dry milk plus
water to make 3½ cups*
½ *teaspoon salt*
1½ *cups whole-grain cornmeal,
preferably yellow*
1 *tablespoon butter or margarine*
1 *whole egg*
4 *egg whites*
¼ *pound Swiss or Cheddar cheese,
grated*
1 *ounce Parmesan or Romano
cheese, grated (¼ cup)*
1 *teaspoon hot red pepper flakes
(optional)*
Vegetable oil
3 *tablespoons sesame seeds*

1. Preheat the oven to 350°F.

2. Rinse a medium-size saucepan with cold water and add the milk and salt. Heat covered over medium heat to just under a boil.

3. Pour the cornmeal into the milk in a slow steady stream, whisking or stirring constantly to prevent lumps. Continue to whisk or stir until the mixture is thick and bubbly, about 5 minutes. With a wooden spoon, beat in the butter. Remove the pan from the heat.

4. Beat the egg and egg whites well and stir into the cornmeal with a wooden spoon, blending well. Fold in the cheeses and red pepper, if desired.

5. Oil a 1½-quart casserole. Pour the cornmeal mixture into the casserole. With a spatula dipped in cold water, smooth the surface. Sprinkle with the sesame seeds and bake for 45 minutes.

6. Spoon immediately onto plates and serve hot.

2 Calcium servings; 1 Protein serving; 1 Whole-Grain serving.

Variation: To make Broccoli-Cheese Spoon Bread, add 3 cups coarsely chopped raw or frozen broccoli along with the cheeses in step 4.

2 Calcium servings; 1 Protein serving; 1 Whole-Grain serving; 1 Green Leafy serving.

DATE-NUT BREAD

A dense, hearty quick bread. Enjoy as part of a cottage cheese or yogurt and fruit lunch, or with milk as a snack.

Makes 1 loaf

1 cup pitted, coarsely chopped dates
¾ cup plus 2 tablespoons apple juice
   concentrate
¼ cup vegetable oil
2 egg whites
1 cup whole-wheat flour
½ cup wheat germ
1 tablespoon baking powder
1 teaspoon ground cinnamon
½ cup coarsely chopped walnuts
1 teaspoon vanilla extract
Vegetable cooking spray

1. Preheat the oven to 350°F.

2. Combine the dates and juice concentrate in a medium-size saucepan and bring to a boil. Remove from the heat and let stand for 10 minutes. Stir in the oil and let cool to room temperature.

3. Beat in the egg whites thoroughly.

4. Mix the flour, wheat germ, baking powder, and cinnamon in a bowl. Add the date mixture and stir just until combined.

5. Stir in the walnuts and vanilla. Pour the batter into a 9 x 5 x 3-inch loaf pan coated with vegetable cooking spray. Bake until a toothpick inserted into the center comes out clean, 45 to 50 minutes.

6. Cool slightly before removing from the pan. Cool completely on a wire rack before slicing.

¹/₇ loaf = 1 Whole-Grain serving; 1 Other Fruit serving.

PECAN-OATMEAL BREAD

A nutty taste and a crumbly texture, lightly spiced.

Makes 1 loaf

1 cup apple juice concentrate,
   heated
1 cup rolled oats
1 whole egg
2 egg whites
¼ cup vegetable oil
½ cup whole-wheat flour

¼ cup wheat germ
2 teaspoons ground cinnamon
2 teaspoons baking soda
1 cup raisins
½ cup chopped pecans
Vegetable cooking spray

1. Preheat the oven to 350°F.

2. Pour the hot juice concentrate over the oats; let stand until cool.

3. Beat the egg, egg whites, and the oil together in a medium-size mixing bowl. Combine the flour, wheat germ, cinnamon, and baking soda in a small bowl; stir into the egg mixture. Beat in the oats and juice mixture and then fold in the raisins and pecans.

4. Pour the batter into a 9 x 5 x 3-inch loaf pan coated with vegetable cooking spray. Bake until a toothpick inserted in the center comes out clean, 40 to 50 minutes.

5. Cool slightly before removing from the pan. Cool completely on a wire rack before slicing.

⅛ **loaf = 1 Whole-Grain serving; 1 Other Fruit serving.**

ZUCCHINI BREAD

Very moist and just sweet enough. The whole grains team tastily with the unpeeled zucchini to double your roughage.

Makes 1 loaf

1 whole egg
4 egg whites
¼ cup vegetable oil
1 cup apple juice concentrate
1 teaspoon vanilla extract
2 cups grated unpeeled zucchini
1 cup whole-wheat flour
½ cup wheat germ
2 teaspoons baking soda
1½ teaspoons baking powder
2 teaspoons ground cinnamon
1 cup raisins
½ cup chopped walnuts
Vegetable cooking spray

1. Preheat the oven to 350°F.

2. Beat the egg and egg whites in a large bowl until thickened. Beat in the oil, juice concentrate, and vanilla. Fold in the zucchini.

3. Combine the flour, wheat germ, baking soda, baking powder, and cinnamon in a small bowl. Add to the zucchini mixture and stir until just blended. Fold in the raisins and walnuts.

4. Pour the batter into a 9 x 5 x 3-inch loaf pan coated with vegetable cooking spray. Bake until a toothpick inserted into the center comes out clean, about 1¼ hours.

5. Cool slightly before removing from the pan. Cool completely on a wire rack before slicing.

⅛ **loaf = 2 Other Vegetable and Fruit servings; 1 Whole-Grain serving.**

ORANGE BISCUITS

Flaky and fragrant, serve these buttered with a savory meal or slathered with fruit-only marmalade at teatime or coffee break.

Makes about 12 biscuits

1 cup whole-wheat flour
⅓ cup unbleached white flour
2½ teaspoons baking powder
¼ teaspoon salt
⅔ cup wheat germ
1½ teaspoons grated orange peel
5 tablespoons cold butter or
  margarine
½ cup orange juice concentrate plus
  water to make ⅔ cup
1 tablespoon apple juice concentrate

1. Preheat the oven to 425°F.

2. Sift the flours, baking powder, and salt together into a mixing bowl. Add the wheat germ, orange peel, and butter and work with a pastry blender or two knives until the mixture resembles meal. Stir in the juice concentrates and water. The dough should be smooth and soft; add more water if necessary.

3. Turn the dough out onto a lightly floured board and knead 30 seconds. Roll out ¾ inch thick and cut 2-inch rounds with a biscuit cutter or glass. Arrange the dough rounds on a baking sheet. Bake until puffed and golden, 10 to 15 minutes. Serve warm.

2 biscuits = 1²/₃ Whole-Grain servings.

BANANA MUFFINS

Bananas past their prime for slicing into cereal are at the peak of perfection for baking into these naturally sweet muffins.

Makes 18 muffins

3 very ripe bananas, about 1½ cups
  purée
½ cup plus 2 tablespoons apple
  juice concentrate
1 tablespoon orange juice
  concentrate
2 tablespoons vegetable oil
1 teaspoon fresh lemon juice
1¼ cups whole-wheat flour
¾ cup wheat germ
1½ teaspoons ground cinnamon
2 teaspoons baking powder
¾ cup raisins or chopped dates
½ cup coarsely chopped walnuts
2 egg whites
Vegetable cooking spray

1. Preheat the oven to 375°F.

2. Process the bananas, juice concentrates, oil, and lemon juice in a blender until smooth. Combine the flour, wheat germ, cinnamon, and baking powder in a mixer bowl.

3. Stir the banana mixture into the dry ingredients to make a thick batter; then stir in the raisins and walnuts.

4. Beat the egg whites until stiff. Gently beat into the batter, using the lowest speed on an electric mixer.

5. Spoon the batter into 18 muffin cups coated with vegetable cooking spray. Bake for 20 to 25 minutes. Remove from the tins immediately.

2 muffins = 1½ Whole-Grain servings; 1 Other Fruit serving.

BRAN MUFFINS

The most delicious weapons in your high-fiber fight against irregularity. Always keep a batch in your freezer.

Makes about 18 muffins

⅔ cup raisins
1 cup apple juice concentrate
¼ cup orange juice concentrate
1½ cups whole-wheat flour
½ cup wheat germ
1½ cups unprocessed bran
2 teaspoons baking soda
½ cup chopped nuts
1 teaspoon ground cinnamon
1½ cups low-fat buttermilk
2 egg whites, slightly beaten
⅓ cup instant nonfat dry milk
2 tablespoons melted margarine or
 butter, cooled
Vegetable cooking spray

1. Preheat the oven to 350°F.

2. Simmer the raisins with ¼ cup of the apple juice concentrate and all the orange juice concentrate in a small saucepan over low heat, stirring constantly, about 5 minutes.

3. Combine the flour, wheat germ, bran, baking soda, nuts, and cinnamon in a mixing bowl. Stir to mix thoroughly.

4. In another bowl, beat together the remaining apple juice concentrate, the buttermilk, egg whites, milk, and margarine. Combine the flour mixture with the buttermilk mixture, blending thoroughly in a few quick strokes. Fold in the raisins and their cooking liquid.

5. Fill muffin tins coated with vegetable cooking spray to two-thirds full. Bake until a toothpick inserted in the center of a muffin comes out clean, about 20 minutes. Remove from the tins immediately.

1 muffin = 1 Whole-Grain serving; ½ Other Fruit serving.

BRANBERRY-NUT MUFFINS

The cranberries add intriguing taste and fiber to this classic.

Makes 16 muffins

2 cups raw cranberries
1¼ cups apple juice concentrate
2 tablespoons orange juice
  concentrate
¾ cup raisins
1½ cups whole-wheat flour
1½ cups unprocessed bran
½ cup wheat germ
½ cup chopped walnuts
1½ teaspoons baking soda
1¾ cups low-fat buttermilk
2 egg whites, slightly beaten
2 tablespoons vegetable oil
Vegetable cooking spray

1. Simmer the cranberries, ½ cup of the apple juice concentrate, and all the orange juice concentrate in a small saucepan until the cranberries are tender, about 10 minutes. Stir in the raisins and set aside to cool.

2. Preheat the oven to 350°F.

3. Combine the flour, bran, wheat germ, walnuts, and baking soda in a mixing bowl. Beat the buttermilk, egg whites, remaining apple juice concentrate, and oil together in a separate bowl. Add the liquid ingredients to the dry ingredients and blend well with a few strokes. Fold in the cranberries and raisins with their cooking liquid.

4. Spoon the batter into 16 muffin cups coated with vegetable cooking spray. Bake until browned, 20 to 25 minutes. Remove from tins immediately.

1 muffin = 1 Whole-Grain serving; ¾ Other Fruit serving.

CORN BERRY MUFFINS

With a glass of milk and a slice of cheese, these whole-grain muffins serve deliciously as an on-the-run breakfast.

Makes 12 muffins

1 cup whole-grain cornmeal
½ cup whole-wheat flour
¼ cup wheat germ
1½ teaspoons baking soda
⅔ cup low-fat buttermilk
¼ cup plus 3 tablespoons apple juice
  concentrate
2 egg whites, lightly beaten
¼ cup vegetable oil
1⅔ cups fresh or frozen blueberries
  (or raisins)
Vegetable cooking spray

1. Preheat the oven to 400°F.

2. Combine the cornmeal,

flour, wheat germ, and baking soda in a mixing bowl. Beat the buttermilk, juice concentrate, egg whites, and oil in a separate bowl. Add the liquid ingredients to the dry ingredients and blend well with a few strokes.

3. Fold in the blueberries or raisins until distributed evenly.

4. Spoon the batter into 12 muffin cups coated with vegetable cooking spray. Bake until lightly browned, about 20 minutes. Remove from the tins immediately.

2 muffins = 1 Whole-Grain serving.

HOT CROSS BUNS

D on't wait until Easter to bake these fragrant yeast buns.

Makes 14 to 18 buns

1 cup plus 3 tablespoons apple juice concentrate
½ cup orange juice
1 tablespoon butter or margarine
½ cup currants or raisins
2 tablespoons diced unsweetened dried apples, apricots, peaches, pears, or pineapple
½ teaspoon ground cinnamon
⅛ teaspoon ground nutmeg
1 package active dry yeast
2 tablespoons lukewarm water (105° to 115°F)
2⅓ cups whole-wheat flour
⅓ cup wheat germ
1 teaspoon grated lemon peel
Vegetable oil
Vegetable cooking spray
1 package (3 ounces) cream cheese

1. Heat 1 cup of the apple juice concentrate and orange juice in a small saucepan to boiling. Add the butter, fruits, and spices, and stir to melt the butter. Let cool to lukewarm.

2. Dissolve the yeast in the warm water in a medium-size mixing bowl. Stir the cooled juices and fruit into the yeast mixture. Stir in 1⅓ cups of the flour, the wheat germ, and lemon peel. Knead in the remaining flour to make a soft dough. Form into a ball and place in an oiled bowl, turning to oil all sides. Let rise covered in a warm place until doubled in bulk, about 1 hour.

3. Punch the dough down on a floured board and shape into 14 to 18 small balls. Place these, well spaced, on baking sheets coated with vegetable cooking spray. Let rise covered in a warm place until about doubled.

4. Preheat the oven to 425°F.

5. When the buns have risen, bake them until golden brown, 15 to 20 minutes.

6. Soften the cream cheese with the 3 tablespoons of apple juice concentrate until it is the texture of frosting. Use additional juice concentrate if needed. Put the mixture in a cake decorating bag or gun and, when the buns are cool, pipe crosses on each.

2 buns = 1 Whole-Grain serving; 1 Other Fruit serving.

OATMEAL WALNUT MUFFINS

A hearty, slightly spicy, whole-grain muffin perfect with peanut butter.

Makes 12 muffins

½ cup whole-wheat flour
¼ cup wheat germ
2 teaspoons baking powder
1 teaspoon baking soda
1 teaspoon ground cinnamon
¾ teaspoon ground ginger
*   (optional)*
¼ teaspoon ground nutmeg
*   (optional)*
1 cup rolled oats, lightly toasted
⅔ cup low-fat buttermilk
⅓ cup plus 2 tablespoons apple juice
*   concentrate*
2 egg whites
¼ cup vegetable oil
½ cup chopped dried apricots
¼ cup chopped walnuts
Vegetable cooking spray

1. Preheat the oven to 375°F.

2. Combine the flour, wheat germ, baking powder, baking soda, and spices. Stir the oats, buttermilk, and all the juice concentrate together in a mixing bowl. Add the egg whites, oil, apricots, and walnuts, and mix well. Stir in the dry ingredients just until blended.

3. Spoon the batter into 12 muffin cups coated with vegetable cooking spray. Bake until golden brown, about 25 minutes. Remove from the tins immediately.

2 muffins = 1 Whole-Grain serving; ½ Other Fruit serving + some iron.

Soups

Soups are mood foods. Depending upon their flavor, temperature, and texture, they can be warming when you're chilly, comforting when you're sad or sick, energizing when you're exhausted, and refreshing when you're overheated. Soup can whet the appetite for a meal or serve as a meal in itself. It provides important fluids, and if prepared with nutritious ingredients, it can fill one or more of the Daily Dozen requirements in a single satisfying bowlful.

BROCCOLI-CHEESE-BREAD SOUP

Over five daily requirements fulfilled in one hearty bowlful.

Serves 4

1 tablespoon vegetable oil
3 medium onions, thinly sliced
2 medium cloves garlic , minced
1½ teaspoons apple juice
  concentrate
2⅔ cups chopped broccoli (fresh or
  frozen)
Salt and pepper to taste
6 ounces low-fat Swiss cheese,
  grated
6 ounces low-fat Cheddar cheese,
  grated
4 slices whole-wheat bread, frozen
  and sliced horizontally to make 8
  thin slices
1 quart Vegetable or Chicken Stock
  (page 242)

1. Preheat the oven to 375°F.

2. Heat the oil over medium heat in a nonstick skillet. Add the onions and garlic and sauté until golden. Stir in the juice concentrate and cook until the onions are nicely glazed, 2 to 3 minutes.

3. Add the broccoli and sauté until crisp-tender. Add salt and pepper to taste.

4. Combine the cheeses in a bowl. Arrange 3 slices of the bread in a 2-quart nonstick casserole. Spread with a third of the broccoli mixture. Top with a third of the cheese. Repeat layers of bread, broccoli, and cheese.

5. Heat the stock to boiling and pour over all. Taste and adjust seasonings. Brown in the oven for 10 minutes. Let the soup cool for a few minutes before serving or tongues may be burned on the hot cheese.

2 Calcium servings; 1 Protein serving; 1 Green Leafy serving; 1 Whole-Grain serving.

PUMPKIN-PEAR-CHEDDAR SOUP

Fall's bounty in a bowl, this nourishing soup can be prepared year round with canned pumpkin.

Serves 6

1 tablespoon vegetable oil
1 medium onion, chopped
2 large pears, peeled, cored, and chopped
2 cups unsweetened unseasoned solid-pack pumpkin
2 cups unsweetened pear juice
4 ounces low-fat Cheddar cheese, grated
Salt and white pepper to taste

1. Heat the oil over medium-low heat in a 2-quart saucepan. Add the onion and sauté until just softened.

2. Stir in the pears and cook for 2 minutes. Stir in the pumpkin and pear juice and simmer for 5 minutes.

3. Stir in the cheese; then season to taste and serve.

2 Yellow Vegetable servings; 1 Other Fruit serving; ½ Calcium serving.

HAZELNUT-PUMPKIN SOUP

The vitamin A comes elegantly and richly attired in this savory, nicely textured soup.

Serves 6

1 tablespoon vegetable oil
1 leek, thoroughly rinsed, patted dry, and chopped (white bulb only)
2 carrots, chopped
1 rib celery, chopped
½ cup chopped hazelnuts
1 can (16 ounces) unsweetened, unseasoned solid-pack pumpkin
4 cups Vegetable Stock or Chicken Stock (page 242)
Salt and pepper to taste

1. Heat the oil over medium-low heat in a nonstick medium-size saucepan. Add the leek, carrots, celery, and hazelnuts and sauté until the vegetables are softened.

2. Stir in the pumpkin and then the stock. Simmer for 10 minutes. Season to taste and serve.

2+ Yellow Vegetable servings.

CREAM OF TOMATO SOUP

Almost as effortless as opening a can, but with far more satisfying and nourishing results.

Serves 3

1 tablespoon margarine or butter
2 tablespoons whole-wheat flour
1¾ cups evaporated skim milk
3 cups tomato or vegetable juice
4 tablespoons tomato paste
Salt and pepper to taste
Dash of fresh or dried oregano, or to taste (optional)
Dash of fresh or dried basil, or to taste (optional)
1¼ cups low-fat cottage cheese
Parmesan cheese or wheat germ (optional)

1. Melt the margarine or butter over very low heat in a saucepan. Add the flour and blend, stirring constantly, for 2 minutes.

2. Gradually blend in the evaporated skim milk. Continue to cook over low heat, stirring occasionally, until thickened.

3. Stir in the tomato or vegetable juice, the tomato paste, and the seasonings to taste, until smooth. Continue cooking over low heat, stirring frequently, for 5 minutes. Serve warm, topped with the cottage cheese, and a sprinkling of Parmesan cheese and/or wheat germ, if desired.

1 Protein serving; 1 Calcium serving; 1 Vitamin C serving; 1 Green Leafy serving (¾ serving if vegetable juice is used).

CAULIFLOWER CREAM

Quick and easy way to have your milk and vitamin C, too.

Serves 4

3 cups small cauliflower florets
1 tablespoon vegetable oil
1 teaspoon margarine
1 medium-large onion, chopped
2 ribs celery, chopped
3 cups evaporated skim milk
Salt and pepper to taste
Freshly grated nutmeg
Fresh chives, chopped (optional)

1. Steam the cauliflower, cov-

ered, over boiling water until just tender. Purée in a blender or food processor.

2. Heat the oil and margarine in a nonstick 2-quart pan. Add the onion and celery and sauté until soft and golden but not brown.

3. Stir in the milk and the cauliflower. Season to taste with salt, pepper, and nutmeg. Simmer over low heat for 5 minutes. Do not boil.

4. Serve warm, garnished with chives, if desired.

1½ Calcium servings; 1 Vitamin C serving.

Variation: For Cream of Broccoli Soup, substitute an equal amount of broccoli for the cauliflower.

1½ Calcium Servings; 1 Vitamin C serving; 1 Green Leafy serving.

GREEN VICHYSSOISE

The addition of spinach or broccoli lends a lovely green hue and a serving of green leafies to this French favorite.

Serves 4

1 tablespoon margarine or vegetable oil
1 medium leek, thoroughly rinsed, patted dry, and chopped (white bulb only)
2 medium shallots, minced
1 cup Vegetable Stock or Chicken Stock (page 242)
2 medium potatoes (about 8 ounces total), diced
1 package (9 or 10 ounces) frozen chopped spinach or broccoli (thawed)
2 cups evaporated skim milk or 2 cups skim milk and ⅔ cup nonfat dry milk
Salt and pepper to taste

1. Heat the margarine or oil over medium-low heat in a 2-quart saucepan. Add the leek and shallots and sauté until softened.

2. Add the stock and potatoes. Raise the heat, bring to a boil, and cook for 5 minutes.

3. Add the spinach and bring back to a boil. Reduce the heat, and simmer just until the potatoes are tender. Purée in a blender or food processor until smooth.

4. Return the purée to the saucepan and stir in the milk. Simmer for 4 minutes; do not boil. Season to taste and serve warm or refrigerate and serve cold.

1 Calcium serving; 1 Green Leafy serving; 1 Other Vegetable serving; if broccoli is used, 1 Vitamin C serving.

HEARTY VEGETABLE–PASTA SOUP

This hearty soup—Italian in both colors and flavors—takes little more time to prepare than the instant variety, and can provide a complete main course that is both warming and filling at the end of a busy day.

Serves 4

1 can (28 ounces) tomatoes in purée
1½ cups water
½ cup chopped fresh parsley
1 tablespoon chopped fresh basil or 1 teaspoon dried, or to taste
½ teaspoon dried marjoram
4 ounces high-protein macaroni elbows or pasta shells
2 cups small broccoli florets
8 ounces small fresh mushrooms, caps only
1 can (16 ounces) chickpeas, drained
¼ cup grated Parmesan cheese
4 ounces low-fat Swiss or similar cheese, grated

1. Combine the tomatoes, water, and herbs in a 2½-quart pan. Simmer over medium heat for 5 minutes. Add the pasta, raise the heat, and bring to a boil. Cook for 5 minutes less than package directions recommend.

2. Add the broccoli, mushrooms, and chickpeas. Simmer until the macaroni is tender but firm to the bite and the broccoli is crisp tender.

3. Ladle the soup into four bowls. Top each serving with a quarter of the cheeses and serve.

1 Protein serving; 1 Green Leafy serving; 1 Vitamin C serving; 1 Calcium serving; 1 Whole-Grain serving.

Variations: To make this soup with tuna, drain 1 can (6 to 7 ounces) water-packed tuna and add to the soup during the last 5 minutes cooking time. This will provide an extra ½ Protein serving.

To make this soup with cottage cheese, add ¾ cup low-fat cottage cheese to each bowlful. This will provide 1 additional Protein serving. Or if you're gaining weight too quickly, substitute the cottage cheese for the other cheeses, but remember that means you won't be getting a full calcium serving.

To make this soup for vegans, substitute 1 pound slivered tofu for the cheese. This will provide an equivalent protein serving plus a calcium serving if the tofu is prepared with calcium (many are).

MISO NOODLE SOUP

A speedy one-pot soup-stew that satisfies like a meal.

Serves 4

2 tablespoons vegetable oil
2 cups small broccoli florets
1 cup thinly sliced scallions (white
   bulb plus 2 inches of green stems)
1 red bell pepper, cored, seeded, and
   finely sliced
8 ounces fresh mushrooms, thinly
   sliced
5 cups water
8 ounces buckwheat noodles
6 to 10 tablespoons white miso paste
   (see Note)
Powdered oriental soup mix
   without MSG (see Note)
2½ pounds silken tofu (bean curd),
   sliced (see Note)
Black sesame seeds (goma; see Note)

1. Heat the oil over medium heat in a wok or nonstick Dutch oven. Add the broccoli, scallions, red pepper, and mushrooms, and stir-fry the vegetables until barely tender. Remove to a large soup tureen and set aside in a warm place.

2. Add the water to the wok. Bring it to a boil and add the noodles.

3. When the noodles are almost done, remove a cup of the hot cooking water and mix with the miso and soup mix in a small bowl. Return the mixture to the simmering noodles and add the tofu.

4. Cook until the noodles are just tender. Pour the mixture over the vegetables in the tureen. Sprinkle with sesame seeds and serve hot.

2 Green Leafy and Yellow Vegetable servings; 1 Protein serving; 1 Whole-Grain serving.

Variations: Instead of or in addition to the tofu, add leftover fish, chicken, or beans to the soup.

Note: All of the oriental ingredients are available in specialty food stores and in some supermarkets. If you have difficulty finding them, omit the soup mix, substitute ordinary tofu for the silken, and white sesame seeds for the black. If you wish to make your own Oriental stock, boil konbu (kobu) kelp in 5 cups water.

RED PEPPER GAZPACHO

A summer soup that can be at once cooling and fiery.

Serves 6

2 cans (16 ounces each) tomatoes in
   purée
1 jar (8 ounces) pimientos, drained
2 small cucumbers, peeled, seeded,
   and cut into 1-inch chunks
4 medium red bell peppers, cored,
   seeded, and sliced
1 large red onion, quartered
⅓ cup red wine vinegar, or to taste
1 tablespoon vegetable oil
Salt
Dash of Tabasco sauce, or to taste

Diced red bell pepper (optional)

1. Place all the ingredients except the diced pepper in a blender or food processor and process until finely chopped but not puréed. Taste and adjust seasonings.

2. Refrigerate for several hours. Garnish with the diced red pepper, if desired.

2 Vitamin C servings; 2 Yellow Vegetable servings.

GAZPACHO VERDE

Serves 4

1½ cups low-fat buttermilk
3 tablespoons tarragon vinegar, or
   to taste
2 tablespoons vegetable oil
Dash of Tabasco sauce, or to taste
Pinch cayenne pepper
Salt and pepper to taste
1 medium yellow onion, coarsely
   chopped
1 clove garlic, core removed, minced
2 medium green bell peppers, cored,
   seeded, and sliced
2 medium cucumbers, seeded and
   cut into 1-inch chunks
2 cups (tightly packed) arugula
1 cup (tightly packed) watercress
2 tablespoons mayonnaise
4 hard-cooked egg whites, minced

1. Whisk the buttermilk, vinegar, oil, Tabasco, cayenne, and salt and pepper together in a small bowl.

2. Combine the vegetables in a medium-size bowl and pour the buttermilk mixture over them.

3. Process in batches in a food processor or blender until smooth. Stir in the mayonnaise. Refrigerate for at least 4 hours before serving. Garnish with the minced egg white.

1 Green Leafy serving; 1 Vitamin C serving; 1 Fat serving; ½ Calcium serving.

VEGETABLE STOCK

Makes about 3 quarts

2 leeks, thoroughly rinsed, patted
  dry, and sliced (white bulbs only)
3 carrots, diced
3 ribs celery, sliced
1 parsnip, sliced
5 onions, chopped
4 cloves garlic, crushed
2 to 3 sprigs thyme, or ½ teaspoon
  dried thyme
6 sprigs parsley
1 bay leaf
2 tablespoons fresh lemon juice or
  tarragon vinegar
10 peppercorns
4 quarts water
Salt to taste
1 tablespoon vegetable oil

1. Combine all the ingredients except for 2 cups of chopped onions and the vegetable oil in a large stock pot and bring to a boil over high heat. Lower the heat and simmer, covered, for 3 hours.

2. Meanwhile, heat the oil over medium heat in a nonstick skillet. Add the onions and sauté until golden brown. Set aside.

3. Strain the stock through a colander lined with cheesecloth and return it to the stock pot. Add the sautéed onions and simmer for 20 to 25 minutes. Strain the stock again and refrigerate.

CHICKEN STOCK

Makes about 3 quarts

4 pounds chicken bones with some
  meat on them
Chicken giblets (not the liver)
2 leeks, thoroughly rinsed, patted
  dry, and sliced (white bulb only)
3 carrots, diced
3 ribs celery, sliced
1 parsnip, sliced
2 onions, chopped
3 cloves garlic, crushed
1 bay leaf
6 sprigs parsley
1 sprig thyme or ½ teaspoon dried
  thyme

1 tablespoon fresh lemon juice or
  tarragon vinegar
12 peppercorns
4 quarts water
Salt to taste

1. Combine all the ingredients in a large stock pot and bring to a boil over high heat. Lower the heat and simmer, covered, for 2½ hours.

2. Allow the stock to cool then strain it through a colander lined with cheesecloth. Refrigerate and skim off any remaining fat.

Vegetarian Main Dishes

Although eating less meat is laudable from most nutritional points of view, it can raise a significant problem for the pregnant: Vegetarian meals often don't provide enough quality protein to help a fetus develop and its mother remain healthy. Here are several exceptions to that generalization—vegetarian dishes that not only supply enough protein, but substantial quantities of other Daily Dozen requirements as well.

BEAN AND BROWN RICE SALAD

Prepare this dish the night before to let flavors mingle. Add a green salad and fresh fruit and you've got a complete dinner, or serve it as a side dish with fish or poultry.

Serves 4 as a main dish or 8 as a side dish

¾ cup dry white wine
4 cups cooked brown rice
1 can (16 ounces) dark red kidney beans, drained
1 can (16 ounces) chickpeas, drained
⅔ cup finely minced red onion
1 cup finely diced red bell pepper
1 cup finely diced green bell pepper
⅓ cup coarsely chopped walnuts or whole pine nuts
2 tablespoons vegetable oil
¼ cup tarragon vinegar
¼ cup unsweetened apple juice
¼ teaspoon dry mustard
Salt and pepper to taste

1. Bring the wine to a boil, then lower the heat and simmer for 5 minutes. Set aside to cool.

2. Combine the rice, beans, chickpeas, onion, peppers, and nuts in a glass or stainless-steel bowl.

3. Whisk the remaining ingredients with the wine until blended. Pour the dressing over the mixture and toss until well coated. Refrigerate until cold, preferably overnight.

¼ recipe = 1 Protein serving; 1 Whole-Grain serving; 1 Vitamin C serving; ½ Yellow Vegetable serving.

BROCCOLI-MUSHROOM SFORMATO

This delicious Italian classic, adjusted here for a lower fat content, is a Best-Odds meal in itself. Serve hot or at room temperature.

Serves 6

4 cups chopped broccoli
¼ teaspoon salt, plus additional to taste
2 tablespoons vegetable oil
1 large onion, diced
1 whole clove garlic, peeled
½ cup finely chopped fresh parsley
8 ounces fresh mushrooms, sliced
1 whole egg
4 egg whites
Freshly ground pepper
10 ounces low-cholesterol Swiss cheese, grated
1 ounce Parmesan cheese, grated
6 slices whole-wheat bread
2 tablespoons walnut pieces

1. Sprinkle the broccoli with salt to taste and steam over medium-low heat until barely tender.

2. Heat 1 tablespoon of the oil over medium heat in a nonstick skillet. Add the onion and garlic and sauté until the onion is softened. Remove the garlic clove when it is golden brown.

3. Add the parsley and mushrooms to the skillet and sauté over medium heat just until the mushrooms begin to soften, 4 to 5 minutes. Stir in the broccoli.

4. Preheat the oven to 375°F.

5. In a small bowl, beat the egg, egg whites, ¼ teaspoon salt, the pepper, and cheeses together lightly. Pour over the broccoli and mushroom mixture and mix well.

6. Line the inside of a nonstick 2-quart casserole with waxed paper. Oil the waxed paper with the remaining 1 tablespoon oil.

7. Process the bread and nuts in a food processor or blender to fine crumbs. Line the bottom and sides of the casserole evenly with about two-thirds of the crumbs, pressing the crumbs to the waxed paper with your hands. Pour the broccoli mixture into the casserole and top with the remaining crumbs.

8. Bake until the eggs are set and the crumbs well toasted, 20 to 25 minutes. Unmold onto a serving platter and carefully remove the waxed paper.

1 Protein serving; 1½ Calcium servings; 1 Green Leafy serving; 1 Vitamin C serving; 1 Whole-Grain serving.

CHICKPEA AND NUT LOAF

A dinner entree loaf with a crunchy texture that doesn't get lost in the cooking.

Serves 4

1 tablespoon vegetable oil
1 large onion, chopped
1 can (16 ounces) chickpeas,
   drained and chopped
½ cup chopped walnuts, peanuts,
   almonds, or cashews (see Note)
2 carrots, grated (about 1 cup)
1 cup thinly sliced celery
1 cup chopped fresh mushrooms
1 cup chopped fresh or frozen
   (thawed) green beans
½ cup wheat germ
1¼ cups whole-wheat bread crumbs
   (about 3 slices bread)
4 egg whites
1 teaspoon dried thyme or dried
   rosemary
Salt and pepper to taste

1. Preheat the oven to 400°F.

2. Line the bottom and sides of a 9 x 5 x 3-inch nonstick loaf pan with waxed paper.

3. Heat the oil over medium heat in a nonstick skillet. Add the onion and sauté until nicely browned. Combine the onion with the remaining ingredients in a large bowl and transfer the mixture into the prepared loaf pan.

4. Bake until nicely browned, about 1½ hours. Unmold the loaf onto a nonstick cooking sheet and remove the waxed paper. Return it to the oven and bake until the top and sides are brown, about 10 minutes.

1 Protein serving; 1 Yellow Vegetable serving; 1 Other Vegetable serving.

Variations: For Chickpea and Nut Patties, shape the mixture into patties and bake on a lightly oiled nonstick cookie sheet until browned. Turn and brown the second side. Serve on whole-wheat buns.

For Cheese-Nut Loaf, combine ½ cup grated Parmesan cheese with the onion, then add to the remaining ingredients.

Note: If you use English (not black) walnuts or cashews, add 2 additional tablespoons wheat germ to compensate for lower protein content.

CHICKPEA AND VEGETABLE CURRY

Rich in flavor, and rich in nutrients—fulfilling a full five requirements with every savory plateful.

Serves 4

1 cup raw brown rice
1 tablespoon vegetable oil
1 teaspoon black or white mustard
  seeds
1 cup chopped onion
1 teaspoon fresh lemon juice
¾ teaspoon ground coriander
1 teaspoon ground cumin
¾ teaspoon turmeric
½ teaspoon ground red pepper
½ teaspoon paprika
2 fresh or canned tomatoes, cut into
  1¼-inch cubes
2 tablespoons chopped fresh
  coriander (optional)
2 teaspoons slivered fresh ginger
1 to 2 jalapeño peppers, seeded and
  chopped (optional; see Note)
⅔ cup Vegetable Stock (see page
  242) or water
Salt to taste
3 cups broccoli florets and stems
3 cups cauliflower florets and stems
2 cans (16 ounces) chickpeas,
  drained
1 red bell pepper, cored, seeded, and
  thinly sliced
Chopped fresh parsley or coriander
  for garnish
2 ounces pine nuts (pignoli)

1. Cook the brown rice according to package directions. Meanwhile, heat the oil over medium heat in a large nonstick skillet. Add the mustard seeds and cover the pan. Cook, shaking the pan constantly, until you hear the seeds pop. Add the onion and sauté until lightly browned.

2. Reduce the heat. Add the lemon juice and spices and blend thoroughly. Add the tomatoes, coriander, ginger, jalapeño peppers, stock, and salt to taste. Stir thoroughly. Add the broccoli, cauliflower, chickpeas, and bell pepper; stir to distribute the sauce evenly.

3. Cover the skillet and cook over low heat until the vegetables are cooked but not mushy, 15 to 20 minutes.

4. Garnish with the parsley or coriander; sprinkle with pine nuts.

2 Vitamin C servings; 1 Protein serving; 1 Whole-Grain serving; 1 Green Leafy serving.

Note: The oil and fumes from fresh chiles can cause a burning sensation to sensitive eye, nose, and mouth tissue. When handling chiles keep your hands away from your face. Wash them well in soap and water before continuing with the recipe.

VEGETARIAN SAUSAGE

Hearty home-style sausage that will do your family's hearts good—and won't break any Best-Odds rules. These also make savory accompaniments to Cassoulet Tofu or breakfast eggs.

Makes 12 patties

1 cup textured vegetable protein
  (available in health food stores)
1 teaspoon dried thyme
1 teaspoon dried sage
1 teaspoon turmeric
½ teaspoon ground coriander
¼ teaspoon ground black pepper
1 cup boiling water
¼ cup whole-wheat flour
3 egg whites, lightly beaten
1½ teaspoons vegetable oil

1. Mix the vegetable protein and spices together in a bowl. Pour the boiling water over the mixture and allow it to stand until the water is absorbed, about 5 minutes. Stir in the flour and egg whites. Taste the mixture and correct the seasonings, if necessary.

2. Heat the oil over medium heat in a nonstick skillet. Shape the vegetable protein mixture into small patties and brown on both sides.

The amount of protein in this dish will depend on the type of textured vegetable protein you use.

MEAL IN A KUGEL

This is a variation of a recipe that won a prize in a national kugel (noodle pudding) contest. The prize was for good taste, but it just as easily could have been for good nutrition. You'll find it winning at brunch, lunch, or supper, as the main event or as a satisfying side show.

Serves 4

8 ounces whole-wheat or high-
  protein noodles
2 tablespoons margarine, butter, or
  vegetable oil
1 onion, diced
1 large clove garlic, finely minced
8 ounces fresh mushrooms, sliced
2 cups coarsely chopped broccoli
2 cups coarsely chopped cauliflower
2 cups low-fat cottage cheese
6 ounces low-fat Cheddar cheese,
  grated
1½ teaspoons dried tarragon
½ teaspoon dry mustard
Pepper to taste

1. Preheat the oven to 350°F.

2. Cook the noodles according

to package directions until tender but still firm to the bite.

3. Heat the butter in a nonstick skillet. Add the onion and garlic and sauté over medium until the onion is translucent. Add the mushrooms and sauté 2 minutes.

4. Toss together the noodles, mushroom mixture, and remaining ingredients, except for ¼ cup of the grated cheese. Taste and adjust seasonings, if necessary.

5. Pour the mixture into an oiled nonstick 13 x 9-inch baking pan and press it firmly into the pan. Sprinkle with the remaining cheese. Bake until the top is lightly browned and bubbly and the vegetables are crisp-tender, about 30 minutes.

1 Protein serving; 1 Whole-Grain serving; 1 Calcium serving; 1 Green Leafy serving; 1 Vitamin C serving; 1 Other Vegetable serving.

CASSOULET WITH TOFU

A vegetarian variation of the cassoulet of France and the couscous of North Africa (sans the couscous), this meal-in-one has everything including good taste. And, unlike its foreign cousins, it doesn't take two days to prepare.

Serves 6

1 tablespoon vegetable oil
1 large onion, diced
2 cloves garlic, minced
1½ pounds tofu, frozen for several
    hours (see Note), sliced
2 medium carrots, sliced
2 medium turnips, sliced
1 teaspoon turmeric
½ teaspoon ground ginger
½ teaspoon black pepper
Salt to taste
2 cups Vegetable Stock (page 242),
    or water, or tomato juice
Vegetarian Sausage (page 247)
2 medium zucchini, sliced
1 can (6 ounces) tomato paste

1 small cabbage, cut into 6 wedges
1 large red bell pepper, cored,
    seeded, and sliced
1 large green bell pepper, cored,
    seeded, and sliced
½ cup chopped fresh parsley
1 can (16 ounces) chickpeas,
    drained
1 can (16 ounces) fava beans or
    other white beans, drained

1. Heat the oil over medium heat in a large heavy pot. Add the onion and garlic and sauté until golden. Add the tofu and brown slightly.

2. Add the carrots, turnips, seasonings, and stock. Bring to a boil. Reduce the heat and simmer, covered, until the vegetables are almost tender, about 40 minutes.

3. Meanwhile, prepare the vegetarian sausage.

4. Add the remaining ingredients except the sausage to the pot and simmer for 15 minutes more.

5. Add the sausage and simmer for 2 to 3 minutes more.

Serve hot. This dish can also be served over couscous.

1½ Protein servings; 1 Yellow Vegetable serving; 2 Vitamin C servings; 1 Other Vegetable serving; ½ Calcium serving.

Note: Freezing tofu gives it a chewier, more meaty texture. Drain the tofu and wrap tightly in a plastic bag before freezing. Rinse with fresh water before using.

BEST-ODDS PIZZA

For those who think that pizza takes a great deal of time and effort, this recipe will come as a delicious revelation. Prepare the filling and a green leafy salad while the pizza bakes, then put your feet up and have a drink (Best-Odds, of course).

Makes two 10-inch pizzas; serves 4

Dough
1 envelope quick-rising yeast
1 cup lukewarm water (110°to 115°F)
1½ tablespoons vegetable oil
1 teaspoon salt
2 to 2¼ cups whole-wheat flour, as needed
Vegetable cooking spray or vegetable oil

Filling
2 cups tomato sauce (no sugar added), jarred or homemade
10 ounces part-skim or light mozzarella cheese, shredded
¼ cup grated Parmesan cheese
Sautéed sliced mushrooms (optional)
Sautéed sliced onions (optional)
Sautéed sliced red or green bell peppers (optional)

1. In large mixing bowl, dissolve the yeast in the water. Stir. Add the oil, salt, 2 cups whole-wheat flour. Mix well. Knead until the dough is smooth and elastic, about 2 minutes. Add additional flour, if needed.

2. Put the dough in a large bowl coated with vegetable cooking spray or lightly coated with oil. Cover with a damp towel and let rest for 5 minutes. Prepare the filling.

3. Preheat the oven to 400°F.

4. Coat 2 cookie sheets with vegetable cooking spray or oil and set aside.

5. Punch down the dough and divide it into 2 equal pieces. Form each piece into a ball. Roll and stretch 1 ball of dough into a 10-inch round. Place it on a cookie sheet and set it aside while you roll out the second ball. Place it on the second cookie sheet.

6. Top each crust with half the filling ingredients. Bake until the cheese is melted and the crust is brown, about 25 minutes. Serve immediately. (Each pie feeds two hungry eaters; they may be frozen, unbaked.)

1 Protein serving; 2½ Whole-Grain servings; 1 Vitamin C serving; 1 Calcium serving.

PESTO FOR PASTA OR DIP

Removing the cores from the garlic and sautéing the cloves lightly before adding them to the other ingredients makes this pesto free from distressing digestive aftereffects.

Serves 4 with pasta

1 tablespoon vegetable oil
4 medium cloves garlic, cores removed, thinly sliced
4 cups loosely packed combination fresh basil and parsley leaves or all parsley plus 2 tablespoons dried basil
4 ounces pine nuts (pignoli)
4 ounces (1 cup) Parmesan cheese, grated
1½ cups low-fat cottage cheese
Salt and freshly ground black pepper to taste

1. Heat the oil in a nonstick skillet. Reduce the heat, add the garlic, and sauté until soft but not brown.

2. Place the garlic, basil and parsley (or parsley and dried basil, if using), pine nuts, Parmesan, and cottage cheese in a blender and blend until smooth. Add a bit of water if the mixture is very thick. Season to taste with salt and pepper.

3. Serve over hot pasta and steamed vegetables or use as a dip for vegetables or crackers.

¼ recipe = 1 Protein serving; 1 Calcium serving; 1 Green Leafy serving.

TOFU AND PEPPERS

A speedy vegetarian supper in a skillet.

Serves 2

¼ cup whole-wheat flour
Salt and pepper to taste
12 ounces herbed tofu, thinly sliced
(see Note)
1 tablespoon vegetable oil
2 green bell peppers, cored, seeded,
and thinly sliced
2 red bell peppers, cored, seeded,
and thinly sliced
3 tablespoons sesame seeds

1. Mix together the flour, salt and pepper and dust the tofu with the seasoned flour.

2. Heat the oil over medium heat in a nonstick skillet. Add the peppers and sauté for 2 minutes. Add the tofu slices and brown lightly on both sides. Sprinkle with the sesame seeds and check seasonings. Serve hot.

1 Protein serving; 2 Vitamin C servings; 1 Green Leafy serving; ½ Calcium serving (or 1 Calcium serving if the tofu has added calcium as most do).

Note: If you can't find herbed tofu, use plain tofu and add a teaspoon of your favorite herb to the recipe.

TOFU STROGANOFF

A perfect dish for full-time vegetarians, mothers-to-be with a temporary aversion to meat, and for meat-eaters who'd like a change of pace.

Serves 6

2 tablespoons vegetable oil
1 medium onion, chopped
12 ounces fresh mushrooms, sliced
¼ cup whole-wheat flour
Salt and pepper to taste
2 pounds firm tofu, frozen for
several hours (see Note, page
249), sliced
½ cup dry white wine
Nutmeg to taste, preferably freshly
grated
12 ounces spinach noodles

1 tablespoon butter
1 cup low-fat buttermilk or yogurt

1. Heat 1 tablespoon of the oil over medium heat in a heavy nonstick pan. Add the onion and sauté until softened. Add the mushrooms and sauté until softened. Remove to a bowl.

2. Mix together the flour, salt and pepper and dust the tofu with the seasoned flour. Add the remaining oil to the pan and

heat. Add the tofu and brown lightly on both sides. Return the onions and mushrooms to the pan. Add the wine and nutmeg, salt and pepper to taste. Simmer for 5 minutes, turning the tofu slices occasionally to be sure that all the tofu is covered with sauce.

3. Cook the noodles according to package directions. Drain, rinse with hot water, and toss with the butter.

4. Just before serving, stir the buttermilk into the tofu mixture and adjust seasonings. Serve hot.

1 Protein serving; 1 Whole-Grain serving; 1 Other Vegetable serving.

VEGETARIAN CHILI

This hearty dish offers complete vegetable protein in tasty Tex-Mex garb. Set the spice alarm to your own taste. Serve with corn muffins (see Note) or a crusty whole-wheat loaf and a leafy green salad.

Serves 6

Chili

2 tablespoons vegetable oil
1½ cups chopped onions
2 cloves garlic, minced
3 green or red bell peppers, cored, seeded, and diced
1 pound tofu, frozen for several hours (see Note, page 249)
1 can (28 ounces) tomatoes in purée
¼ cup chili powder, or to taste
1 tablespoon dried oregano
1 teaspoon salt, or to taste
¼ teaspoon cayenne, or to taste
⅛ teaspoon freshly ground black pepper
2 teaspoons apple juice concentrate
1 can (6 ounces) tomato paste
1 can (20 ounces) dark red kidney beans, drained
1 can (10½ ounces) pinto beans, drained

Toppings

2 large red or green bell peppers, cored, seeded, and finely diced
1 red onion, chopped
3 ounces low-fat Cheddar or Monterey Jack cheese, shredded
Jalapeño peppers or other chiles, chopped

1. Heat the oil over medium-low heat in a nonstick skillet. Add the onions, garlic, and bell peppers and sauté until the onion is softened, about 5 minutes. Crumble the tofu into the skillet and stir. Increase the heat to medium and cook until the onions and tofu are browned.

2. Stir in the tomatoes with purée, chili powder, oregano, salt, cayenne, pepper, juice concentrate, and tomato paste. Bring to a boil over high heat.

Reduce the heat and simmer for 30 minutes, adding water or tomato purée if the chili becomes too thick.

3. Stir in the beans and simmer for another 30 minutes. Serve with any of the listed toppings.

1 Protein serving; 1 Vitamin C serving; if red peppers are used, 1 Green Leafy serving

Note: For a perfect accompaniment, omit the blueberries from Corn Berry Muffins (page 232) and add ¼ cup finely chopped jalapeño peppers.

MACARONI CASSEROLE PLUS

For those who yearn for the nostalgia of Mom's macaroni and cheese but wish to remain true to their Daily Dozen.

Serves 4

8 ounces high-protein macaroni
2½ tablespoons margarine
2 cups sliced fresh mushrooms
2 tablespoons whole-wheat flour
2 cups evaporated skim milk
6 ounces low-fat Swiss cheese,
  grated
2⅔ cups broccoli florets
2 cans (6 to 7 ounces) water-packed
  tuna, drained and flaked; or 2
  pounds firm-style tofu, frozen for
  several hours (see Note, page 249)
½ cup whole-wheat bread crumbs

1. Preheat the oven to 350°F.

2. Cook the macaroni according to package directions until barely tender. Rinse with hot water and set aside.

3. Heat 2 tablespoons of the margarine over medium heat in a nonstick skillet. Add the mushrooms and sauté for 3 minutes. Blend in the flour until smooth. Lower the heat and gradually stir in the evaporated milk. Continue cooking and stirring until smooth and slightly thickened, about 5 minutes.

4. Stir in the grated cheese and cook, stirring constantly, until the cheese melts. Stir the cheese sauce into the macaroni. Add the broccoli and tuna or tofu and toss until evenly distributed. Transfer the mixture into a nonstick casserole.

5. Melt the remaining ½ tablespoon margarine and blend well with the bread crumbs. Spread the mixture over the top of the casserole.

6. Bake until the top is golden, about 30 minutes. Serve hot.

2 Protein servings; 1 Calcium serving; 1 Whole-Grain serving; 1 Green Leafy serving; ½ Other Vegetable serving.

Main Courses

Most likely there isn't much wrong with the main courses you ordinarily make so that with a few alterations, your favorite mains can become Best-Odds mains. These delicious alternatives are specially designed to provide concentrated nutrition.

CREAMY FISH AND CHEESE CASSEROLE

Complement this casserole with a green leafy salad and brown rice and await the compliments of your dining companions.

Serves 4

1 tablespoon butter or margarine
1 medium onion, chopped
1 large shallot, minced
2 large red bell peppers, cored, seeded, and thinly sliced
4 ounces fresh mushrooms, sliced
2 tablespoons whole-wheat flour
1 can (12 ounces) evaporated skim milk
⅓ cup nonfat dry milk
¼ cup chopped fresh parsley
Salt and pepper to taste
Freshly grated nutmeg to taste
6 ounces low-fat Cheddar or Swiss cheese, shredded
1 pound fish fillets or steaks, cut into 1½-inch chunks
2 ounces pimiento, chopped
2 slices whole-wheat bread

1. Melt the butter over medium heat in a nonstick skillet. Add the onion and shallot and sauté until translucent. Add the bell pepper and sauté for 3 minutes. Add the mushrooms and sauté another 2 minutes.

2. Blend in the flour and cook for 2 minutes, stirring constantly. Add the evaporated and dry milks and cook, stirring constantly, over medium heat until thick. Stir in the parsley and salt, pepper, and nutmeg to taste.

3. Preheat the oven to 350°F.

4. Add the cheese to the skillet and cook, stirring constantly, until it melts. Stir in the fish and pimiento. Turn the mixture into a 1½-quart nonstick casserole.

5. Process the bread in a food processor or blender to coarse crumbs. Sprinkle over the top of the casserole. Bake for 30 minutes.

2 Protein servings; 2 Calcium servings; 1 Vitamin C serving; 1 Green Leafy serving.

PASTA WITH SALMON

Can't tolerate milk? This casserole will help you meet your calcium requirement—and plenty of others, besides.

Serves 4

1 can (1 pound) salmon, with skin and bones (see Note)
4 cups small broccoli florets and peeled sliced stems
2 medium carrots, thinly sliced
8 ounces high-protein pasta shells
1 tablespoon vegetable oil
1 medium onion, finely diced
1 large clove garlic, finely minced
1 cup Vegetable Stock (page 242)
½ cup dry white wine
2 teaspoons dried basil, or to taste
Freshly ground black pepper to taste
⅓ cup slivered or sliced almonds, lightly toasted
Grated Parmesan cheese (optional)

1. Mash the salmon with the bones and skin. Steam the broccoli and carrots separately until barely tender. Set aside.

2. Cook the pasta according to package directions.

3. While the pasta is cooking, heat the oil over medium-low heat in a nonstick skillet. Add the onion and garlic and sauté until softened. Add the stock, wine, basil, and black pepper and bring to a boil. Reduce the heat and simmer for 5 minutes.

4. Add the broccoli, carrots, and salmon and toss lightly over low heat until heated through.

5. Drain the pasta and rinse with hot water. Combine with the salmon mixture in a large serving bowl. Sprinkle with the almonds and serve hot. Pass the grated cheese.

1½ Calcium servings; 1 Protein serving; 2 Green Leafy and Yellow vegetable servings; 1 Vitamin C serving; 1 Whole-Grain serving.

Note: The new mild-tasting water-packed canned salmon is prepared without skin and bones. Although it is lower in calories, may look pretty, and may even please the palates of those who reject the fishier tasting varieties, it won't provide any calcium. It will also be low in the fish oils that are believed to help prevent heart attack.

PREGNANT CHEF'S SALAD

Accompany this salad with a whole-grain bread and fruit to bring the Daily Dozen tally to 8½ requirements filled.

Serves 4

1 head romaine or other dark green leafy lettuce
3 carrots, shredded
3 small potatoes, boiled or steamed in their jackets, sliced
3 small red or green bell peppers, cored, seeded, and sliced
1 cup sliced fresh mushrooms
1 can (6 to 7 ounces) water-packed tuna, drained and flaked, or 6 ounces cooked, fresh turkey, julienned
4 ounces Swiss cheese, julienned
3 hard-cooked eggs, quartered
¼ cup grated Parmesan cheese
3 tablespoons sesame seeds
Italian Vinaigrette (page 265)

1. Rinse and dry the lettuce, tear into bite-size pieces, and place in a large salad bowl. Add the carrots, potatoes, peppers, and mushrooms and toss to combine.

2. Mound the tuna in the center of the salad. Sprinkle the Swiss cheese around the tuna and garnish with the eggs.

3. Sprinkle the salad with the Parmesan cheese and sesame seeds. Pour the vinaigrette over all. Toss. Serve at once.

1½ Calcium servings; 1 Protein serving; 1 Green Leafy and 1 Yellow Vegetable serving; 1 Vitamin C serving; 1 Other Vegetable serving.

QUICK-FIX FISH

For many, preparing fresh fish at home presents a challenge they're unwilling to accept. It shouldn't, for virtually no food can be cooked more quickly and more easily. Try this recipe for preparing any type of fish—fillet or steak. You can vary the herbs, if you like, use horse-radish instead of mustard, or add ¼ cup grated Parmesan cheese.

Serves 4

2 tablespoons mayonnaise
¼ cup grainy mustard
2 tablespoons white wine vinegar or white wine
1½ teaspoons dried tarragon or

2 tablespoons chopped fresh
4 ocean fish fillets or steaks (6 to 8 ounces each), such as snapper, sea bass, trout, flounder, cod, or tilefish
Salt and pepper to taste
¾ cup dry white wine, or as needed

1. Preheat the oven to 325°F.

2. Mix the mayonnaise, mustard, vinegar, and half the tarragon thoroughly in a small bowl.

3. Rinse and thoroughly dry the fish. Arrange the fillets in a single layer in a nonstick baking dish and sprinkle with salt and pepper. Spread the mayonnaise mixture over the fillets and sprinkle with the remaining tarragon. Pour the wine around the fish.

4. Bake until the fish is lightly browned and flakes with a fork. The cooking time will vary with the type of fish and how thick the fillets are.

2 Protein servings.

QUICK-FIX CHICKEN

Of all the many ways to prepare the versatile chicken, those which offer the fastest route from butcher shop to table are probably the most appealing to expectant mothers in a hurry for a nourishing dinner. This is a quick-fix, never-fail way of preparing chicken, with a choice of flavors.

Serves 4

4 large chicken breast halves
and
2 tablespoons mayonnaise
*¼ cup mustard, preferably with
   seeds*
1 tablespoon apple juice concentrate
or
2 tablespoons mayonnaise
*¼ cup mustard, preferably with
   seeds*
2 tablespoons dry white wine
½ teaspoon dried tarragon
or
*¼ cup fruit-only apricot and/or
   peach preserves*
*1 tablespoon mustard, preferably
   with seeds*
1 teaspoon dry white wine

or
*¼ cup fruit-only apricot and/or
   peach preserves or fruit-only
   orange marmalade*
½ teaspoon garlic powder
¼ teaspoon black pepper
*1 teaspoon cider vinegar or dry
   white wine or apple juice
   concentrate*
and
*1 cup chicken stock or 1 cup dry
   white wine*

1. Preheat the oven to 325°F.

2. Skin the chicken breasts and remove all visible fat. Rinse and pat dry. Arrange meat side up in a nonstick baking pan just large enough to hold them.

3. Mix your choice of ingredi-

ents until smooth and spread on the chicken breasts. Pour the stock over and around the breasts.

4. Bake until the breasts are just cooked on the inside and lightly browned outside, 20 to 30 minutes. Serve hot.

1 or more Protein servings, depending on the size of the chicken breast.

QUICK-FIX CHICKEN AU GRATIN

Just as speedy, just as satisfying.

Serves 4

4 large chicken breast halves
2 tablespoons fresh lemon juice
1 tablespoon flour
4 tablespoons Dijon mustard
½ teaspoon Worcestershire sauce or
     steak sauce
1 garlic clove, finely minced
1 tablespoon mayonnaise
½ cup whole-wheat bread crumbs

1. Remove the skin and all visible fat from the chicken breasts. Rinse and pat dry. Brush with lemon juice and then sprinkle with the flour. Place the chicken meat side up in a nonstick baking pan, just large enough to hold it.

2. Combine 2 tablespoons of the mustard, the Worcestershire sauce, and garlic and spread the mixture evenly over the chicken. Cover the chicken with foil, and, if possible, refrigerate for 1 hour or more.

3. Preheat the oven to 350°F.

4. Bake, still covered, for 25 minutes. Then combine the remaining mustard with the mayonnaise and spread over the chicken. Coat each breast evenly with the bread crumbs. Bake, uncovered, until nicely browned, about 10 minutes.

1 or more Protein servings, depending on the size of the chicken breast.

TUNA-PASTA PRIMAVERA

It's usually the sauce on the pasta that adds unnecessary calories. Here's one sauce that adds nutrients instead.

Serves 4

8 ounces whole-wheat or high-
  protein fusilli (corkscrew pasta)
1 tablespoon vegetable oil
1 teaspoon (core removed) minced
  garlic
¼ cup chopped fresh basil or 2
  teaspoons dried
¼ cup chopped fresh parsley (plus 2
  tablespoons if basil is dried)
1 large red bell pepper, cored,
  seeded, and cut into 1-inch strips
1 large green bell pepper, cored,
  seeded, and cut into 1-inch strips
2 cups broccoli florets, cut into 1-
  inch pieces
1 teaspoon dried oregano
1 cup cauliflower florets, cut into 1-
  inch pieces
1 teaspoon dried thyme
1 cup zucchini, cut into 1-inch
  matchsticks
1 cup Italian Vinaigrette (page 264)
1 can (6 to 7 ounces) water-packed
  tuna, drained
2 ounces Parmesan cheese, grated
¼ cup pine nuts (pignoli)

1. Cook the pasta according to package directions until tender but still firm.

2. Heat the oil over medium heat in a nonstick skillet. Add the garlic, basil, and parsley and sauté for 2 minutes. Add the peppers and sauté just until they begin to soften. Remove from the heat.

3. Place the broccoli in a steamer over boiling water, sprinkle with oregano, and steam until barely tender. Immediately transfer to a large bowl. Place the cauliflower in the steamer, sprinkle with thyme, and steam until barely tender. Immediately add to the broccoli. Steam the zucchini for 2 or 3 minutes. Do not permit it to become translucent. Add it to the broccoli and cauliflower.

4. Stir the pepper mixture into the vegetables; then toss with the pasta. Add the vinaigrette, tuna, Parmesan, and pine nuts and toss until all the ingredients are well coated. Serve warm or chill and serve cold.

1 Protein serving; 1 Whole-Grain serving; 2 Vitamin C servings; 1 Green Leafy serving; ½ Calcium serving.

SALMON MOUSSE

Protein, calcium, and significant amounts of other nutrients in an elegant, yet easy-to-fix package. Particularly refreshing on a warm summer night. Just add a salad and whole-grain bread, and your meal is complete.

Serves 4

1½ tablespoons unflavored gelatin
1 can (16 ounces) tomatoes in purée
1 can (1 pound) salmon, with bones and skin (see Note, page 255)
⅔ cup low-fat yogurt
2 tablespoons mayonnaise
¼ cup chopped fresh dill
¼ cup chopped fresh parsley
1 red bell pepper, cored, seeded, cut into chunks
1 tablespoon chopped onion (optional)
1 tablespoon fresh lemon juice, or to taste
¼ cup slivered almonds
Vegetable cooking spray

1. In a small saucepan, soften the gelatin in ⅓ cup purée from the canned tomatoes. Put the remaining tomatoes and purée in a blender or food processor.

Add the salmon, yogurt, mayonnaise, dill, parsley, half the red pepper, onion, and lemon juice and process until smooth. Blend in two batches, if necessary. Transfer to a bowl.

2. Heat the gelatin mixture over medium heat until it dissolves and stir into the salmon mixture. Finely dice the remaining red pepper and stir it and the almonds into the salmon mixture.

3. Coat a 1-quart ring or other type mold with vegetable cooking spray. Pour the salmon mixture into the mold. Cover and refrigerate to chill until firm.

1 Protein serving; 1 Vitamin C serving; 1 Green Leafy serving; 1 Calcium serving

Vegetable Side Dishes

Unlike Popeye, many of us never learned to enjoy our vegetables "straight." Not to worry. If you're among those who prefer disguising vegetables rather than eating them in recognizable forms, you can hide them in loaves, soups, or casseroles; bury them under sauces or au gratin crumbs; smother them with dips or salad dressing; or present them incognito in any of the following ways.

CARROT AMBROSIA

Maybe this is why Bugs Bunny would do anything for a carrot fix.

Serves 4

1 tablespoon margarine or butter
¼ cup pineapple juice concentrate
¼ cup orange juice concentrate
Pinch of salt
Freshly ground black pepper to taste
1 pound fresh or frozen whole baby
  carrots (preferably Belgian)

Combine the margarine, juice concentrates, salt, and pepper to taste in a saucepan. Heat over medium-low heat until the margarine melts; then add the carrots. Bring to a boil. Reduce the heat and cook until the carrots are tender. Serve hot.

2 Yellow Vegetable servings.

VEGETABLES IN CHEESE SAUCE

Serves 4

4 servings any vegetable (see Food
  Selection Groups, page 58)
1 tablespoon margarine
1 tablespoon whole-wheat flour
1½ cups evaporated skim milk or
  1½ cups skim milk stirred with
  ½ cup nonfat dry milk
4 ounces low-fat Cheddar cheese,
  grated

Salt and white pepper to taste
Freshly grated nutmeg to taste

1. Steam the vegetable until just tender.

2. Melt the margarine over low heat in a small saucepan (preferably nonstick). Stir in the flour, stirring constantly for 2 or 3 minutes. Gradually stir in the

milk and cook, stirring constantly, until thick and smooth. Add the grated cheese and cook until it melts.

3. Add seasonings to taste.

Pour the sauce over the vegetable and serve.

1 Calcium serving; 1 Vegetable serving (depending on the vegetable used).

THREE-VEGETABLE BAKE

Prepare this entire loaf to get three vegetable servings at once or make just one layer. Either way, vegetables never tasted so good.

Serves 4

Vegetable cooking spray
½ cup whole-wheat bread crumbs
3 tablespoons sesame seeds
1 tablespoon margarine, melted
4 egg whites
1 cup evaporated skim milk or 1 cup skim milk stirred with ⅓ cup nonfat dry milk
Salt and pepper to taste
2½ cups chopped broccoli
4 medium shallots, chopped
¼ cup grated Parmesan cheese
2 medium potatoes
2 medium carrots, sliced
¼ teaspoon dried basil

1. Line a 9 x 5 x 3-inch loaf pan with waxed paper and spray the paper with vegetable cooking spray. Combine the bread crumbs, sesame seeds, and margarine and press evenly onto the bottom and sides of the loaf pan.

2. Beat together the egg whites, skim milk, and salt and pepper to taste. Set aside.

3. Steam the broccoli until barely tender and chop finely. Combine with half the shallots. Spread the broccoli evenly in the bottom of the loaf pan. Sprinkle with a little Parmesan.

4. Steam the potatoes and slice. Layer the potatoes over the broccoli; sprinkle with the remaining shallots and a little more Parmesan.

5. Preheat the oven to 350°F.

6. Steam the carrots and spread evenly over the potatoes. Sprinkle with the basil. Press down to remove any air pockets. Beat the remaining Parmesan into the egg mixture and pour over all the vegetables, lifting the edges a bit to allow the mixture to run down.

7. Bake for 25 minutes. Unmold and serve hot.

1 Green Leafy serving; 1 Vitamin C serving; 1 Other Vegetable serving; 1 Calcium serving.

NO CLEAN-UP VEGETABLES

These vegetables cook in the oven while you bake the fish or roast the chicken and leave you with no pots to scour.

Serves 2

2 servings any vegetable or
   combination of vegetables (see
   Food Selection Groups, page 58)
Vegetable cooking spray
Grated Parmesan or low-fat cheese

1. Preheat the oven to 350°F.

2. Slice the vegetables or break them into bite-size pieces.

3. With vegetable cooking spray, coat a square of foil large enough to hold the vegetables. Place the vegetables on the foil and sprinkle with the cheese. Seal the packet by folding the foil and crimping the edges securely.

4. Bake until just tender, 10 to 20 minutes, depending on the vegetable. Test for doneness by poking a toothpick through the foil.

Depending on which vegetable is used, 1 Green Leafy and Yellow Vegetable or 1 Other Vegetable serving.

VEGETABLES ITALIAN STYLE

The quickest way to bring extraordinary taste out of ordinary vegetables.

Serves 4

4 servings green leafy vegetable
   (page 58), cut into bite-size pieces
2 tablespoons vegetable oil
2 cloves garlic, core removed,
   minced
Salt and pepper to taste

1. Steam the vegetable just until it is almost tender. Do not cook it fully. Set aside.

2. Heat the oil over medium-low heat in a nonstick pot large enough to hold the vegetables. Add the garlic and cook for 2 minutes. Add the vegetables and quickly stir-fry until the vegetables are just tender. Add salt and pepper to taste. Serve immediately.

Depending on which vegetable is used, 1 Green Leafy and Yellow Vegetable or 1 Other Vegetable serving.

Salad Suggestions & Dressing Recipes

Fresh salads of all kinds are so popular nowadays and it should come as no surprise that they are bountiful sources of Daily Dozen requirements. Add to your bowl whatever you are short of on a particular day. Green Leafy or Yellows (broccoli, lettuce, or carrots, for example); Vitamin C foods (oranges, cantaloupe, peppers); Other Vegetables and Fruits (potatoes, green beans, mushrooms, apples, pears, grapes); in fact, just about any fruit or vegetable is good in a salad. So, too, are Protein foods (tuna, chicken, turkey, beef, ham, fish, tofu, chick-peas, pignoli); Calcium foods (Parmesan cheese, chunks of Cheddar or Swiss) and even Whole Grains (whole-wheat croutons, bite-size shredded wheat, a sprinkling of wheat germ). The combinations of flavors and textures are endless. Be bold. Go for variety. One of the following dressings will be, no doubt, the perfect topping for your experiment.

ITALIAN VINAIGRETTE

Makes ¾ cup

½ teaspoon dried oregano
½ teaspoon dried basil
¼ teaspoon dried marjoram
2 tablespoons chopped fresh parsley
1 clove garlic, core removed
2 tablespoons vegetable oil
½ cup Vegetable Stock (page 242), boiling, or 1 vegetable bouillon cube dissolved in ½ cup boiling water
2 tablespoons wine vinegar
Salt and freshly ground black pepper to taste

1. Combine the herbs, garlic, and oil in a small bowl. Let stand 15 minutes to 1 hour.

2. Add the boiling stock to the herb mixture. Whisk in the vinegar. Season to taste with salt and pepper and whisk again. Cool to room temperature before serving or store, covered, in the refrigerator.

½ recipe = 1 Fat serving.

SWEET TANGY MUSTARD DRESSING

Makes ¾ cup

¼ cup apple juice concentrate
¼ cup cider vinegar
¼ cup vegetable oil
2 teaspoons Dijon or Pommery
  mustard

Place all the ingredients in a small bowl and whisk until blended.

¼ recipe = 1 Fat serving.

GARLIC-AVOCADO DRESSING

Makes about 1⅓ cups

1 small avocado, peeled, pitted, cut
  into chunks
2 tablespoons fresh lemon juice
3 tablespoons cider vinegar
1 large clove garlic, core removed
¼ teaspoon ground cumin
  (optional)

½ cup Vegetable Stock (page 242) or
  1 bouillon cube dissolved in ½
  cup water

Place all the ingredients in a blender or food processor and process until smooth.

½ recipe = 1 Other Vegetable and Fruit serving; 1 Fat serving.

BUTTERMILK-DILL DRESSING

Makes about 1½ cups

1 cup low-fat buttermilk
¼ cup low-fat cottage cheese
2 tablespoons minced onion
2 tablespoons minced fresh parsley
2 tablespoons minced fresh dill
1 tablespoon mayonnaise
1 clove garlic, core removed,
  crushed

Place all the ingredients except the garlic in a food processor or blender and process until smooth. Stir in the garlic and refrigerate for at least 2 hours to allow the flavors to blend.

¼ recipe = ¼ Calcium serving.

Puddings and Other Desserts

Puddings and gelatins have always been considered "nutritious"—the wholesome among desserts. But, unfortunately, all have a great nutritional minus: sugar. We've solved that problem deliciously.

BAKED BROWN RICE PUDDING

Just like grandma used to bake, but with a delicious whole-grain difference. A delight for dessert or topped with yogurt or cottage cheese for a sweet breakfast treat.

Serves 6

1 cup raw brown rice
3 eggs
4 egg whites
3 cups evaporated skim milk
1 cup apple juice concentrate
¾ cup chopped raisins
1 teaspoon vanilla extract
½ teaspoon salt
Dash of ground cinnamon, or to taste
Dash of freshly grated nutmeg, or to taste (optional)
1 teaspoon margarine or butter, room temperature
Vegetable cooking spray
½ cup whole raisins

1. Cook the rice according to package directions.

2. Preheat the oven to 325°F.

3. Beat the eggs and egg whites lightly together. Add the milk, juice concentrate, chopped raisins, vanilla, salt, and spices to taste; blend well.

4. Use the margarine to grease the bottom of a 2-quart baking dish coated with vegetable cooking spray. Spread the rice evenly in the bottom of the dish and sprinkle with the whole raisins. Pour the liquid mixture over the rice and raisins.

5. Bake until set, about 50 to 60 minutes. Refrigerate until cold before serving.

1½ Other Fruit serving; 1 Whole-Grain serving; 1 Calcium serving; ⅔ Protein serving.

Variation: For a really low cholesterol rice pudding, substitute 1 whole egg and 7 egg whites for the eggs and egg whites in the main recipe.

CREAMY BROWN RICE PUDDING

The cafeteria favorite, with a few Best-Odds modifications.

Serves 6

1 cup raw brown rice
10 tablespoons apple juice
  concentrate
1½ cups evaporated skim milk
1 egg
3 egg whites
½ teaspoon cinnamon, or to taste
½ cup raisins or currants
Slivered almonds (optional)

1. Cook the rice according to package directions, substituting 6 tablespoons of the juice concentrate for 6 tablespoons of the water.

2. Beat all the remaining ingredients, including the remaining juice concentrate, but not the almonds lightly, together in a medium saucepan.

3. Fold the cooked rice into the milk mixture, blending well. Cook, stirring frequently, over medium-low heat until thickened, 8 to 10 minutes.

4. Spoon into individual serving bowls and chill. If desired, sprinkle with the almonds before serving.

1 Whole-Grain serving; ½ Calcium serving; ⅔ Other Fruit serving; some Iron.

HARVEST PUDDING

A harvest of Best-Odds requirements with a pumpkin pie taste. Enjoy it for dessert, as a snack, even topped with yogurt for breakfast.

Serves 8

2 cups canned unsweetened solid-pack pumpkin
1⅓ cups apple juice concentrate
1½ teaspoons ground cinnamon, or to taste
3 egg whites
½ cup raisins, chopped
1 medium apple, peeled, cored, and coarsely chopped
1 medium pear, peeled, cored, and coarsely chopped
½ cup fresh cranberries (optional)

1⅔ cups rolled oats
6 tablespoons wheat germ
1 tablespoon margarine or butter, melted
¼ cup coarsely chopped walnuts or pecans

1. Preheat the oven to 350°F.

2. Place the pumpkin, ¾ cup of the juice concentrate, ½ teaspoon of the cinnamon, and the egg whites in a bowl; beat together until well blended. Stir in

the raisins, apple, pear, and cranberries.

3. Combine the remaining apple juice concentrate and cinnamon, the rolled oats, wheat germ, margarine, and nuts in another bowl; blend until crumbly. Stir half the oat mixture into the pumpkin mixture.

4. Transfer the pumpkin mixture into a 9-inch nonstick baking dish. Sprinkle the remaining oat mixture evenly over the top.

5. Bake until the crumbs are light brown and the pudding is set, 30 to 40 minutes. Serve warm or cold with unsweetened whipped cream, Best-Odds Ice Cream (page 289), or evaporated skim milk, if desired.

2 Yellow Vegetable servings; 1 Other Fruit serving; 1 Whole-Grain serving.

PURE FRUIT GELS

There's always room on the Best-Odds Diet for these naturally sweetened and naturally flavored gels. Refreshing and not too filling, they're particularly appealing when a queasy tummy won't welcome anything else.

APPLE-BANANA GEL
Serves 4

1½ tablespoons unflavored gelatin
2 cups water
1 cup apple juice concentrate
1 cup sliced bananas

1. Stir the gelatin into ⅓ cup of the water; let stand 1 minute to allow the gelatin to soften. Bring the remaining water to a boil, add the gelatin, and stir until thoroughly dissolved.

2. Stir in the juice concentrate. Turn the mixture into a 1½-quart nonstick mold or individual serving dishes. Refrigerate just until the gelatin begins to set. Stir in the bananas and chill until firm.

1½ Other Fruit servings.

PINEAPPLE-ORANGE GEL
Serves 4

1½ tablespoons unflavored gelatin
1½ cups water
1 cup orange juice concentrate
1 can (20 ounces) crushed pineapple in unsweetened juice
1 to 2 tablespoons apple juice concentrate, if needed
¼ cup chopped nuts (optional)

1. Stir the gelatin into ½ cup of the water; let stand 1 minute to soften. Meanwhile, bring the remaining water to a boil, add the gelatin, and stir until thoroughly dissolved.

2. Add the juice concentrate and crushed pineapple with its juice; stir to combine. Taste and if additional sweetness is needed, add 1 or 2 tablespoons apple juice concentrate.

3. Pour the mixture into a nonstick mold and refrigerate until the gelatin just begins to set. Stir in the nuts, if desired, and chill until firm.

2 Vitamin C servings; 1 Other Fruit serving.

Pies

Slice up some good nutrition with your next slice of pie. Bake these delicious favorites or try some of your own filling recipes using the Wheat-Germ or Shreddie Crusts, or a crumb crust made from Best-Odds Cookies. Sweeten fruit fillings with juice concentrates, and flavor them with cinnamon and other spices to taste.

WHEAT-GERM PIE CRUST

The flaky texture that comes with an all-white-flour crust is completely compensated for by the nutritional value of the wheat germ.

Makes dough for two-crust 9-inch pie

1 cup unbleached white flour
1 cup wheat germ
½ cup unsalted butter or
margarine, cold
¼ cup ice water

1. Combine the flour and wheat germ in a mixing bowl. Cut in the butter until the mixture resembles coarse meal. Mix in just enough of the ice water so that the dough holds together. Handle the dough as little as possible.

2. Turn the dough out onto a floured board. Divide into two pieces, one slightly larger than the other. Form both pieces quickly into balls. Wrap each ball in waxed paper and refrigerate for 1 hour at least.

3. Dust the larger ball with flour (leave the smaller ball in the refrigerator while you work with the larger). Roll it into a circle about ⅛ inch thick. Line a 9-inch pie plate with the dough. Trim the edge.

4. Fill the pie. Roll out the remaining dough for the top crust. Place it carefully over filling and press both crusts together to seal at the edge. Trim the excess dough and flute the rim. Bake as directed in the pie recipe of your choice.

PUMPKIN PIE

As classic—and as wholesome—as the Macy's parade.

Makes 9-inch pie

Crust

2 tablespoons margarine
⅓ cup apple juice concentrate
¾ cup whole-wheat flour
½ cup wheat germ
¼ cup chopped pecans

Filling

1 whole egg
2 egg whites
1 can (16 ounces) unsweetened solid-pack pumpkin
1 teaspoon ground cinnamon, or to taste
½ teaspoon ground ginger, or to taste
½ teaspoon freshly grated nutmeg, or to taste
1 cup raisins
¾ cup plus 2 tablespoons apple juice concentrate
⅔ cup plus 2 tablespoons evaporated skim milk
2 teaspoons vanilla extract
1 tablespoon unflavored gelatin

1. To make the crust: Heat the margarine and juice concentrate until the margarine melts. Blend the margarine mixture with the flour, wheat germ, and pecans until smooth. Press into a deep 9-inch pie plate.

2. Preheat the oven to 425°F.

3. To make the filling: Mix the egg, egg whites, pumpkin, and spices in a large mixing bowl. Process the raisins, juice concentrate, ⅓ cup plus 2 tablespoons skim milk, and the vanilla in a blender or food processor until smooth. Add to the pumpkin mixture and mix until well blended.

4. Stir the gelatin into the remaining ⅓ cup milk; let stand 1 minute to soften the gelatin. Stir thoroughly into the pumpkin mixture.

5. Pour the mixture into the pie shell. Bake 15 minutes. Reduce the heat to 350°F and bake until set, 40 to 45 minutes. Cover with aluminum foil if the pie begins to brown too quickly. Cool completely before serving.

⅛ pie = 3 + Yellow Vegetable servings; 1 Whole-Grain serving; 1 Other Fruit serving.

PUMPKIN CHIFFON PIE

A lighter version of the Thanksgiving standby.

Makes 9-inch pie

½ Wheat-Germ Pie Crust dough
(page 269)
2 envelopes unflavored gelatin
¾ cup plus 3 tablespoons apple juice
concentrate
1 can (16 ounces) unsweetened
solid-pack pumpkin
1 teaspoon ground cinnamon
½ teaspoon ground nutmeg
1 teaspoon vanilla extract
2 large egg whites
¼ teaspoon cream of tartar
1 tablespoon orange juice
concentrate

1. Preheat the oven to 425°F.

2. Roll out the pie dough and line a 9-inch pie plate with it. Trim and flute the edge. Prick the bottom with a fork and fill the shell with raw rice or beans. Bake 8 minutes, then carefully shake out the rice and continue baking until the crust is golden brown, about 2 to 4 minutes more.

3. Stir the gelatin into ¼ cup apple juice concentrate in a small saucepan; let stand 1 minute to soften the gelatin. Heat to boiling and then remove from the heat; stir to dissolve the gelatin.

4. Stir the pumpkin, ½ cup plus 1 tablespoon apple juice concentrate, the spices, and vanilla into the gelatin. Refrigerate to chill just until the mixture begins to thicken. Do not let it set.

5. Beat the egg whites with the cream of tartar until stiff; beat in the remaining 2 tablespoons apple juice concentrate and the orange juice concentrate. Beat in the pumpkin mixture just until smooth; do not overbeat. Pour the mixture into the crust and chill until set, about 2 hours.

⅛ pie = 2 Yellow Vegetable servings; 1 Whole-Grain serving; 1 Fat serving.

Note: If you are gaining weight too quickly, prepare the filling without the crust. Serve it in sherbert glasses.

NATURE-SWEETENED APPLE PIE

As American as the others, but a lot more nutritious. If you are gaining weight too quickly, bake this filling crustless, in a lightly oiled nonstick casserole or in the Shreddie Crust (page 285).

Makes two-crust 9-inch pie

Wheat-Germ Pie Crust (see page 269)
7 medium baking apples
½ cup apple juice concentrate, or to taste
⅓ cup broken walnut pieces
½ cup raisins
½ teaspoon lemon juice
1 teaspoon ground cinnamon, or to taste
1 tablespoon cold margarine or butter, cut into pieces

1. Preheat the oven to 450°F.

2. Roll out the pie dough for the bottom pie shell. Line a 9-inch pie plate with it. Set aside.

3. Peel, core, and cut the apples into ¼-inch slices. Toss them with the juice concentrate, walnuts, raisins, lemon juice, and cinnamon in a large mixing bowl. Stir the apples until syrup is formed and the apples are well coated.

4. Mound the apples high in the pie shell, drizzling the syrup from the bowl over them. Dot with the margarine. Roll out the top crust and lay it over the apples. Seal, trim, and flute the edge. Make a design in the crust with a sharp knife or prick it with a fork to allow steam to escape.

5. Bake for 10 minutes. Reduce the heat to 350°F and bake until golden brown, 35 to 45 minutes longer. If the pie begins to brown too quickly, cover it with foil. Let cool 30 minutes before serving.

⅛ **pie = 1 Whole-Grain serving; 1 Other Fruit serving; 1 Fat serving.**

Cookies

If you share the Sesame Street Cookie Monster's addiction, this collection can help you get through pregnancy with nary a withdrawal pain. Here are crispy, crunchy, chewy, and cakey cookies all made with nourishing ingredients and without sugar, and all capable of taming the cookie monster in you and in those you love.

CRANBERRY CRUNCH BARS

Tart-sweet, and crumbly.

Makes 18 to 25 bars

1 cup apple juice concentrate
¼ cup orange juice
1 tablespoon cornstarch
1 teaspoon ground cinnamon
1½ cups currants or chopped
    raisins
5 tablespoons orange juice
    concentrate
Grated zest of 1 orange
1 cup coarsely chopped cranberries
1½ cups whole-wheat flour
½ cup wheat germ
1 cup rolled oats
Vegetable cooking spray
½ cup chopped nuts

1. Stir together ½ cup of the apple juice concentrate, the orange juice, cornstarch, and cinnamon in a saucepan until smooth. Add the currants and cook over low heat for 5 minutes, stirring occasionally.

2. Stir in the orange juice concentrate, orange zest, and cranberries. Set aside to cool.

3. Preheat the oven to 350°F.

4. Combine the flour, wheat germ, and oats in a large bowl. Stir in the remaining ½ cup apple juice concentrate until the mixture resembles coarse crumbs. Spread half the mixture in a 9-inch square pan coated with vegetable cooking spray and press it down evenly. Spread the filling evenly over the flour mixture. Stir the nuts into the remaining flour mixture and pat over the filling as evenly as possible.

5. Bake until lightly browned, 30 to 40 minutes. Cool before cutting.

2 bars = 1+ Whole-Grain serving; 1 Other Fruit serving; some Iron.

NO-BAKE FRUIT AND NUT BALLS

A quick fix for the sweet tooth and a quick lift for a sagging energy level.

Makes about 35 balls

2 cups mixed chopped unsweetened
    dried fruit, such as dates, raisins,
    apples, apricots, peaches, pears,
    papaya, pineapple
½ cup chopped nuts or Grape Nuts

¾ cup rolled oats, or as needed
¼ cup apple juice concentrate, or as
    needed

Combine the fruit, nuts, and ¾ cup oats in a bowl; stir in enough juice concentrate to moisten the mixture. Form into small balls, pressing very firmly. If the balls don't hold together, add more juice or more oats. Re-frigerate to chill the balls before serving.

⅛ recipe = 1 Other Fruit serving; some Iron.

FUDGE BROWNIES

For confirmed chocoholics, nine months without chocolate could be devastating. Thanks to these rich, cakelike, yet nutritious confections, it needn't come to that.

Makes about thirty-five 2 x 2 inch brownies

1 cup whole-wheat flour
½ cup wheat germ
2 teaspoons baking soda
1½ cups apple juice concentrate
½ cup butter or margarine
6 tablespoons unsweetened cocoa
½ cup low-fat buttermilk
1 whole egg
2 egg whites
2 teaspoons vanilla extract
½ cup coarsely chopped walnuts

1. Preheat the oven to 350°F.

2. Combine the flour, wheat germ, and baking soda in a large bowl.

3. Combine the juice concentrate, butter, and cocoa in a small saucepan. Bring to a boil, stirring frequently. Add to the dry ingredients and beat until smooth. Add the buttermilk, egg, egg whites, and vanilla and beat just until mixed. Gently fold in walnuts.

4. Pour the batter into a floured and greased 15 x 10-inch jelly-roll pan. Bake until a toothpick inserted into the center comes out clean, about 20 to 25 minutes. Cool before cutting.

3 brownies = 1 Whole-Grain serving.

CAROB BROWNIES

For those who enjoy brownies with a glass of milk, but who don't want to compromise their calcium absorption by eating chocolate, this is a chewy treat.

Makes about thirty-two 1 x 2-inch brownies

3 tablespoons butter or margarine
½ cup plus 1 tablespoon apple juice concentrate
⅔ cup raisins
1 teaspoon vanilla extract
⅔ cup whole-wheat flour
1½ teaspoons baking powder
¼ cup unsweetened carob powder
½ cup chopped walnuts
Vegetable cooking spray

1. Combine the butter or margarine, juice concentrate, and raisins in a small saucepan and cook over very low heat for 10 minutes. Remove from the heat and add the vanilla.

2. Mix together the flour, baking powder, carob powder, and walnuts in a medium-size bowl. Add the juice mixture, and blend quickly but thoroughly.

3. Pour the batter into an 8-inch square pan that has been coated with vegetable cooking spray. Bake until a toothpick inserted into the center comes out clean, about 10 minutes. Let cool in the pan, then cut into squares.

1/12 recipe = ½ Other Fruit serving.

FIG BARS

Naturally sweetened, whole-grain bars that satisfy like the originals.

Makes about 36 cookie bars

1 tablespoon fructose
4 tablespoons butter or margarine
1 cup plus 2 tablespoons apple juice concentrate
1½ cups whole-wheat flour
1 cup wheat germ
1½ teaspoons vanilla extract
1 pound dried figs
2 tablespoons ground almonds or other nuts
Vegetable cooking spray

1. Preheat the oven to 350°F.

2. Cream the fructose and butter together in a mixer bowl. Heat ½ cup plus 2 tablespoons of the juice concentrate over medium heat until warm. Add the juice to the butter mixture and continue to cream.

3. Add the flour, wheat germ, and vanilla, and mix to form a dough. Divide the dough evenly in two, forming each half into a rectangular bar. Wrap them separately in waxed paper, and refrigerate to chill for 1 hour.

4. Meanwhile, combine the figs and remaining juice concentrate in a saucepan, and cook together over low heat until figs are soft. In a blender, purée the figs with the juice. Pour the purée into a small bowl and stir in the almonds until smooth.

5. Coat a large, preferably

nonstick, cookie sheet with vegetable cooking spray. Place one rectangle of dough on the sheet and roll it out until it is very thin. Even out the edges as much as possible. Spread the fig mixture over the dough.

6. Place the second rectangle of dough between two sheets of waxed paper that are the size of the cookie sheet. Roll out the dough to fill out the waxed paper. Remove one sheet and place the dough as neatly as possible over the fig mixture. Press down lightly, and even out the ends with a sharp knife. Remove the remaining waxed paper.

7. Bake until lightly browned, 15 to 30 minutes. Cut into squares or diamond shapes while still hot.

½ **recipe = 1+ Whole-Grain serving; 1 Other Fruit serving; some Iron.**

RAISIN-OATMEAL COOKIES

Wash these chunky cookies down with a glass of milk and enjoy after-school memories any time of the day or night.

Makes about 60 cookies

4 cups rolled oats
1¼ tablespoons ground cinnamon
¾ cup nonfat dry milk
½ cup wheat germ
¾ cup butter or margarine, room
temperature
1 whole egg
2 egg whites
1 cup apple juice concentrate
1 cup raisins, chopped
½ cup whole raisins
½ cup unsweetened carob chips
(available in health food stores;
optional)

1. Preheat the oven to 325°F.

2. Combine the oats, cinnamon, dry milk, and wheat germ in a medium-size bowl.

3. Beat the butter, egg, egg whites, and juice concentrate together in a large bowl. Stir in the dry ingredients until blended. Stir in the raisins and carob chips.

4. Drop the batter by rounded teaspoonful on ungreased cookie sheets. Bake until the edges are firm, 10 to 12 minutes. Cool briefly on the cookie sheet; then remove to wire rack to cool completely.

4 cookies = 1 Whole-Grain serving; ⅔ Other Fruit serving.

PEANUT BUTTER BALLS

These high-energy, low-effort cookies would be at home on a trail in the Rocky Mountains, but they also make delicious suburban or city snacking

Makes about 30 balls

½ cup peanut butter
¼ cup nonfat dry milk
¾ cup plus ⅓ cup prepared
    unsweetened or homemade
    granola (page 218)
¼ cup wheat germ
¼ cup apple juice concentrate

Mix all the ingredients thoroughly in a medium-size bowl. Shape into 1-inch balls. Refrigerate to chill before serving.

$1/10$ **recipe = ½ Whole-Grain serving; ⅓ Protein serving.**

SPICE COOKIES

A cakey cookie with lots of spice and perfect with a glass of milk.

Makes 3 dozen cookies

1½ cups whole-wheat flour
¾ cup wheat germ
1 teaspoon baking powder
1 teaspoon baking soda
½ teaspoon ground cloves or
    allspice
1¼ teaspoons ground ginger
1½ teaspoons ground cinnamon
1 cup apple juice concentrate
¼ cup vegetable oil
2 egg whites

1. Mix the flour, wheat germ, baking powder, baking soda, and spices in a bowl.

2. Beat the juice concentrate,

oil, and egg whites together at slow speed in a large mixer bowl. Gradually mix in the dry ingredients. Wrap the dough in waxed paper and refrigerate until cold.

3. Preheat the oven to 375°F.

4. With wet hands, shape the dough into 1-inch balls. Place on a nonstick cookie sheet and press down with a fork to flatten. Bake 8 to 10 minutes. Cool completely on a wire rack.

3 cookies = 1 Whole-Grain serving.

OATMEAL FRUIT-NUT BARS

Chewy and satisfying.

Makes about 30 bars

¾ cup rolled oats
¾ cup finely chopped nuts
¼ cup wheat germ
1 teaspoon ground cinnamon
⅓ cup apple juice concentrate
¾ cup pitted dates
¾ cup raisins
6 tablespoons orange juice
  concentrate
2 teaspoons grated orange zest
  (optional)

1. Preheat the oven to 350°F.

2. Process the oats in a blender or food processor to the consistency of coarse meal. Mix the oats, nuts, wheat germ, and cinnamon in a large bowl. Stir in the apple juice concentrate until mixture is crumbly.

3. Reserve ½ cup of the oat mixture; press the remaining mixture evenly into a nonstick 8-inch square baking pan.

4. Process the dates, raisins, orange juice concentrate, and orange zest in the blender or food processor until the fruit is chopped but not puréed. Spread the fruit mixture evenly over the oat layer. Top with the reserved oat mixture and press it down firmly.

5. Bake until lightly browned, 25 to 30 minutes. Cool completely. Cut into squares or bars.

⅛ recipe = 1 Whole-Grain serving; 1 Other Fruit serving; some Iron.

Note: If you are gaining weight too quickly, substitute wheat flakes for the nuts.

FRUITY OATMEAL COOKIES

A different oatmeal cookie; chewier and stickier than the rest.

Makes about thirty 2-inch cookies

10 dates, pitted
6 tablespoons apple juice
  concentrate
2 tablespoons vegetable oil
1½ cups rolled oats (or a mixture of
  oats and raw wheat flakes)
1 cup raisins

¼ to ½ cup chopped nuts
Dash of ground cinnamon, or to
  taste
1 egg white

1. Place dates and juice concentrate in a saucepan, and simmer together until fruit softens.

2. Purée the date mixture in a blender or food processor, then pour into a mixer bowl. Add the oil, oats, raisins, nuts, and cinnamon; stir thoroughly.

3. Beat the egg white lightly in a separate bowl; fold gently into the batter.

4. Drop the batter in tablespoonsful onto a nonstick cookie sheet that has been lightly greased with oil; flatten each mound with the back of a fork. Bake for 10 to 12 minutes.

⅛ **recipe = 1 Whole-Grain serving; 1 Other Fruit serving.**

Cakes

To "take the cake," you don't have to take the excess sugar and fat, or the refined flour. Almost any bakery favorite can be baked better with whole grains, fruits, and nuts on the inside, creamy but nutritious frostings and naturally-sweet fillings on the outside. Every cake lover will find a new friend here.

CARROT-PINEAPPLE CAKE

A vegetable-hater's sweet revenge. One scrumptious slice serves up an entire day's requirement of yellow vegetables.

Makes one 9-inch layer cake

2 cups shredded carrots
⅓ cup plus 2 tablespoons water
2 cups apple juice concentrate (you will use slightly less than this amount)
1½ cups raisins
Vegetable cooking spray
2 cups whole-wheat flour
½ cup wheat germ
1 tablespoon plus 1 teaspoon baking soda
1 tablespoon ground cinnamon
½ teaspoon ground ginger (optional)
¼ cup vegetable oil
2 whole eggs
4 egg whites
1 tablespoon vanilla extract
¾ cup drained unsweetened crushed pineapple
⅔ cup chopped walnuts
Cream Cheese Frosting (recipe follows)

1. Combine the carrots, water, and ⅔ cup of the apple juice concentrate in a large saucepan. Simmer covered over low heat until the carrots are tender. Purée the mixture in a blender or food processor until smooth. Add ¾ cup of the raisins and process until the raisins are chopped. Cool.

2. Preheat the oven to 350°F. Line two 9-inch cake pans with waxed paper and spray the paper with vegetable cooking spray.

3. Combine the flour, wheat germ, baking soda, and spices in a large mixer bowl. Add 1¼ cups juice concentrate, the oil, eggs, egg whites, and vanilla; beat well. Fold in the pineapple, carrot purée, walnuts, and remaining ¾ cup raisins. Pour the batter into prepared cake pans.

4. Bake until a knife inserted in the center comes out clean, 35 to 40 minutes. Cool layers completely on wire racks; then frost with cream cheese frosting.

1/12 recipe = 2 Yellow Vegetable servings; 1 Whole-Grain serving; 1 Other Fruit serving.

CREAM CHEESE FROSTING

8 ounces cream cheese or low-fat Neufchatel, at room temperature
3 tablespoons apple juice concentrate
2 teaspoons vanilla extract
½ cup finely chopped raisins
1 cup drained unsweetened crushed pineapple
1½ teaspoons unflavored gelatin
2 tablespoons pineapple juice concentrate

1. Place the cream cheese, apple juice concentrate, vanilla, raisins, and pineapple in a food processor; process until smooth.

2. Stir the gelatin into the pineapple juice concentrate; let stand 1 minute to allow the gelatin to soften. Heat to boiling and stir to dissolve the gelatin.

3. Beat the gelatin mixture into the cream cheese mixture until well blended. Refrigerate until frosting begins to set.

ANGELIC DEVIL'S FOOD CAKE

Angels never had it so good; a rich, deeply chocolate cake that won't make you lose your halo.

Makes one 9 x 13-inch cake

1¼ cups whole-wheat flour
½ cup wheat germ
2 teaspoons baking powder
2 teaspoons baking soda
¾ cup unsweetened cocoa

¼ cup vegetable oil
1¾ cups apple juice concentrate
½ cup strong brewed decaffeinated coffee
1 whole egg
2 egg whites
1 teaspoon vanilla extract

1. Preheat the oven to 325°F.

2. Place the flour, wheat germ, baking powder, baking soda, cocoa, oil, juice concentrate, and coffee in a large mixer bowl; beat until smooth. Add the egg, egg whites, and vanilla and beat until thoroughly mixed.

3. Pour the batter into a lightly floured and greased 9 x 13-inch baking pan. Bake until the top springs back when lightly pressed, about 35 minutes. Cool slightly in pan before turning out onto a rack to cool completely.

$^1/_{10}$ **recipe = 1 Whole-Grain serving.**

CAROB PARTY CAKE

Celebrate any occasion—from the start of a new job to the start of a new trimester—with this rich-tasting cake.

Makes two 8-inch square cakes

1 cup whole-wheat flour
⅓ cup wheat germ
¼ cup nonfat dry milk
1 tablespoon baking powder
⅔ cup unsweetened carob powder
⅔ cup skim milk
1⅓ cups apple juice concentrate
1 tablespoon vanilla extract
4 egg whites
½ cup raisins or chopped dried apricots
½ cup chopped walnuts
Vegetable cooking spray
Unsweetened whipped cream (optional)

1. Preheat the oven to 350°F.

2. Combine the flour, wheat germ, dry milk, and baking powder in a large bowl. Stir in the carob powder, milk, juice, and vanilla.

3. Beat the egg whites until stiff; fold them into the batter. Fold in the raisins and walnuts.

4. Pour the batter into two nonstick 8-inch square baking pans, coated with vegetable cooking spray. Bake until the top springs back when lightly pressed, 20 to 25 minutes. Turn out onto racks and cool completely. Frost, if desired, with unsweetened whipped cream.

$^1/_8$ **recipe = 1 Whole-Grain serving; 1 Other Fruit serving; some Iron.**

APPLE-NUT CAKE

Makes one 9-inch square cake

1 whole egg
4 egg whites
1 teaspoon vanilla extract
¼ cup vegetable oil
1¼ cups apple juice concentrate
1½ cups whole-wheat flour
¾ cup wheat germ
2 teaspoons baking soda
2 teaspoons ground cinnamon
¾ cup raisins
¾ cup walnuts, coarsely chopped
3 cups peeled, coarsely diced
   Cortland apples
1 tablespoon bourbon or apple juice
   concentrate
Vegetable cooking spray

1. Preheat the oven to 325°F.

2. Beat the egg and egg whites in a large mixer bowl un-til thickened. Beat in the vanilla, oil, and 1¼ cups juice concentrate.

3. Stir together the flour, wheat germ, baking soda, and cinnamon in another bowl. Add to the egg mixture and stir until blended. Fold in the raisins, nuts, apples, and bourbon.

4. Pour the batter into a 9-inch square baking pan coated with vegetable cooking spray. Bake until a toothpick inserted into the center comes out clean, about 1¼ hours. Let cool in the pan for 10 minutes; then remove to a wire rack to cool completely.

¹/₁₂ recipe = 1 Whole-Grain serving; ¾ Other Fruit serving.

FRIENDLY FRUITCAKE

Season's greetings without the season's indiscretions. This holiday favorite is best prepared 2 weeks or more in advance.

Makes 1 ring or 6 small loaves

1 cup raisins
¾ cup dried apricots, coarsely
   chopped
⅓ cup water
1 cup orange juice concentrate
¾ cup chopped dried apple slices
1 cup coarsely chopped pitted dates
2 cups fresh whole-wheat bread
   crumbs

¾ cup rolled oats
⅔ cup apple juice concentrate
½ cup chopped nuts, such as
   pecans, walnuts, and/or almonds
¼ cup sunflower seeds
Grated zest of 1 orange
Vegetable cooking spray
⅓ cup orange juice
1 tablespoon rum extract

1. Preheat the oven to 350°F.

2. Simmer the raisins, apricots, water, and ⅔ cup of the orange juice concentrate in a small saucepan for 5 minutes.

3. Thoroughly combine the simmered fruit mixture with the remaining ingredients through the orange zest (and including the remaining orange juice concentrate) in a large bowl. Press into a 2-quart nonstick ring mold or individual 3 x 5½-inch loaf pans, coated with vegetable cooking spray.

4. Bake the ring cake for 55 minutes or the small cakes for 35 minutes. Unmold onto a wire rack and cool completely.

5. Place the cake on a square of foil lined with a square of cheesecloth, each large enough to wrap around the cake. Stir together the orange juice and rum extract and pour the mixture evenly over the fruitcake. Wrap the cake tightly in the cheesecloth, then in the foil. Refrigerate at least several days or up to 2 weeks. Pour additional juice over the cake every few days.

¹/₁₂ **recipe = 1½ Other Fruit serving; 1 Whole-Grain serving; some Iron.**

HARVEST CAKE

Enjoy before, during, and after the fall—and don't forget to credit yourself with two Yellow Vegetable servings.

Makes two 8-inch square cakes

1 cup raisins
1½ cups apple juice concentrate
¼ cup vegetable oil
1 whole egg
3 egg whites
2 cups tightly packed finely shredded carrots
2 cups whole-wheat flour
½ cup wheat germ
1½ teaspoons ground cinnamon, or to taste
1 teaspoon ground cloves (optional)
1 teaspoon freshly grated nutmeg (optional)
2½ teaspoons baking powder

¾ teaspoon baking soda
1 small apple, peeled, cored, and finely diced (about ⅔ cup)
1 small pear, peeled, cored, and finely diced (about ⅔ cup)
1 cup coarsely chopped pecans
Vegetable cooking spray

1. Preheat the oven to 350°F.

2. Chop half the raisins. Combine all the raisins, the juice concentrate, and the oil in a small saucepan. Bring to a boil. Reduce the heat and simmer 1 minute. Transfer to a large mixing bowl and cool.

3. Beat the egg and egg whites together and stir them and the carrots into the raisin mixture.

4. Combine the flour, wheat germ, cinnamon, cloves and nutmeg (if desired), baking powder, and baking soda in a separate bowl; gradually stir into the carrot mixture, blending well. Fold in the apple, pear, and pecans.

5. Pour the batter into two nonstick 8-inch square baking pans coated with vegetable cooking spray. Bake on the middle rack of the oven until a toothpick inserted into the center comes out clean, 35 to 45 minutes. Cool for 10 minutes before removing to a wire rack to cool completely.

$1/12$ **recipe = 2 Yellow Vegetable servings; 1 Whole-Grain serving; 1 Other Fruit serving.**

CHEESECAKE

If Sara Lee were expecting. . . .

Makes one 10-inch cheesecake

2½ tablespoons unflavored gelatin
1¼ cups plus 2 tablespoons apple juice concentrate
1 cup evaporated skim milk
2 teaspoons vanilla extract
3 cups low-fat pot-style cottage cheese
2 egg whites
¼ teaspoon cream of tartar
Shreddie Crust (recipe follows)

1. Stir the gelatin into ½ cup of the juice concentrate to soften. Set aside. Bring the milk to a boil, add the gelatin mixture, and stir until the gelatin is thoroughly dissolved.

2. Stir the vanilla and ¾ cup juice concentrate into the milk mixture.

3. Place the cottage cheese in a blender or food processor, add some of the liquid mixture, and process until smooth. (If using a blender, process in two batches.) Mix the cheese and juice mixtures until smooth. Pour into a bowl and refrigerate to chill just until slightly set. Do not allow it to become firm.

4. Beat the egg whites with the cream of tartar and remaining 2 tablespoons juice concentrate until stiff. Quickly beat the egg white mixture into the gelatin mixture, being careful not to deflate the whites.

5. Pour into the shreddie crust and refrigerate to chill until firm.

$1/12$ **recipe = ½ Protein serving; ½ Other Fruit serving; ⅓ Calcium serving.**

Variations: Add any of the following in Step 3 before refrigerating the cheese mixture: ⅓ cup ground nuts; ½ cup blueberries; ¾ cup well-drained unsweetened crushed pineapple

SHREDDIE CRUST
Makes 10-inch pastry shell

2 cups bite-size shredded wheat
* biscuits*
¼ cup nuts, whole or pieces
* (walnuts, pecans, almonds,*
* hazelnuts)*
½ cup apple juice concentrate
Vegetable cooking spray

1. Preheat the oven to 350°F.

2. Process the shredded wheat in a blender or processor until finely ground. Add the nuts and process until ground. Add the juice concentrate and process until well mixed.

3. Shape the dough into a ball and place it in the middle of a nonstick 10-inch pie plate coated with vegetable cooking spray. Pat down and cover with a sheet of waxed paper. With your fingers, press the dough to line the pan evenly.

4. Bake until lightly browned, 8 to 10 minutes. Cool completely.

¹/₁₂ recipe = ¼ Whole-Grain serving.

PUMPKIN-PECAN CAKE

Rich in taste and vitamin A and the availability of canned pumpkin makes it a year-round treat.

Makes one 9-inch square layer cake

Vegetable cooking spray
¼ cup vegetable oil
1 whole egg
2 egg whites
1¾ cups apple juice concentrate
⅔ cup chopped raisins
1½ cups whole-wheat flour
½ cup wheat germ
2½ teaspoons baking powder
½ teaspoon baking soda
1 teaspoon ground cinnamon
½ teaspoon ground allspice
* (optional)*

¼ teaspoon ground ginger
* (optional)*
1 cup canned unsweetened solid-
* pack pumpkin*
⅔ cup finely chopped pecans
1 cup unsweetened apple butter
Pecans, roughly chopped (optional)

1. Preheat the oven to 350°F. Coat two nonstick 9-inch cake pans with vegetable cooking spray.

2. Beat the oil, egg, and egg

whites together in a large mixer bowl. Heat ¾ cup of the juice concentrate with the raisins until raisins soften. Set aside to cool.

3. Combine the flour, wheat germ, baking powder, baking soda, and spices thoroughly. Add the flour mixture with the remaining 1 cup juice concentrate to the egg mixture; stir just until blended. Fold in the pumpkin, finely chopped pecans, and raisins with liquid.

4. Pour the batter into the pre-

pared pans. Bake until a knife inserted into the center comes out clean, 35 to 40 minutes. Cool for 10 minutes. Remove from the pans to large plates and refrigerate until cold.

5. Spread 1 cake layer with all of the apple butter. Sprinkle the roughly chopped pecans over the apple butter. Top with the second layer.

⅛ recipe = 2 Yellow Vegetable servings; 1 Whole-Grain serving; 1 Other Fruit serving.

CHOCOLATE PUDDING CAKE

A delicious hybrid. For the chocolate allergic, carob powder may be substituted for cocoa.

Serves 8

3 tablespoons butter or margarine
2 teaspoons vanilla extract
½ cup skim milk, at room
    temperature
½ cup whole-wheat flour
¼ cup wheat germ
⅓ cup plus 3 tablespoons
    unsweetened cocoa or carob
    powder
1 tablespoon baking powder
2 tablespoons hot water mixed with
    enough apple juice concentrate to
    make 1⅔ cups
¼ cup sliced almonds
Unsweetened whipped cream
    (optional)

1. Preheat the oven to 350°F.

2. Place the butter in a deep 2-quart casserole and put it in the oven to melt the butter. Remove the dish from the oven. Mix the butter, vanilla, and milk in a small bowl and set aside.

3. Mix the flour, wheat germ, 3 tablespoons cocoa, and the baking powder in the casserole. Stir in the milk mixture just until blended. Sprinkle evenly with ⅓ cup cocoa. Pour the water mixed with the apple juice concentrate over the batter. Do not mix the batter.

4. Bake on the middle oven rack until a crust forms, about 20 minutes. Sprinkle with the almonds; bake until a toothpick inserted in the cake layer only comes out clean, about 10 to 15 minutes longer (the bottom layer will be loose and syrupy).

5. Cool before serving. Serve with unsweetened whipped cream, if desired.

1 Whole-Grain Serving.

GINGERBREAD

Light in texture, heady with spice, and a full whole-grain serving in every portion.

Makes one 9-inch square cake

1 cup whole-wheat flour
½ cup wheat germ
2 teaspoons baking soda
1½ teaspoons ground ginger
1 teaspoon ground cinnamon
2 egg whites, lightly beaten
1 cup apple juice concentrate
¼ cup vegetable oil
Vegetable cooking spray

1. Preheat the oven to 350°F.

2. Mix the flour, wheat germ, baking soda, and spices in a large mixing bowl. Add the egg whites and ½ cup of the juice

concentrate; stir to blend.

3. Heat the remaining juice concentrate until hot. Add it to the batter with the oil and mix until smooth.

4. Pour the batter into a non-stick 9-inch square pan coated with vegetable cooking spray. Bake until the top springs back when lightly touched and the sides have begun to pull away from the pan, about 35 minutes. Cool completely before cutting.

⅛ recipe = 1 Whole-Grain serving; ½ Other Fruit serving.

NUT TORTE

A light, nutty cake with a European flavor. Frosted with unsweetened whipped cream, it's at home on any Viennese dessert table.

Makes one 8-inch square layer cake

1⅓ cups apple juice concentrate
2 teaspoons vanilla extract
2 tablespoons vegetable oil
1 cup wheat germ
1½ teaspoons baking powder
¾ cup finely chopped nuts

7 egg whites, room temperature
½ cup fruit-only preserves, warmed
Unsweetened whipped cream
Toasted sliced almonds or chopped walnuts or hazelnuts

1. Preheat the oven to 325°F. Line two nonstick 8-inch square cake pans with waxed paper.

2. Combine the juice concentrate, vanilla, and oil in a large mixing bowl. Add the wheat germ, baking powder, and nuts; stir just to mix.

3. Beat the egg whites in a large mixer bowl until stiff but not dry. Gently fold into the wheat-germ mixture just until the whites disappear.

4. Pour the batter into the prepared pans. Bake until the cake springs back when lightly pressed, 30 to 35 minutes.

5. Invert the pans onto two large plates and carefully peel off the waxed paper while still warm. Let cool. Spread the top of 1 layer with half the preserves and then with a small amount of whipped cream. Sprinkle with some of the almonds. Place the other layer on top and spread it with the remaining preserves. Cover the top and sides with the remaining whipped cream and sprinkle with the remaining almonds. Refrigerate until ready to serve.

⅛ **cake = 1 Whole-Grain serving; ½ Protein serving; ½ Other Fruit serving.**

CHEWY OATMEAL CAKE

An easy-to-make, homey cake, slightly crumbly in texture.

Makes one 9-inch square cake

¾ *cup whole-wheat flour*
½ *cup wheat germ*
1½ *teaspoons baking soda*
1 *teaspoon ground cinnamon*
¼ *teaspoon ground nutmeg*
1½ *cups heated apple juice*
　　concentrate
1 *cup rolled oats*
⅓ *cup butter or margarine, room*
　　temperature
1 *whole egg*
2 *egg whites*
1 *teaspoon vanilla extract*
Vegetable cooking spray

1. Preheat the oven to 350°F.

2. Combine the flour, wheat germ, baking soda, and spices in a small bowl.

3. Pour the hot juice concentrate over the oats in another small bowl; cover and let stand 20 minutes.

4. Beat the butter in a mixer bowl at high speed until light and fluffy. Beat in the egg, egg whites, and vanilla. Add the oat mixture and mix well. Add the flour mixture and stir until thoroughly combined.

5. Pour the batter into a 9-inch square pan coated with vegetable cooking spray. Bake until the top springs back when lightly pressed, about 50 minutes. Cool completely before cutting.

$^1/_{10}$ **cake = 1 Whole-Grain serving; ½ Other Fruit serving.**

Frozen Desserts

These sorbets are as different from ices as juice is from soda. Enjoy them often. The same, too, with the ice cream recipes. The myth that commercial ice creams provide ample calcium or protein is done away with in "The Great Ice Cream War" on page 66, but that doesn't mean you can't scream for ice cream while you're pregnant. Best-Odds homemade ice creams are nutritious treats you can enjoy every day of your entire pregnancy. Unlike their commercial cousins, they are high in protein and calcium—and low in fat. Although sorbets are not rich in calcium and protein, they are very low in calories and high in vitamins and minerals. They refresh without over burdening the belly. Frozen dessert-makers are now available within almost everyone's price range, some selling for as low as $30.

When preparing a frozen dessert, it is very important to taste and add additional juice concentrate as needed. Before freezing, the flavor should be more intense than you like because it will lighten as air is mixed in and the volume of the dessert increases.

Add additional taste, texture, and nutrition by topping your sorbet or ice cream with any or all of the following sundae-makers: wheat germ, nuts, raisins, Best-Odds cookie or cake crumbs, fresh berries or other fruits, or fruit-only preserves.

CANTALOUPE SORBET

Serves 4 to 6

3 cups puréed cantaloupe (about 1 large melon)
1 orange, peeled and seeded (optional)
¼ to ½ cup apple or orange juice concentrate or combination of both

1 egg white
3 tablespoons apple juice concentrate

1. Process the cantaloupe, orange, and ¼ cup juice concentrate in a blender or food processor until smooth. Taste for flavor and sweetness and add juice

concentrate as needed. Pour the mixture into an ice-cream maker and begin freezing.

2. Beat the egg white and 3 tablespoons apple juice concentrate until stiff. Fold into the sorbet when the mixture has begun to thicken. Continue freezing until the sorbet is ready.

¼ **recipe = 2 Yellow Fruit servings.**

Variations: For any other fruit sorbet, substitute approximately 3 cups puréed ripe fruit. Any one of the following or, better still, a combination of two or more will make an excellent sorbet: blueberries, strawberries, cherries, melon, mangoes, pineapple, oranges, grapefruit, bananas, grapes, peaches, nectarines, apples, or pears.

BANANA-SPICE ICE CREAM

Serves 2 to 4

2 very ripe medium bananas, puréed (about 1 cup)
⅓ cup plus 3 tablespoons apple juice concentrate, or to taste
2 teaspoons vanilla extract
1 can (12 ounces) evaporated skim milk
2 tablespoons half-and-half
½ teaspoon ground cinnamon, or to taste
⅛ teaspoon ground ginger, or to taste
Freshly grated nutmeg to taste
1 egg white

1. Process all the ingredients except the egg white and 3 tablespoons apple juice concentrate in a blender or food processor until smooth. Taste for spices and sweetness and adjust, if necessary.

2. Pour the mixture into an ice-cream maker and begin to freeze according to manufacturer's directions.

3. Beat the egg white and 3 tablespoons apple juice concentrate until stiff. Fold it into the ice cream when it begins to thicken and continue freezing until the ice cream reaches the desired consistency.

¼ **recipe = 1 Other Fruit serving; ¾ Calcium serving.**

Variations: For Banana-Rum Raisin Ice Cream, reduce the vanilla to 1 teaspoon, add 1 teaspoon rum extract, omit the spices, and add ⅓ cup raisins when the mixture is almost frozen.

For Pumpkin-Spice Ice Cream, substitute ¾ cup canned unsweetened solid-pack pumpkin for the bananas. Reduce the vanilla to 1½ teaspoons, and increase the juice concentrate to ½ cup. Taste and adjust spices and sweetness.

¼ recipe = 2 Yellow Vegetable servings; ¾ Calcium serving; ½ Protein serving; ½ Other Fruit serving.

COFFEE ICE CREAM

Serves 2 to 4

1 can (12 ounces) evaporated skim milk
½ cup very strong brewed decaffeinated coffee
Instant decaffeinated coffee to taste
½ cup plus 3 tablespoons apple juice concentrate, or to taste
2 tablespoons half-and-half
2 teaspoons vanilla extract
1 egg white

1. Process all the ingredients except the egg white and 3 tablespoons apple juice concentrate in a blender or food processor until smooth. Taste for flavor and sweetness and adjust, if necessary.

2. Pour the mixture into an ice-cream maker and begin to freeze according to manufacturer's directions.

3. Beat the egg white and 3 tablespoons apple juice concentrate until stiff. Fold into the ice cream when it begins to thicken and continue to freeze until ice cream reaches the desired consistency.

¼ recipe = ¾ Calcium serving; ½ Protein serving.

Variation: For Mocha Ice Cream, process 3 tablespoons unsweetened carob powder with ingredients in Step 1.

BANANA-BERRY YOGURT POPS

Makes 6

2 very ripe bananas, cut into chunks
1 cup berries, fresh or frozen
1½ cups low-fat yogurt
2 tablespoons apple, pineapple, or orange juice concentrate

Process all the ingredients in a blender or food processor until smooth. Pour the mixture into six pop molds or 5-ounce paper cups. Place in freezer. If using cups, insert popsicle sticks when the mixture is firm enough to hold them upright. Freeze until completely frozen.

2 pops = 1 Other Fruit serving; ½ Calcium serving.

BERRY ICE CREAM

Serves 2 to 4

1½ cups fresh or frozen
    unsweetened strawberries,
    blueberries, raspberries, or
    combination
1 can (12 ounces) evaporated skim
    milk
½ cup plus 3 tablespoons apple juice
    concentrate, or to taste
2 tablespoons half-and-half
2 teaspoons vanilla extract
2 tablespoons fruit-only preserves in
    compatible flavor (optional)
1 egg white

1. Process all the ingredients except the egg white and 3 tablespoons juice concentrate in a blender or food processor until smooth. Taste for flavor and sweetness and adjust, if necessary.

2. Pour the mixture into an ice-cream maker and begin to freeze according to manufacturer's directions.

3. Beat the egg white and 3 tablespoons juice concentrate until stiff. Fold into the ice cream when it begins to thicken and continue to freeze until the ice cream reaches the desired consistency.

¼ recipe = ¾ Calcium serving; ½ Protein serving; ½ Vitamin C serving (if strawberries are used) or ½ Other Fruit serving (if other berries are used).

Variation: For Peach Ice Cream, substitute sliced very ripe peaches for the berries.

FROZEN TOFU

Unlike commercial tofu "ice creams," this one is actually good for you. A perfect lunch when nothing else appeals, it is also a treat for those who can't eat dairy ice creams.

Serves 4

1 pound tofu
½ cup apple juice concentrate
1 very ripe banana
1 pint berries or 2 cups sliced fruit,
    coarsely puréed
2 teaspoons vanilla extract
2 egg whites (optional)
3 tablespoons apple juice
    concentrate (optional)

3 tablespoons unsweetened apple-
    sauce (optional)

1. Purée the tofu, juice concentrate, and banana in a blender or processor. Add the berries or fruit and vanilla, and blend until smooth.

2. Pour the mixture into an ice-cream maker and begin to freeze according to manufacturer's directions.

3. Beat the egg whites, if desired, to soft peaks. If you are adding the egg whites, add the apple juice concentrate and applesauce and continue beating until stiff.

4. Fold the egg whites into

the tofu mixture when it begins to thicken and continue to freeze until it reaches the desired consistency.

1 Protein serving; ⅔ Calcium serving; 2 Other Fruit servings (or 1 Other Fruit and 1 Vitamin C serving if strawberries or other vitamin C fruit is used).

FROZEN JUICE POPS

Mix fresh juice (orange, apple, grape, or other favorite) with a little juice concentrate and freeze in pop molds or 5-ounce paper cups. Add sticks to the cups when the juice pops are almost frozen hard.

FROZEN FRUIT

FROZEN GRAPES

For an easy and refreshing frozen snack, just rinse, dry, and stem red or green seedless grapes; freeze in a plastic bag.

FROZEN BANANAS

Peel and slice bananas; freeze in a plastic bag. For carob-coated bananas, make a paste of unsweetened carob powder and milk and dip peeled bananas— in the paste; freeze on a waxed-paper-lined tray.

FROZEN BERRY YOGURT

Serves 4

4 cups nonfat or low-fat plain yogurt
2 cups strawberries, blueberries, or
  other berries, fresh or frozen
½ cup apple juice concentrate

Process all the ingredients in a blender or food processor until smooth. Freeze in an ice-cream

maker according to manufacturer's directions.

¼ recipe = 1 Calcium serving; 1 Vitamin C serving (if strawberries are used); 1 Other Fruit serving (if other berries are used); ½ Protein serving.

Party Foods

If you fear the party will be over even before it gets started because you have to strike the usual high-fat, low-nutrition party fare from your buffet, spread out these munchies, and you'll have nothing to worry about. Choose unusual vegetables for colorful crudités to accompany dips, and a wide assortment of whole-grain crackers or breads cut finger-size to cover with spreads and cheeses.

BLUE CHEESE DIP

A skinny dip with all the richness and flavor of its high-fat cousins. Try it as a potato topper, too.

Makes about 1½ cups

1 cup low-fat cottage cheese
¼ cup low-fat buttermilk
2 tablespoons mayonnaise
2 ounces blue cheese
Freshly ground black pepper to taste

1. Combine the cottage cheese, buttermilk, and mayonnaise in a blender or food processor and process until smooth.

2. Mash the blue cheese with a fork and blend it into the cottage cheese mixture. Add the pepper and serve with the vegetables suggested for Dilly Salmon Dip (following page) or whole-grain crackers.

¹/₆ recipe = ⅓ Protein serving; ⅓ Calcium serving.

SEASONED POPCORN

Everybody's favorite high-fiber snack, dressed up for a party.

Makes 6 cups

1 to 2 tablespoons butter
¼ teaspoon ground cumin
1 teaspoon chili powder
¼ teaspoon salt, or to taste
¼ cup grated Parmesan cheese
6 cups popped popcorn, preferably air popped

1. Melt the butter over very low heat in a small saucepan. Stir in the cumin, chili powder, and salt, and cook to blend the flavors, 2 minutes.

2. Just before serving, toss the seasoned butter and the cheese with the popcorn. Store any leftovers in plastic bags in a cool, dry place.

Variation: For Curried Popcorn, substitute ¼ teaspoon ground coriander and 1 tea- spoon curry powder for the cumin and chili powder. Omit the cheese.

Note: Popcorn doesn't offer much nutrition, but is fiber-rich and fun to eat.

SHREDDIE MIX

You probably won't be able to stop with just one handful, but with this nutritious party mix there's no reason to.

Makes about 6½ cups

3 tablespoons margarine
1 tablespoon Worcestershire sauce
1 teaspoon garlic powder (optional)
1 teaspoon onion powder (optional)
½ teaspoon salt, or to taste
1 teaspoon dried thyme, dried oregano, or ground cumin
4 cups bite-size shredded wheat biscuits
½ cup unsalted mixed nuts
2 cups whole-wheat sesame sticks or pretzels

1. Preheat oven to 300°F.

2. Melt the margarine over low heat in a small saucepan. Stir in the seasonings and cook for 1 minute.

3. Combine the shredded wheat, nuts, and sesame sticks on a large baking sheet. Sprinkle with the margarine mixture and toss well to mix. Spread evenly on the baking sheet.

4. Bake for 5 minutes. Stir, respread, and bake 5 minutes more. Repeat one more time. Serve hot or at room temperature.

Variations: Use any of the following combinations of seasonings instead of the thyme:
1 teaspoon curry powder and ½ teaspoon ground coriander, or 1 teaspoon chili powder and ½ teaspoon ground cumin.

DILLY SALMON DIP

Party dips are often heavy on the fat; this one is heavy on the protein and calcium. It's great with vegetables or hearty whole-grain bread, but prepare it ahead so that the flavors have time to blend. Dilly Salmon Dip does double duty as a sauce over pasta, and vegetables served at room temperature.

Makes about 2½ cups

*1 can (1 pound) salmon, with bones
and skin (see Note, page 255)*
*1 small cucumber, peeled, seeded,
and cut into chunks*
*¼ cup chopped fresh dill (or 1
teaspoon dried dill and ¼ cup
fresh parsley)*
2 to 4 tablespoons minced onion
2 tablespoons mayonnaise
1 tablespoon lemon juice or to taste
Salt and pepper to taste

1. Place all the ingredients in a blender or food processor and process until smooth.

2. Refrigerate to chill for at least 2 hours. Serve with one or more of the following: raw or lightly steamed broccoli, cauliflower, asparagus, snow peas, green beans; raw zucchini, endive leaves, cucumber, cherry tomatoes, celery, carrots; thin slices whole-grain cocktail bread.

⅛ **recipe = ½ Protein serving;
½ Calcium serving.**

CHEESEBALL

High in taste, low in fat. Serve with whole-grain crackers and cocktail bread, and a variety of raw vegetables or fruit.

Makes 1 small cheeseball or log

*6 ounces low-fat Cheddar cheese,
diced*
*¼ cup low-fat pot-style cottage
cheese*
*½ cup tightly packed chopped fresh
parsley*
*¼ cup finely chopped onion, or to
taste*
*1 to 2 teaspoons Worcestershire
sauce (vegetarians substitute
steak sauce)*
¾ teaspoon dry mustard, or to taste
2 tablespoons melted margarine
1 tablespoon milk
2 tablespoons minced pimiento
¼ cup chopped walnuts or pecans

1. Place the Cheddar, cottage cheese, 2 tablespoons of the parsley, the onion, Worcestershire sauce, mustard, margarine, and milk in a blender or food processor and process until smooth, adding more milk if the mixture is too stiff to blend.

2. Transfer the mixture to a bowl and stir in the pimiento. Refrigerate to chill the cheese until it can be shaped, about 30 minutes.

3. Combine the remaining parsley and the nuts on a plate. Form the cheese into a ball or log and roll it in the parsley mixture.

¹/₆ **recipe = ½ Calcium serving.**

Drinks

Water's hard to beat for refreshment, but for variety fill your Daily Dozen fluid quota, with these, or invent your own liquid concoctions. Blend fruit juices and puréed fruits (grapefruit juice with strawberries, for example); add herbs or spices to vegetable juices (fresh basil to tomato, perhaps); or blend fruit juice concentrates with hot water for something warm and comforting.

HOLIDAY WASSAIL BOWL

A warming, spicy treat that beats the Dickens out of club soda for satisfying the seasonal spirit.

Serves 12

6 small Cortland or McIntosh apples
½ teaspoon cinnamon
5 cups apple cider
¾ teaspoon ground ginger, or to taste
¾ teaspoon freshly grated nutmeg, or to taste
¼ teaspoon ground allspice, or to taste
3 whole cloves, or to taste
1 cinnamon stick
2 cups sherry or Madeira
⅔ cup plus ¼ cup apple juice concentrate
2 tablespoons brandy extract
4 egg whites

1. Preheat the oven to 350°F.

2. Core the apples, leaving them whole and unpeeled. Sprinkle them with ½ teaspoon cinnamon. Pour 2 cups of the cider into a baking pan just large enough to hold the apples. The cider should be at least 1 inch deep; if it isn't, add water. Place the apples in the pan and bake until soft but not mushy, about 45 minutes.

3. Meanwhile, combine 1 cup of the cider and the spices in a small saucepan. Cover and bring to a boil. Reduce the heat and simmer for 10 minutes.

4. Combine the spice mixture, sherry or Madeira, remaining 2 cups cider, and ⅔ cup juice concentrate in a large saucepan. Bring to a boil. Reduce the heat and simmer for 10 minutes, stirring frequently.

5. Strain the mixture and stir in the brandy extract. Keep warm until ready to serve.

6. Just before serving, whip the egg whites and ¼ cup juice concentrate until stiff but not dry. Slip the whites into a punch bowl. Pour the warm cider mixture very slowly over the egg whites, folding gently. Float the apples in the mixture and serve. For the nonpregnant, a splash of brandy can be added to each cup of wassail.

1 Other Fruit serving.

FROTHY EGGNOG

For new lang syne, bring in the year with extra calcium and protein.

Serves 2

2 cups skim milk
1 whole egg
2 egg whites
2 tablespoons apple juice
   concentrate
½ teaspoon vanilla extract
Freshly grated nutmeg to taste

   1. Process all ingredients except the nutmeg in a blender until frothy.

   2. Pour into two glasses. Grate nutmeg over each glass and serve.

1 Calcium serving; ½ Protein serving.

   Variation: For a Double Eggnog, substitute evaporated skim milk for the fresh skim milk or add ⅔ cup nonfat dry milk to the skim milk.

TOFU-FRUIT SHAKE

A fruity and refreshing calcium cocktail for the non-milk drinker.

Serves 1

4 ounces soft tofu
1 small ripe banana or ½ cup
   berries, or 1 large very ripe peach
   (peeled), or 1 cup diced ripe
   cantaloupe, mango, or other
   sweet fruit
⅓ cup fruit-sweetened fruit juice
   (apple, pear, papaya, pineapple,
   grape, or other)
2 tablespoons fruit juice concentrate
   (apple, pineapple, orange, or
   other)

   Combine the ingredients in blender and purée until smooth. Pour into a shallow ice cube tray and chill in freezer for 30 minutes. Return to the blender and purée until light and creamy.

1 Fruit serving (depending on fruit used); ¾ Calcium serving; ⅔ Protein serving.

DOUBLE-THE-MILK SHAKE

Knock off two calcium requirements in every frosty, rich-tasting glassful. Prepare for this drink ahead of time. Cut a peeled banana into chunks, put them in a plastic bag, and freeze for 12 to 24 hours.

Serves 1

1 cup skim or low-fat milk
⅓ cup instant nonfat dry milk
1 frozen, overripe banana, cut into
* chunks*
1 tablespoon apple juice concentrate,
* or to taste*
1 teaspoon vanilla extract
Dash of ground cinnamon, or to
* taste (optional)*

Process all the ingredients in a blender until smooth. Serve at once in a chilled glass.

2 Calcium servings; 1 Other Fruit serving.

Variations: For Berry Milkshake, add ½ cup berries, fresh or frozen (unsweetened), and 1 tablespoon apple juice concentrate, or to taste, before blending. Omit the cinnamon.

For Creamy Orange Milkshake, add 2 tablespoons orange juice concentrate. Omit the cinnamon.

INNOCENT SANGRIA

Serve a pitcher of these at your next fiesta.

Serves 8 (5 ounces each)

3 cups unsweetened grape juice
¾ cup apple juice concentrate
2 tablespoons orange juice
* concentrate*
1 tablespoon fresh lime juice
1 tablespoon fresh lemon juice
1 small lemon, cut into half slices
1 small orange, cut into half slices
1 small McIntosh or Cortland
* apple, unpeeled, cored, and cut*
* into 8 wedges; or 1 large peach,*
* unpeeled, pitted, and cut into 8*
* wedges*
¾ cup seltzer or club soda

1. Combine the fruit juices in a pitcher and stir in the sliced fruit. Refrigerate until cold.

2. Just before serving, add the seltzer or club soda. Serve over ice in wine glasses.

1 Other Fruit serving.

MOCK STRAWBERRY DAIQUIRI

Belly up to your blender for a cool and refreshing summer taste sensation.

Serves 4

2 cups hulled fresh or frozen (not thawed) unsweetened strawberries
1 cup ice cubes
1 tablespoon fresh lime juice
1 teaspoon rum extract, or to taste
¼ cup apple juice concentrate
4 whole strawberries
4 slices fresh lime

Purée all the ingredients except the whole strawberries and lime slices in a blender. Pour into chilled glasses and garnish each drink with a fresh strawberry and a lime slice skewered on a long toothpick.

1 Vitamin C serving.

Variation: For Mock Banana or Peach Daiquiris, substitute 2 very ripe bananas, cut into chunks, or 2 large ripe peaches, cut into wedges (about 2 cups), for the strawberries.

1 Other Fruit serving.

SPARKLING PUNCH FOR LOVERS

Just add candlelight.

Serves 2

2 tablespoons pineapple juice concentrate
2 tablespoons orange juice concentrate
2 teaspoons apple juice concentrate
1 teaspoon fresh lemon juice
¼ teaspoon brandy or rum extract
¼ cup hulled fresh or frozen (not thawed) unsweetened strawberries or raspberries
Seltzer or club soda

Blend the fruit juices and brandy extract in a blender until well mixed. Pour into two 10-ounce cocktail glasses. Add 2 ice cubes to each glass. Top with the berries and fill glasses with seltzer or club soda.

1 Other Fruit serving.

VIRGIN V-8

Tangier, and with a greater nutritional tally, than ordinary tomato.

Serves 2

2 cups V-8 juice
Juice of 1 lemon
2 teaspoons Worcestershire sauce
  (vegetarians substitute steak
  sauce)
Pinch of salt
Dash of pepper
2 inner celery ribs with leaves

Pour all the ingredients except the celery over ice cubes in a cocktail shaker. Shake until cold. Pour into 2 tall glasses and garnish with the celery.

1 Green Leafy and Yellow serving; 1 Vitamin C serving.

WINTER WARMTH IN A MUG

The perfect accompaniment to a roaring fire.

Serves 2

2 cups unsweetened cranberry-apple
  juice
¼ lemon stuck with 2 cloves
½ whole nutmeg
2½ cinnamon sticks

Combine all the ingredients except 2 of the cinnamon sticks in a saucepan. Heat over low heat for 5 minutes; do not boil. Strain and serve in warm mugs with the cinnamon sticks.

1 Other Fruit serving.

HOT ORANGE TEA

Worried about caffeine in regular teas? Try Hot Orange Tea.

Serves 1

3 tablespoons thawed orange juice
  concentrate
Boiling water
1 fresh orange slice (optional)

Pour the juice concentrate into a cup and fill it with boiling water. Garnish, if you like, with the orange slice.

1 Vitamin C serving.

Variation: For Hot Spiced Fruit Tea, stir your tea with a cinnamon stick or boil the water with a clove and a dash of nutmeg. Spice your tea to taste.

Quick Fixes

If you are too exhausted to fuss in the kitchen at the end of a long, hard day, fit all of the Daily Dozen in before bedtime with a selection from these quick fixes.

QUICK-FIX PROTEIN

❖ ¾ cup low-fat cottage cheese with fruit, fruit-only preserves, a tomato, or minced chives (1 Calcium serving)

❖ 1 cup plain low-fat yogurt plus ¼ cup low-fat cottage cheese with fruit-only preserves

❖ 3 to 3½ ounces tuna or salmon mashed with 2 tablespoons low-fat yogurt and ½ tablespoon mayonnnaise

❖ 1 whole egg and 2 egg whites scrambled with 1 thin slice cheese (about ½ ounce)

QUICK-FIX CALCIUM

❖ Double-the-Milk shake (2 Calcium Servings)

❖ 1½ ounces low-fat Swiss cheese or Cheddar with whole-grain crackers or a sliced pear or apple (1 Other Fruit serving)

❖ 1½ ounces low-fat Swiss cheese or Cheddar melted in a whole-wheat pita or on a slice of whole-grain bread (1 Whole-Grain serving)

❖ Best-Odds Ice Cream

❖ ¾ cup plain low-fat yogurt sweetened with fruit-only preserves or fruit juice concentrate

❖ 1 cup Best-Odds Café au Lait: Stir ⅓ cup nonfat dry milk into strong decaffeinated coffee

QUICK-FIX VITAMIN C

❖ 6 ounces orange or grape-fruit juice

❖ 1 Virgin V-8 (page 301)

❖ ¼ red or ½ green bell pepper

❖ 1 large tomato, sprinkled with pepper and a squeeze of lemon juice

❖ ½ cup strawberries or ¼ cantaloupe (1 Yellow Fruit serving)

QUICK-FIX WHOLE GRAINS

❖ 1 slice whole-grain bread with peanut butter and fruit-only preserves

❖ ½ whole-wheat English muffin with fruit-only preserves

❖ 1 slice whole-grain bread, toasted, lightly spread with butter or margarine, and sprinkled with cinnamon and a few chopped raisins

❖ 2 tablespoons wheat germ, sprinkled on whatever you're eating next—low-fat yogurt, fruit, Best-Odds ice cream, cereal, soup, a casserole

❖ 2 Best-Odds Muffins or any other Best-Odds baked goods that provides 1 Whole-Grain serving

❖ 1 cup Shreddie Mix

QUICK-FIX GREEN LEAFIES OR YELLOWS

❖ ½ small carrot

❖ ⅛ cantaloupe

❖ ¼ cup canned, unsweet-ened solid-pack pumpkin mixed with ¼ cup apple juice, 1 table-spoon apple juice concentrate, and a dash of cinnamon (2 +Yellow Vegetable servings)

❖ 6 ounces V-8 (Tomato-Plus does not supply the same nutri-ents)

❖ 1 stalk broccoli with Blue Cheese Dip or dip of 1 table-spoon mayonnaise, 2 table-spoons plain low-fat yogurt, and 2 tablespoons mustard

QUICK-FIX PROTEIN AND WHOLE GRAINS

❖ 3 to 3½ ounces water-packed tuna or salmon with ½ tablespoon mayonnaise and 2 tablespoons plain low-fat yogurt on a small whole-wheat pita or 1 slice of whole-grain bread

❖ 1 cup plain low-fat yogurt, 2 tablespoons apple juice concen-trate, and 2 tablespoons wheat germ. Add 1 sliced banana (1 Other Fruit serving) or add ¾ cup low-fat cottage cheese (for a total of 2 Protein servings)

❖ 1 slice whole-grain bread or a small whole-wheat pita filled with 3 ounces low-fat cheese, sliced chicken, or turkey

QUICK-FIX PROTEIN AND GREEN LEAFIES OR YELLOWS

❖ 1½ cups V-8, heated quickly, and topped with ¾ cup low-fat cottage cheese

❖ ¾ cup low-fat cottage cheese blended with 2 table-spoons canned unsweetened solid-pack pumpkin, ¼ cup un-sweetened applesauce, 2 table-spoons apple juice concentrate, and cinnamon, to taste

QUICK-FIX PROTEIN AND VITAMIN C

❖ ¾ cup low-fat cottage cheese or 1½ cups plain low-fat yogurt (1½ Calcium servings) plus ⅔ cup strawberries or ¼ cantaloupe (1 Yellow Fruit serving), diced

❖ ¾ cup low-fat cottage cheese and 1 large sliced tomato, sprinkled with chives

PART FOUR

Appendix

For Your Information

Do you want to know how the daily dozen translates into a sample menu or what amounts of vitamins and minerals an ideal prenatal supplement should contain? What's really in the junk food you secretly favor? Which of the chemicals that find their way into your cuisine are safe, which are questionable, and which are off limits? How to ask for skim milk in French, wheat germ in Italian, or fruit juice in German? If the answer to any of these is yes, then this ready reference section is for you.

PUTTING IT ALL TOGETHER

Squeezing the Daily Dozen into your daily schedule may seem a tricky maneuver—especially since you have more to do each day than eat. But they actually fit neatly into any kind of lifestyle, as you can see from reading through the sample menus below. The Daily Dozen servings are shown in parenthesis; the recipes can be located in the Recipe Index.

For the Working Mother-to-Be

How does the Daily Dozen fit into a working expectant mother's schedule? Easily. Add up this working day's diet and you'll find it provides the Daily Dozen and more.

Before rising:
1 whole-wheat bread stick or brown-rice cake to prevent nausea (½ Whole-Grain)
1 cup hot water with lemon if it enhances regularity (1 Fluid)

Breakfast:
1 ounce of shredded wheat with ⅓ cup Great Granola, ½ cup strawberries
1 cup skim milk (2 Whole-Grain; 1 Calcium; 1 Fluid; ½ Protein)

or

Mixed Medley for a Sweet Tooth (2 Whole-Grain; 1 Calcium; 1 Other Fruit; ½ Protein)
1 cup decaffeinated tea (hot or iced) with lemon or milk, sweetened to taste with orange or apple juice concentrate, as desired (1 Fluid)
Pregnancy vitamin supplement

Desktop Snack:
1 Best-Odds Bran or Oatmeal-Walnut Muffin (½ Whole-Grain), pre-cut and spread with fruit-only preserves
1 cup café au lait (⅓ cup nonfat dry milk stirred into 1 cup decaffeinated coffee) or 1 glass skim milk (1 Calcium; 1 Fluid; ⅓ Protein)

Lunch:
Tuna Salad on whole-wheat bread with sliced tomato (1 Protein; 2 Whole-Grain; 1 Fat; ½ Vitamin C)
1 glass water, seltzer, or Perrier (1 fluid)
¼ cantaloupe (1 Vitamin C; 1 Yellow Fruit)

Desktop snack:
1 small can V-8 juice (1 Green Leafy; 1 Vitamin C; 1 Fluid)
Whole-grain snack sticks (½ Whole-Grain)

Cocktail time:
1 glass Innocent Sangria (1 Other Fruit; 1 Fluid)
Seasoned Popcorn

Dinner:
Cream of Broccoli Soup (1½ Calcium; 1 Vitamin C, 1 Green Leafy; 1 Fluid; ½ Protein)
Quick-Fix Chicken (about 5 ounces meat without skin; 1½ Protein)
Baked potato with 1 pat margarine or butter (1 Other Vegetable; ⅓ Fat)
Arugula and red pepper salad with Italian Vinaigrette sprinkled with pine nuts (1 Green Leafy; 1 Iron; 1 Yellow; 1 Fat)
1 glass seltzer with lime (1 Fluid)

Bedtime snack:
Best-Odds peach or banana ice cream (1 Other Fruit; ¾ Calcium; ¼ Protein)
Sliced toasted almonds

For the Expectant Mother On the Go

Traveling is always a perfect excuse for letting your diet slide. But it's an excuse your baby won't accept—especially since he or she can't even enjoy the view of San Francisco Bay or the bargains on woolens in Canada! Keep both your palate and your baby happy when you're away from home with creative menu selections and snack purchasing.

Before leaving home:
1 glass orange juice (if you're on

the road, you can pack a container in the ice bucket in your room the night before (1 Vitamin C; 1 Fluid)

Coffee Shop Breakfast:
½ cup fresh strawberries or ½ grapefruit (1 Vitamin C)

2 poached eggs on 2 slices whole-wheat toast (1 Protein; 2 Whole-Grain)

1 pat butter, served on the side (⅓ Fat)

1 glass skim milk (if the coffee shop doesn't serve it, pick it up at a nearby grocer's and have it later; 1 Calcium; ⅓ Protein; 1 Fluid)

1 cup decaffeinated coffee or tea (1 Fluid)

Pregnancy vitamin supplement

Handbag snack:
2 ounces Swiss cheese (1½ Calcium; ⅔ Protein)

1 fresh yellow peach (½ Yellow Fruit)

Deli lunch:
Turkey sandwich on whole-wheat bread with mustard (1 Protein; 2 Whole-Grain)

Cole slaw (1 Vitamin C)

1 cup decaffeinated coffee or tea, hot or iced (1 Fluid)

Handbag snack:
Whole-wheat pretzels (½ Whole-Grain)

4 dried apricots halves (1 Yellow Fruit; some Iron)

1 can V-8 juice (1 Vitamin C; 1 Green Leafy; 1 Fluid)

Italian restaurant dinner:
Caesar salad (1 Green Leafy; ½ Calcium; 1 Fat)

Veal Piccata (1½ Protein)

Vegetable of the day (any one will do; you've had your Daily Dozen of vegetables already)

1 glass non-alcoholic wine or juice or Mineral Water (1 Fluid)

Unsweetened fresh berries or melon, if desired

Bedtime in a hotel room:
Enjoy a half-pint of skim milk and some dried fruits and nuts (1 Calcium; 1 Fluid; 1 Other Fruit; some Iron; ½ Protein)

On Weekends

Getting your Daily Dozen isn't hard work—even on the weekend.

On rising:
1 glass fruit juice (1 Other Fruit or 1 Vitamin C; 1 Fluid)

Breakfast Snack:
¼ cantaloupe (1 Yellow Fruit; 1 Vitamin C) or Pumpkin-Pecan Cake (1/16th = 1 Yellow Fruit)

¾ cup cottage cheese (1 Protein; ½ Calcium)

2 tablespoons wheat germ (1 Whole Grain)

1 cup decaffeinated tea (hot or iced), with lemon or milk, sweetened to taste with orange or apple juice concentrate (1 Fluid)

Pregnancy vitamin supplement

Brunch:
Crunchy Oatmeal-Pecan Waffles (1 Protein; 1 Calcium; 1 Whole-Grain)
Fruited Yogurt (extra Calcium and Protein)
1 cup decaffeinated coffee or tea (1 Fluid)

Snack:
Banana or Berry Double-the-Milk Shake (2 Calcium; 1 Other Fruit; 1 Fluid; ⅔ Protein)

Cocktail party:
1½ to 2 ounces cheese (no need to tote a scale; an eyeball approximation will suffice; 1 Calcium; ½ Protein)
Whole-grain crackers (tuck a few into your evening bag in case none are offered; ½ Whole-Grain)
Carrots and other raw vegetables with dip (1 Yellow Vegetable; Other Vegetables)
2 juice spritzers (equal amounts of juice and club soda, with a twist; 2 Fluid; 1 Other Fruit)

Late supper:
Red Pepper Gazpacho (2 Vitamin C, 2 Yellow Vegetable; 1 Fluid)
Pregnant Chef's Salad (1½ Calcium, 1 Protein, 1 Green Leafy, 1 Yellow Vegetable; 1 Vitamin C; 1 Other Vegetable; 1 Fat)
1 slice whole-wheat bread (1 Whole-Grain)
1 pat butter or margarine (⅓ Fat)
1 glass water or seltzer (1 Fluid)

At bedtime:
Creamy Brown Rice Pudding (1 Whole-Grain; ½ Calcium; some Iron)

For the Milk Hater

Yes, you can get through a day of pregnancy—everyday, in fact—without ever drinking a glass of milk.

Before rising:
1 brown rice cake (½ Whole-Grain)
1 glass water (1 Fluid)

Breakfast:
Cheesy Hot Cereal (2 Whole-Grain; 2 Calcium; 1 Protein)
1 cup decaffeinated coffee or tea (1 Fluid)
Pregnancy vitamin supplement

Snack:
1 Corn Muffin with Blueberries (½ Whole-Grain) spread with fruit-only blueberry preserves
1 glass orange juice (1 Vitamin C; 1 Fluid)

Lunch:
Swiss cheese and pear omelet (1 Protein; 1 Fruit; 1 Calcium; 1 Fat)
1 slice whole-grain bread with ½ pat butter (1 Whole-Grain; ⅙ Fat)
1 cup decaffeinated coffee or tea or 1 glass seltzer (1 Fluid)

Snack:
Peeled, sliced apple spread with 2 tablespoons peanut butter (1 Other Fruit; 1 Fat; ⅓ Protein)

1 cup Hot Orange Tea (1 Fluid)

Cocktail hour:
Raw vegetables (extra Vegetables)
Blue Cheese Dip (extra Protein and Calcium)
Cranberry-apple juice spritzer (1 Fluid)

Dinner:
Cream of Tomato Soup (1 Calcium; 1 Vitamin C)
Salmon Mousse (1 Protein; 1 Calcium; 1 Vitamin C; 1 Yellow Vegetable) or Salmon Casserole (2 Green Leafy and Yellow, 1½ Calcium; 1 Protein; 1 Vitamin C; 1 Whole-Grain)
Mixed dark greens with Butter-Milk Dill Dressing (1 Green Leafy)

Bedtime:
Cottage cheese sundae—¾ cup cottage cheese topped with seasonal fruits, fruit-only preserves, 2 tablespoons wheat germ, and chopped walnuts or almonds (1 Protein; 1 Fruit; 1 Whole-Grain; ½ Calcium)

JUNK FOOD: WHAT'S IN IT FOR YOU AND YOUR BABY?

The following examples of fast foods come from a variety of major chains. Although nutritional values vary somewhat from chain to chain, these are typical. The junk foods evaluations are from *Nutritive Value of Food* a USDA publication for typical recipes. Note that the best of these foods provide no more than 1 or 2 Best-Odds servings; many provide none at all. The percentages are of daily requirement in pregnancy.

	Calories	% of Protein	Fat	Sodium	Best-Odds Servings
For typical serving of	2,200*	100 gms	75 gms**	3,300 mg	
Main Dishes					
Big Burger	29%	29%	43%	28%	1¼ Protein/Iron #
Cheeseburger	13%	14%	17%	16%	⅔ Protein/Iron #
Big cheeseburger	24%	30%	41%	37%	1¼ Protein/⅔ Calcium/Iron #
Hot dog	16%	11%	29%	23%	½ Protein/Iron #
Fish sandwich	29%	18%	61%	22%	¾ Protein/Iron #
Fried chicken: Breast	9%	16%	8%	17%	⅔ Protein/Iron #
Legs (2)	10%	24%	9%	13%	1 Protein/Iron #
Chicken Sandwich	12%	10%	17%	14%	½ Protein/Iron #
Chicken fillet	23%	27%	35%	12%	1 Protein/Iron #
Pizza (slice)	15%	19%	15%	27%	1 Protein/1 Calcium
French fries (2 oz.)	10%	3%	16%	3%	1 Other Vegetable
Pies & Cakes					
Chocolate cake	11%	3%	11%	5%	0
Cherry pie	12%	2%	18%	13%	1 Other Fruit
Danish pastry	10%	4%	16%	7%	0
Doughnut	10%	3%	16%	6%	0

For typical serving of	Calories 2,200*	% of Protein 100 gms	Fat 75 gms**	Sodium 3,300 mg	Best-Odds Servings
Candy (1 oz.)					
Caramels	5%	1%	4%	2%	0
Milk chocolate	7%	2%	12%	***	0
Fudge	5%	1%	4%	2%	0
Hard candy	5%	0	0	***	0
Peanut bar	7%	5%	4%	***	0
Cookies					
Brownie with nuts	11%	3%	7%	4%	0
Chocolate chip	6%	1%	11%	3%	0
Oatmeal-raisin	4%	1%	6%	2%	0
Sandwich-type	5%	1%	10%	3%	0
Beverages					
Colas	4%	0	0	NA	0
Ginger ale	3%	0	0	NA	0
Milk shake	15%	11%	9%	8%	1 calcium/½ Protein

*2,200 calories is a typical daily requirement for an average-size pregnant woman. You may need more or less.

**75 grams of fat represents about 31 percent of your caloric intake, the approximate amount recommended by many authorities today. Individuals with coronary artery problems should have even less. Also, remember that the fat used in almost all fast-food restaurants is often high in cholesterol and/or saturated fats—the kind of fat it's best for you to avoid.

***Less than 1 percent.

#These foods contain some iron.

Also note: Every item on this list is low in dietary fiber.

CHEMICAL CUISINE

A good part of the American diet is made up of chemicals Grandma never heard of. The following list is adapted from a chart available from the Center for Science in the Public Interest called Chemical Cuisine (see page 319). Though none of the additives listed are known to directly cause damage to the unborn fetus, many are known to be generally hazardous and should be avoided by us all.

Additive	Used for	Comments
Alginate, Propylene Glycol Alginate: Safe	Thickening; stabilizing ice creams, frostings, dairy products, candy, beer, soft drinks, salad dressings.	Made from seaweed that appears safe.
Alpha Tocopherol (Vitamin E): Safe	Antioxidant to keep oil from going rancid.	A vitamin that's refined out of white flour and rice, it's safe and nutritious.

Artificial Colors—Most are synthetics that do not occur in nature. Some are safer than others, but since they are not usually listed by name, and are frequently used in foods of little nutritive value, they are best avoided.

Blue No. 1: Avoid	Beverages, candy, baked goods.	Inadequately tested, possible cancer risk.
Blue No. 2: Avoid	Beverages, candy, pet foods.	FDA asserts reasonably certain not harmful but studies are equivocal.
Citrus Red No. 2: Avoid	Skin of some Florida oranges.	Causes cancer, but dye does not seep into pulp.
Green No. 3: Avoid	Candy, beverages.	Studies equivocal; color rarely used.
Red No. 3: Avoid	Cherries in fruit cocktail, candy, baked goods.	Evidence it causes thyroid tumors, but pressure to ban resisted.
Red No. 40: Caution	Soft drinks, candy, gelatin desserts, baked goods, pet foods, pastry (mostly junk foods).	Key tests flawed; safety uncertain.

Additive	Used for	Comments
Yellow No. 5: Caution	Gelatin desserts, candy, baked goods, pet food.	Widely used, but causes allergic reactions, mostly in aspirin-sensitive people. Must be listed on labels.
Yellow No. 6: Caution	Beverages, candy, sausage, baked goods, gelatin desserts.	May cause tumors; occasional allergic reactions.
Artificial flavoring—Comprised of hundreds of chemicals: Caution	To mimic natural flavors in soft drinks, candy, breakfast cereals, gelatin desserts and other junk foods where the real thing is absent.	Most occur in nature and are probably safe; some may cause hyperactivity in children.
Ascorbic Acid, Vitamin C, Sodium Ascorbate, Erythorbic Acid (not a nutrient): Safe	Antioxidant, nutrient, color stabilizer in oily foods, cereals, soft drinks, cured meats.	Serves important function of preventing formation of nitrosamines.
Aspartame: Caution	Artificial sweetener in desserts, beverages, and other foods.	Questions raised about safety; should be avoided by those with PKU and pregnant women.
Beta Carotene (converted to vitamin A by body): Safe	Coloring/nutrient in margarine, shortening, nondairy whiteners, butter.	A yellow pigment that occurs in many vegetables, fruits, and animal fats, it's safe in moderate amounts.
Brominated Vegetable Oil (BVO): Avoid	Emulsifier, clouding agent in soft drinks.	Residues found in body fat are cause for concern.
Butylated Hydroxyanisole (BHA): Avoid	Antioxidant that prevents rancidity in oils, cereals, potato chips, gum.	Most studies find BHA safe, one found it carcinogenic.

Additive	Used for	Comments
Butylated Hydroxytoluene (BHT): Avoid	Antioxidant that prevents rancidity in oils, cereals, potato chips, gum, and more.	Studies equivocal: either increases or decreases risk of cancer. Residues found in body fat. Better to avoid.
Caffeine: Avoid	Stimulant found naturally in coffee, tea, cocoa; added to soft drinks.	Suspected of causing miscarriage and birth defects; may be related to fibrocystic breast disease.
Calcium (or Sodium) Proprionate: Safe	Preservative that prevents mold growth on baked goods.	The calcium is beneficial; the proprionate safe.
Calcium (or Sodium) Stearoyl Lactylate; Sodium Stearoyl Fumarate: Safe	Dough conditioner, whipping agent in bread doughs, cake fillings, synthetic whipped cream, processed egg whites.	Break down to harmless substances in body. No reproductive studies done.
Carageenan: Caution	Thickening and stabilizing agent in dairy products, ice cream, infant formula.	Derived from seaweed. May be harmful in large amounts. More testing needed.
Casein, Sodium Caseinate: Safe	Thickening and whitening ice cream, ice milk, sherbet, coffee creamers.	A milk protein, it is nutritious and safe.
Citric Acid, Sodium Citrate: Safe	Acid, tart flavoring and chelating agent in ice cream, sherbet, fruit drinks, candy, carbonated beverages, instant potatoes.	Widely used, cheap and safe.
EDTA: Safe	Chelating agent in salad dressing, margarine, processed fruits and vegetables, canned shellfish, and soft drinks.	Important in removing possibly harmful traces of metal from manufacturing process.

Additive	Used for	Comments
Ferrous Gluconate: Safe	Coloring in black olives; nutrient in pills.	Form of iron.
Fumaric Acid: Safe	Tartness in powdered drinks, puddings, gelatin desserts, pie fillings.	Safe source of acidity in foods; but Dioctyl Sodium Sulfosuccinate (DSS), often used with it, is poorly tested.
Gelatin: Safe	Thickening and gelling of powdered dessert mixes, yogurt, beverages, ice cream, cheese spreads.	A protein from animal bones and hooves, it has little nutritive value.
Glycerin ,Glycerol: Safe	Maintaining water content of marshmallows, baked goods, candy.	Part of fat molecules, it is safe.
Gums (Guar, Locust Bean, Arabic, Furcelleran, Ghatti, Karaya, Tragacanth): Safe	Thickening and stabilizing, frozen puddings, ice cream, beverages, dough, salad dressing, cottage cheese, candy, drink mixes, beer.	Derived from natural sources, they are poorly tested, but appear safe.
Hyptyl Paraben: Caution	Preservative in beer, noncarbonated soft drinks.	Studies suggest it is safe, but it has not been tested with alcohol.
Hydrolized Vegetable Protein (HVP): Safe	Enhancing flavor of instant soups, sauce mixes, frankfurters, beef stew.	A vegetable (usually soy) protein chemically broken down into amino acids; may be used to replace real food ingredients.
Lactic Acid: Safe	Checking spoilage, regulating acidity in olives, cheese, frozen beverages.	A natural substance found in almost all living organisms.

Additive	Used for	Comments
Lactose: Safe	A mild sweetener in whipped toppings, breakfast pastries.	A milk sugar, it is safe, although some people have difficulty digesting it.
Lecithin: Safe (but see page 201)	An emulsifier and antioxidant in baked goods, margarine, chocolate, ice cream.	Found commonly in plant and animal tissue, it is safe in amounts used in foods, but may present a risk in pregnancy in the huge doses in supplements.
Mannitol: Safe	A low-calorie sweetener used in a wide variety of foods; also used to keep foods dry.	A carbohydrate poorly absorbed by the body; half as many calories as sugar; considered safe.
Mono- and Di-glycerides: Safe	Emulsifiers, make baked goods soft, prevent staling; keep oil from separating.	Safe, although foods they are used in are often high in refined flour, fat, sugar.
Monosodium Glutamate: Caution	Flavor enhancer in soups, seafood, poultry, cheese, sauces, stews, and more.	Possibly hazardous to infants; causes adverse reactions in many adults. Not recommended in pregnancy.
Phosphoric Acid, (calcium, iron, sodium, aluminum, and ammonium phosphates, sodium acid pyrophosphates): Caution	Many purposes (supplementation, flavoring, leavening, inhibiting discoloration) in many processed foods, soft drinks, baked goods, cereals, cheeses, powdered and dehydrated foods, cured meats.	Safe itself; but excessive use could lead to dietary imbalance and osteoporosis, leg cramps.

Additive	Used for	Comments
Polysorbate 60 (also 65, 80): Safe	Emulsifiers that keep baked goods fresh, dill dissolved in pickles, oil from separating in artificial whipped cream; lets coffee creamers dissolve.	Safe.
Propyl Gallate: Avoid	Antioxidant that retards spoilage of fats in oils, meat products, snack foods, chicken soup base, gum.	Studies suggest possibility of cancer risk.
Quinine: Avoid	Flavoring in tonic water, quinine water, bitter lemon.	Used to cure malaria, this drug is poorly tested as an additive; may cause birth defects.
Saccharin: Avoid	Artificial sweetener in wide range of "diet" products.	Evidence it causes cancer and does not help with weight loss.
Sodium Benzoate: Safe	Preservative in fruit juices, carbonated drinks, pickles, preserves.	Used for over 70 years to prevent growth of microorganisms in food.
Sodium Carboxymethylcellulose (CMC): Safe	Thickening and stabilizing ice cream, beer, icings, pie fillings, diet foods, candy; prevents sugar from crystallizing.	Studies indicate this derivative of acetic acid is safe.
Sodium Nitrite, Sodium Nitrate: Avoid	Preserving, coloring, flavoring bacon, ham, frankfurters, luncheon meats, smoked fish, corned beef; prevents growth of bacteria that cause botulism.	Nitrite can lead to formation of cancer-causing chemicals. Nitrate slowly breaks down into nitrite.

Additive	Used for	Comments
Sorbic Acid, Potassium Sorbate: Safe	Preventing growth of mold and bacteria in cheese, jelly, syrup, cake, wine, dry fruits.	Occurs naturally in berries; may be a safe replacement for nitrite, but needs more testing for wider use.
Sorbitan Monostearate: Safe	An emulsifier that keeps oil and water mixed in puddings, icings, and cakes; prevents discoloration in candy.	Safe.
Sorbitol: Safe	Sweetening dietetic foods and drinks, gum, candy.	A naturally occurring sweetener, it is related to sugar but is metabolized more slowly and does not cause cavities.
Starch, Modified Starch: Safe	Thickening soup, gravy, baby foods.	Chemicals are used to modify starches from corn, flour, potatoes, so they will dissolve in cold water.
Sulfur Dioxide, Sodium Sulfite, Sodium or Potassium Bisulfite, Sodium or Potassium Metabisulfite: Avoid	Preserving; preventing discoloration in cut fruits and vegetables and bacterial growth in wine and beer.	Destroys thiamine; can cause severe allergic reaction, especially in asthmatics.
Vanillin, Ethyl Vanillin: Safe	Giving vanilla flavor to ice cream, baked goods, beverages, chocolate, candy, gelatin desserts.	Synthetic replacement for pure vanilla from the vanilla bean.

For more information write the Center for Science in the Public Interest, 1875 Connecticut Avenue N.W., Suite 300, Washington, DC 20009.

DAILY MINERAL NEEDS FOR THE AVERAGE YOUNG WOMAN: NONPREGNANT, PREGNANT, AND LACTATING

Nutrient	Units	Nonpregnant	Pregnant	Lactating	
Calcium	mg	1,000	1,200 to 1,300	1,500	
Calcium will be withdrawn from maternal skeleton if inadequate quantities consumed to meet needs of fetal skeleton or breast milk production; vitamin D required for absorption. Oxalic acid in spinach, beet greens, and rhubarb interfere with calcium absorption. Small amounts of the calcium in vegetables are lost in the cooking water. Calcium requirements are being reevaluated and can be expected to be revised upward. The pregnancy and lactation figures given here are slightly above the U.S. RDA.					
Phosphorus	mg	800	1,200	1,200	
Must be in balance with calcium; vitamin D required for absorption; small amounts of phosphorus in vegetables are lost in the cooking water.					
Magnesium	mg	300	450	450	
Deficiency not generally a problem except in alcoholics. Deficiency also related to preeclampsia; magnesium is used in treatment.					
Iron	mg	18	48 to 78	48 to 78	
Absorption is enhanced by vitamin C; iron from animal sources is better absorbed than that from vegetable sources. Foods lacking in color are lacking in iron, for example, celery, white bread, sugar vs. spinach, whole-wheat bread, or molasses. Iron cookware adds to the iron content of foods cooked within.					

These figures are based on the RDA (Recommended Dietary Allowances) of the Food and Nutrition Board of the National Academy of Sciences for women 23 to 50. Some experts recommend larger allowances of certain nutrients. Most requirement are greater for women under 23.

Needed For	Sources	Overdose Risks
Strong bones and teeth; muscle contraction; normal heart rhythm; blood clotting; transmission of nerve impulses; enzyme activity.	*Best:* Milk and hard cheeses. *Good:* Green leafies, canned sardines and salmon with bones. *Fair:* Soft cheeses, legumes, shellfish, almonds, soybeans.	Calcium deposits in soft tissue, particularly when individual is immobilized for some reason in pregnancy.
Strong bones and teeth; enzyme activity; building and repairing tissue. Is a part of every human cell.	*Best:* Meat, fish, poultry, eggs. *Good:* Milk, cheese, and other dairy products. *Fair:* May be less absorbable in bran, legumes, and grains.	Too much phosphorus in relation to calcium can result in leg cramps often a problem in pregnancy, and in calcium deficiency.
Metabolism; enzyme action; temperature control; nerve and muscle contraction; protein synthesis.	*Best:* Wheat germ and bran. *Good:* Whole grains, nuts. *Fair:* Some green leafies.	Nervous system disturbances; diarrhea.
Transfer and transport of oxygen.	*Best:* Liver and other organ meats, oysters, black strap molasses. *Good:* Spinach, beans and peas. *Fair:* Lean meats, other shellfish, egg yolks, nuts, dried fruit, other green leafies, whole grains, fish, poultry.	Rare, but include vomiting, cramps, toxic build up in liver.

Nutrient	Units	Nonpregnant	Pregnant	Lactating
Zinc	mg	15	20	25

Need for zinc, especially in pregnancy, is becoming more and more apparent.

Nutrient	Units	Nonpregnant	Pregnant	Lactating
Iodine	mcg	150	175	200

Iodized salt protects against iodine deficiency in a society in which the source of our foodstuffs and thus its iodine content, is unknown.

Nutrient	Units			
Potassium	gm	Not established; estimated 0.8 to 1.3 gms		

Need increased by certain medications (for example, diuretics); exercise, especially in hot weather; vomiting and diarrhea.

Nutrient	Units			
Chromium	mcg	U.S. minimum suggested safe and adequate dose: 50 mcg.		

High intakes of refined sugar and high levels of exercise increase need for chromium and could lead to deficiency; studies are under way to determine if deficiency could lead to gestational diabetes.

Chloride	Estimated: 0.5 gm

A component of salt (sodium-chloride), it may be in short supply in salt restricted diets.

Sodium	Estimated: 0.5 to 3 gm

As above, a component of salt, necessary in pregnancy for maintaining fluid balance. Excess salt is not necessary at any time.

Needed For	Sources	Overdose Risks
Growth; appetite regulation; wound healing; taste; digestion; protein synthesis.	*Best:* Oysters, wheat germ. *Good:* Meat, poultry, legumes, eggs, popcorn, whole grains, fish and seafood.	Nausea, vomiting, dehydration, fatigue, kidney failure, diarrhea, fever.
Healthy thyroid function; production of thyroid hormones.	*Best:* Seafood, seaweed, iodized salt. In other foods content varies according to content in soil or water where grown or where cattle graze.	Over long period, depressed thyroid activity.
Muscle activity and contractions; energy metabolism; nerve functioning; fluid balance; heart rhythm; protein synthesis.	*Best:* Dried fruit, nuts, green leafies, fresh fish, mushrooms, bran, wheat germ, yams, bananas, oranges. *Good:* Many other vegetables, fruits, meats, legumes in moderate amounts.	Heart irregularities.
Metabolism of sugars and fats; cardiovascular health.	*Best:* Whole grains, meats, mushrooms, asparagus, brewer's yeast.	None known.
Regulating electrolyte and fluid balance; formation of gastric juices; digestion.	*Best:* Common salt. *Good:* Animal products.	
Regulating electrolyte and fluid balance; muscle irritability.	*Best:* Common salt. *Good:* Animal products. (Also found in baking powder, foods that have been salted and products to avoid like MSG.)	High blood pressure; stroke.

Nutrient	Units	Nonpregnant	Pregnant	Lactating	
Sulfur	Not established; intake adequate if protein intake is adequate.				
Copper	Not established; estimated 2 to 3 mg.				
Manganese	Not established; estimated 2.5 to 5 mg.				
Fluoride	Not established; estimated 1.5 to 4 mg.				

Needed For	Sources	Overdose Risks
Constituent of all body tissues.	*Best:* Protein foods.	
Formation of red blood cells, nerve and connective tissues; glucose metabolism.	*Best:* Organ meats, nuts, dried peas and beans.	Rare, but high levels in blood have been associated with poor pregnancy outcome.
Bone and pancreas development; use of glucose and fats; synthesis of fats and carbohydrates; muscle contraction.	*Best:* Whole grains, beans, peas, nuts, tea, cloves. Found in lesser amounts in other foods.	Unknown.
Decay-resistant teeth; possibly strong bones.	*Best:* Water, naturally or chemically fluoridated; foods prepared with fluoridated water; fluoride supplements.	Mottled, deformed teeth in baby.

DAILY NUTRIENT REQUIREMENTS FOR THE AVERAGE YOUNG WOMAN: NONPREGNANT, PREGNANT, AND LACTATING

Nutrient	Units	Nonpregnant	Pregnant	Lactating	
Energy	calories	2,000	2,300	2,500	

These estimates are for a moderately active woman who weighs about 125 pounds; you may need more calories, or fewer, depending upon your prepregnancy weight, your level of activity, etc.

Protein	grams	44	74	64	

This nutrient is vital to the development of your baby, particularly his or her brain; the Best-Odds Diet recommends 100 gm daily.

Fat Soluble Vitamins

Vitamin A	IU	4,000	5,000	6,000	

Toxic in doses a little higher than the RDA; stored in the liver.* Best source, betacarotene, which is converted by the body to safe levels of vitamin A and is not toxic.

*Ever since you were a little girl you probably heard that you ought to eat liver—it's good for you. Now we know that as the storage organ for both chemicals (that an animal eats) and vitamin A, it can also be toxic, especially for a developing fetus (see page 201). A little liver once in a great while won't hurt. But don't make it a regular menu item.

These figures are based on the RDA (Recommended Dietary Allowances) of the Food and Nutrition Board of the National Academy of Sciences for women 23 to 50. Some experts recommend larger allowances of certain nutrients. Most requirements are greater for women under 23.

Needed For	Sources	Overdose Risks
Fueling the baby factory in your uterus.	All foods have calories. Fats have more than twice as many calories (9 per gram) as protein (4 per gram) or carbohydrates (4 per gram). Choose from foods that are also high in nutrition.	Obesity, which increases the risk of premature death; complications and discomfort in pregnancy; and complications in childbirth and surgery.
All life processes including tissue growth and repair, brain development, production of breast milk, and building your baby's body. Nearly 100 grams will be deposited in his or her body and in your accessory tissues during pregnancy. Lack may be related to preeclampsia, prematurity, abnormal bleeding, and low IQ in infant.	*Best:* Animal protein (meat, fish, eggs, milk and cheese). *Good:* Soy products. *Fair:* Other plant protein (peas, beans, grains). These should be combined to make complete protein (see page 61).	Possibly related to some types of cancer; also dietary imbalance leading to deficiencies in other nutrients.
Cell growth and development, good eye development and health, healthy skin and mucous membranes, bone growth, reproductive health, fat metabolism, infection resistance.	*Best:* Fish liver oils, liver; green leafy and yellow vegetables, and yellow fruits. *Good:* Egg yolks, butter, oysters. *Fair:* Fortified milk, whole-milk cheeses, margarine.	Yellowing of skin from an excess of carotene, birth defects, bone fragility and pain, nosebleeds, liver and spleen enlargement, dry peeling skin, itching, hair loss, nausea, blurred vision, headache. As little as 50,000 IUs can cause symptoms.

Nutrient	Units	Nonpregnant	Pregnant	Lactating	
Vitamin D	IU	200 to 300	400	400	

Very little vitamin D found naturally in foods.

| **Vitamin E** | IU | 12 | 15 | 16 | |

Deficiency in American adults with normal fat absorption mechanisms has not been documented; it has been suggested that dietary supplementation with vitamin E may retard aging.

| **Vitamin K** | Not established, since vitamin is produced in body; safe and adequate level considered 0.07 to 0.14 mg. | | | | |

Deficiency due to dietary insufficiency has not been demonstrated; may be administered to woman in labor, or to newborn to improve blood clotting.

Water Soluble Vitamins

| **Vitamin C** | mg | 60 | 80 | 100 | |

Not stored in the body so needed daily; unstable to heat and air (except in acids), so prepare vitamin C foods with minimum cooking, in covered utensils; destroyed by aging and drying, so use vitamin C foods fresh.

Needed For	Sources	Overdose Risks
Absorption of calcium and phosphorus in the GI tract and retention and utilization in bones, blood, and other tissues.	*Best:* Sunlight. *Good:* Fish liver oils; fortified milk. *Fair:* Egg yolks, liver, saltwater fish, fortified butter and margarine.	Loss of appetite, vomiting, diarrhea, headache, drowsiness, urinary problems, excessive calcium in the blood and other tissues.
Integrity of cellular and intracellular structures; prevention of destruction of enzymes and intracellular structures. As antioxidant, may render potentially dangerous free radicals harmless. Deficiency can lead to sterility or poor pregnancy outcome.	*Best:* Wheat germ and wheat germ oil, soybean, corn, and cottonseed oil. *Good:* Margarine, mayonnaise, nuts, peanuts and peanut butter. *Fair:* Whole grains, corn, beef liver, fish, eggs.	None known.
Regulation of blood clotting, primarily.	*Best:* Intestinal flora (which produce it). *Good:* Green leafies, pork, whole wheat, oats, bran. *Fair:* Fruits, seeds, tubers, milk, eggs.	Adverse effects only from synthetic vitamin K used.
Support material for bones, vascular system, muscles, cartilage, connective, and other tissue; metabolism; formation of hemoglobin and red blood cells. Need increased by pregnancy, rapid growth, smoking, wounds, fevers, infections and stress.	*Best:* Citrus fruits, strawberries, peppers, cantaloupe, some green leafies, cauliflower. *Good:* Tomatoes. *Fair:* Pineapple, bean and grain sprouts.	Diarrhea, kidney stones, possible dependence by fetus.

Nutrient	Units	Nonpregnant	Pregnant	Lactating	
Thiamin (B₁)	mg	1.1	1.5	1.6	

Absorption impaired in alcoholics; requirement is increased with increased carbohydrate intake. Unstable in heat and light, dissolves in water; prepare thiamin foods with minimal cooking, little water, and in covered utensils.

| **Riboflavin (B₂)** | mg | 1.2 | 1.5 | 1.7 | |

Stable in heat, air, acids, but not in light. Destroyed rapidly in milk stored in glass bottles.

| **Niacin** | mg | 13 | 15 | 18 | |

Stable in heat, light, air, acid. Soluble in hot water, so waterless cooking or steaming is best preparation method for preserving niacin. Requirement increased with caloric intake.

| **Vitamin B₆** | mg | 2 | 2.6 | 2.5 | |

(Pyridoxine, pyridoxal, and pyridoxamine)
Requirement increases with increased protein intake and with certain drug therapies. Considerable loss occurs in cooking, so cooking should be minimal when possible.

Needed For	Sources	Overdose Risks
Carbohydrate metabolism.	*Best:* Pork, peas, liver, wheat germ, yeast. *Fair:* Oysters, avocado, pineapple, citrus fruits, potatoes, milk, whole grains, spinach, tomatoes, bananas, whole grains, beans, peanuts, nuts, seeds.	Allergic reaction in some people.
Adequate tissue function, tissue oxygenation and respiration, protein and energy metabolism.	*Best:* Liver, milk, cottage cheese. *Good:* Eggs, meats. *Fair:* Whole grains, enriched grains, green leafies, beans, and peas.	None known.
The release of energy from carbohydrates and fats; the synthesis of protein and fat; healthy GI tract, skin, and nervous system; cell health.	*Best:* Meats, poultry, fish. *Good:* Mushrooms, legumes, nuts. *Fair:* Grains. Produced in body from tryptophan found in milk and eggs.	Tingling and flushing of skin; itching; digestive upset; low blood pressure; abnormal liver function; activation of ulcers.
Protein metabolism; the conversion of tryptophan to niacin. Also fat and carbohydrate metabolism.	*Best:* Blackstrap molasses, dry brewer's yeast, wheat bran and germ, soybeans, cottonseed meal, brown rice. *Good:* Organ meats, veal, lamb, tomatoes, bananas, salmon. *Fair:* Other fish, beef, cabbage, corn, oats, carrots, potatoes, legumes, poultry.	None known at 10 to 50 times U.S. RDA; severe nervous system dysfunction at much larger doses.

Nutrient	Units	Nonpregnant	Pregnant	Lactating	
Folacin	mg	.4	.8	.5	

Unstable in heat and air. Considerable losses in cooking and storage, so cooking should be minimal when possible.

Biotin	RDA not established for pregnancy; U.S. RDA is .3 mg.				

Consuming considerable quantities of raw egg white inactivates biotin.

Vitamin B$_{12}$	mcg	3.0	4.0	4.0	

Since vitamin occurs only in animal products, lifelong vegetarians may develop a deficiency; stable during normal cooking.

Pantothenic Acid	RDA not established for pregnancy; 4 to 7 mg. recommended, more in pregnancy.				

Widespread in both plant and animal tissue; not destroyed by ordinary cooking.

Needed For	Sources	Overdose Risks
Metabolism; synthesis of essential nucleic acids for normal cell division and replication; growth; formation of red blood cells.	*Best:* Liver, green leafies. *Good:* Lima beans, asparagus, nuts, whole grains, lentils. *Fair:* Oranges, orange juice.	Interferes with some drugs; can mask B_{12} deficiency; gastrointestinal and sleep disturbance possible; irritability and excitement.
Metabolism of proteins, carbohydrates, and fats.	*Best:* Organ meats. *Good:* Egg yolks, chocolate, peanuts, cauliflower, nuts, peas, and mushrooms. *Fair:* Milk. Also produced by intestinal flora.	None known.
Normal red blood cell formation; healthy nervous system; cell function.	*Best:* Organ meats. *Good:* Muscle meats, fish. *Fair:* Milk, eggs, cheese.	None known.
Many body functions including antibody production, adrenal activity, growth, metabolism.	*Best:* Organ meats, yeast, eggs, salmon. *Good:* Broccoli, cauliflower, mushrooms, bran, whole wheat, sweet potatoes, potatoes, lima beans, soybeans, peanuts, peas, oatmeal, beef, chicken, cheese.	Diarrhea and edema, occasionally; may trigger thiamine deficiency.

PARLEZ-VOUS BEST ODDS?

Destination Paris? Madrid? Rome? Frankfurt? Tuck this handy little Best-Odds dictionary into your travel tote to make sure that baby gets the best nutrition while you enjoy the best that international cuisine has to offer.

What to Ask For:	French	
Skim milk	lait écremé	
Nonfat dry milk	lait écremé en poudre	
Cottage cheese, low-fat	fromage frais au lait écremé[1]	
Cheese, low-fat	fromage au lait écremé	
Yogurt, low-fat	yaourt/yogourt au lait écremé	
Without sugar	sans sucre	
Without MSG	sans glutamate mono-sodique	
Whole-wheat bread	pain complet	
Wheat germ	germe de blé	
Oatmeal	flocons d'avoine	
Mineral water	eau minerale	
Decaffeinated coffee	café décafféiné (familiarly: Déca)	
Fruit juice	jus de fruit	
Sauce/gravy	sauce/jus	
Dressing (oil & vinegar)	assaisonnement (vinaigrette)	
Side dish or On the side	Plat d'accompagnie-ment	

Compiled by Michel Thomas, Language Centers, New York and Beverly Hills

Italian	Spanish	German
latte scremato	leche descremada	Magermilch
latte scremato in polvere	Leche en polvo descremada	Fettfreie Trockenmilch
Ricotta scremata[2]	queso bajo de grasa[3]	Quark mager
formaggio magro	queso (bajo de grasa)	Magerkäse
yogurt magro	yogurt (bajo de grasa)	Joghurt (mager)
senza zucchero	sin azucar	ohne Zucker
senza glutamato di monosodio	sin ajinomoto (or) sin monosodio de glutamato	ohne Monosodium glutamat
pane integrale	pan integral (or) pan de trigo	Vollkornbrot
germe di grano	germen de trigo	Weizenkeime
farinata d'avena	cereal de avena	Haferflocken
acqua minerale	agua mineral	Mineralwasser
caffè decaffeinato	café descafeinado	kaffeinfreier Kaffee (familiarly: Kaffee Hag)
succo di frutta	jugo de frutas	Fruchtsaft
salsa/sugo	salsa	Sauce/Sosse
condimento (olio y aceto)	aderezo	Salatsosse
contorno	en otro plato	Beilagen

1. Fromage frais is difficult to find in restaurants. One may substitute "petit suisse à zero pourcent de matières grasses," if obtainable, which resembles lean cream cheese.

2. Ricotta scremata is available in some places in Italy, although not everywhere. Occasionally one may find low-fat farmer or fresh cheeses sold under brand names, but there is no generic name such as "cottage cheese."

3. Low-fat cottage cheese in Mexico has 4 percent fat, equivalent to our regular cottage cheese.

CHOOSING A PRENATAL SUPPLEMENT

There are no standards set either by the FDA or the American College of Obstetrics and Gynecology specifying exactly what should be in a prenatal supplement. Often, your practitioner will prescribe the supplement, and in general prescribed formulas are superior to those bought over the counter.

If you are selecting a vitamin/mineral supplement yourself, look for a formula that contains:

❖ No more than 4,000 or 5,000 IU of vitamin A; amounts over 10,000 IU can be toxic.

❖ 800 to 1,000 mcg (1 mg) of folic acid.

❖ No more than 400 IU of vitamin D.

❖ 200 to 300 mg calcium.* If you're not getting high-calcium foods, you will need additional supplementation to reach the 1,200 mg RDA. Do not take more than 250 mg of calcium (or more than 25 mg of magnesium) *along with* supplementary iron since these minerals interfere with iron absorption. Take any larger doses at least two hours before or after your iron supplement.

❖ Approximately the RDA** for vitamin C (70 mg); thiamine (1.5 mg); riboflavin (1.6 mg); pyridoxine (B6, 2.6 mg); niacinamide (17 mg); vitamin B12 (2.2 mg); vitamin E (10 mg). Most formulas contain 2 to 3 times the RDA of these; there are no known harmful effects from such doses.

❖ Approximately the RDA for zinc (15 mg) and iron (30 mg elemental). ***More iron may be prescribed if you are anemic.

❖ Some preparations may also contain magnesium, copper, biotin, and/or pantothenic acid. Such trace minerals as chromium, manganese, and molybdenum are rarely found in pregnancy supplements.

---

*If the doctor has prescribed larger doses of calcium and magnesium, take them two hours before or after your regular supplement. The calcium may be necessary if you are not getting enough calcium in your diet. Both minerals may help if you are having leg cramps.

**The RDAs (Recommended Dietary Allowances) are listed in the chart beginning on page 320.

***Copper is necessary in any supplement containing zinc, since zinc can interfere with the body's absorption of copper increasing the need for this mineral. Zinc and copper are both necessary in a supplement containing iron, since the iron may interfere with their absorption. Zinc is also necessary if you are taking large doses (1,200 to 1,500 mg) of calcium.

INDEX

RECIPE INDEX